Frontiers in Natural Product Chemistry

# Volume 1

**Prof. Dr. Atta-ur-Rahman**
**Prof. Dr. M. Iqbal Choudhary**
**Dr. Khalid M. Khan**
Karachi, Pakistan

# Frontiers in Natural Product Chemistry

Bentham Science Publishers Ltd.
http://www.bentham.org/fnpc

## Volume 1, 2005

# Contents

# Frontiers in Natural Product Chemistry

## EDITORIAL

This Proceedings volume entitled *"Frontiers in Natural Product Chemistry"* contains a feast of original articles contributed by experts in the interdisciplinary field of natural product science. They include articles on the synthesis of several classes of natural products, isolation and structure elucidation of natural compounds, pharmacology and bioassay screening of natural substances and other related topics. These papers were presented as Plenary and Invited Lectures during the 9th International Symposium on Natural Product Chemistry (9th ISNPC) held in Karachi during January 10-13, 2004. This series of symposia is well reputed for its excellence and focused theme.

The Proceedings volume also contains several good articles on the stereoselective synthesis of bioactive natural products, which have been contributed by leading synthetic chemists based on the recent research work. Besides these, several contributions on the isolation, structural elucidation and pharmacology of plant-based natural products including proteins have been included. The volume also contains articles on a variety of topics including biotechnology and value-addition to natural products. We hope that this compilation of original research articles will add to the useful literature of the natural product chemistry.

We would like to express our thanks to Ms. Afshan Siddiq, Ms. Madiha Rauf, Mr. Liaqat Raza and Mr. Muhammad Tariq for their assistance in the preparation of the index. We are also grateful to Mr. Wasim Ahmad for typing and to Mr. Mahmood Alam for secretarial assistance.

**Prof. Dr. Atta-ur-Rahman**
**Prof. Dr. M. Iqbal Choudhary**
**Dr. Khalid M. Khan**
Karachi, Pakistan

# Contributors

| | |
|---|---|
| Tamio Hayashi | Department of Chemistry, Graduate School of Science, Kyoto University, Sakyo, Kyoto 606-8502, Japan |
| Noel F. Thomas | Department of Chemistry, Faculty of Sciences, Universiti Malaya, 59100 Kuala Lumpur, Malaysia |
| Kiew C. Lee | Department of Chemistry, Faculty of Sciences, National University of Singapore, 117543 Singapore |
| Jean-Frédéric F. Weber | Faculty of Pharmacy, Universiti Teknologi MARA, 40450 Shah Alam, Malaysia |
| Ibtisam Abdul Wahab | Faculty of Pharmacy, Universiti Teknologi MARA, 40450 Shah Alam, Malaysia |
| Khalijah Awang | Department of Chemistry, Faculty of Sciences, Universiti Malaya, 59100 Kuala Lumpur, Malaysia |
| A. Hamid A. Hadi | Department of Chemistry, Faculty of Sciences, Universiti Malaya, 59100 Kuala Lumpur, Malaysia |
| Pascal Richomme | Faculté des Sciences, Université d'Angers, 2, boulevard Lavoisier, 49045 Angers, France |
| E. Winterfeldt | Organic Chemistry Department, Hannover University, Schneiderberg, 1B, D-30167, Hannover, Germany |
| Roberto Ballini | Dipartimento di Scienze Chimiche dell'Università di Camerino, 62032 Camerino, Italy |
| Giovanna Bosica | Dipartimento di Scienze Chimiche dell'Università di Camerino, 62032 Camerino, Italy |
| Dennis Fiorini | Dipartimento di Scienze Chimiche dell'Università di Camerino, 62032 Camerino, Italy |
| Alessandro Palmieri | Dipartimento di Scienze Chimiche dell'Università di Camerino, 62032 Camerino, Italy |
| Hedvig Bölcskei | Gedeon Richter Ltd. H-1475 Budapest, P.O.B. 27 Hungary |
| Lajos Szabó | Institute of Organic Chemistry, Budapest University of Technology and Economics, H-1111 Budapest, Gellért tér 4, Hungary |
| Csaba Szántay | Institute of Organic Chemistry, Budapest University of Technology and Economics, H-1111 Budapest, Gellért tér 4, Hungary |

| | |
|---|---|
| Daniele Passarella | Dipartimento di Chimica Organica e Industriale, Università degli Studi di Milano, Via Venezian, 21 - 20133 Milano, Italy |
| Alessandra Giardini | Dipartimento di Chimica Organica e Industriale, Università degli Studi di Milano, Via Venezian, 21 - 20133 Milano, Italy |
| Giordano Lesma | Dipartimento di Chimica Organica e Industriale, Università degli Studi di Milano, Via Venezian, 21 - 20133 Milano, Italy |
| Alessandra Silvani | Dipartimento di Chimica Organica e Industriale, Università degli Studi di Milano, Via Venezian, 21 - 20133 Milano, Italy |
| Bruno Danieli | Dipartimento di Chimica Organica e Industriale, Università degli Studi di Milano, Via Venezian, 21 - 20133 Milano, Italy |
| Ian Fleming | Department of Chemistry, Lensfield Road, Cambridge CB2 1EW, UK |
| Uma S. Palkar | S.I.E.S College , Sion (W), Mumbai 400022, India |
| Sibtain Ahmed | Molecular Biochemistry Lab., Dept. of Chemistry, University of Agriculture, Faisalabad, Pakistan |
| Nighat Aslam | Molecular Biochemistry Lab., Dept. of Chemistry, University of Agriculture, Faisalabad, Pakistan |
| Farooq Latif | National Institute of Genetic Engineering and Biotechnology, Faisalabad, Pakistan |
| M.I. Rajoka | National Institute of Genetic Engineering and Biotechnology, Faisalabad, Pakistan |
| Amer Jamil | Molecular Biochemistry Lab., Dept. of Chemistry, University of Agriculture, Faisalabad, Pakistan |
| Nurun N. Rahman | Department of Pharmaceutical Chemistry, Faculty of Pharmacy, University of Dhaka, Dhaka-1000, Bangladesh |
| S. Huda | Department of Pharmaceutical Chemistry, Faculty of Pharmacy, University of Dhaka, Dhaka-1000, Bangladesh |
| Khondaker M. Rahman | Department of Pharmaceutical Chemistry, Faculty of Pharmacy, University of Dhaka, Dhaka-1000, Bangladesh |
| Mohammad H. Rahman | Department of Pharmaceutics and Pharmaceutical Technology, Faculty of Pharmacy, University of Dhaka, Dhaka-1000, Bangladesh |

Herbert Budzikiewicz — Institut für Organische Chemie der Universität, Greinstr. 4, 50939 Köln, Germany

Suchada Chantrapromma — Department of Chemistry, Faculty of Science, Prince of Songkla University, Hat-Yai, Songkhla 90112, Thailand

Hoong-Kun Fun — X-ray Crystallography Unit, School of Physics, Universiti Sains Malaysia, 11800 USM, Penang, Malaysia

Surat Laphookhieo — Department of Chemistry, Faculty of Science, Prince of Songkla University, Hat-Yai, Songkhla 90112, Thailand

Saroj Cheenpracha — Department of Chemistry, Faculty of Science, Prince of Songkla University, Hat-Yai, Songkhla 90112, Thailand

Chatchanok Karalai — Department of Chemistry, Faculty of Science, Prince of Songkla University, Hat-Yai, Songkhla 90112, Thailand

J.H.P. Tyman — Centre for Environmental Research, Brunel University, Uxbridge, Middlesex, UB8 3PH, UK

Ignatius Suharto — Faculty of Industrial Technology, Catholic University of Parahyangan (Unpar), Jl Ciumbuleuit 94-96, Bandung 40141, Indonesia

Leonardus B.S. Kardono — Research Center for Chemistry, Indonesian Institute of Sciences (LIPI), Kawasan PUSPIPTEK, Serpong 15314, Indonesia

Atta-ur-Rahman — H.E.J. Research Institute of Chemistry, International Center for Chemical Sciences, University of Karachi, Karachi-75270, Pakistan

M. Iqbal Choudhary — H.E.J. Research Institute of Chemistry, International Center for Chemical Sciences, University of Karachi, Karachi-75270, Pakistan

S. Ghulam Musharraf — H.E.J. Research Institute of Chemistry, International Center for Chemical Sciences, University of Karachi, Karachi-75270, Pakistan

Wolfgang Voelter — Abteilung für Physikalische Biochemie des Physiologisch-chemischen Instituts der Universität Tübingen, Hoppe-Seyler-Str. 4, 72076 Tübingen, Germany

Roland Wacker — Abteilung für Physikalische Biochemie des Physiologisch-chemischen Instituts der Universität Tübingen, Hoppe-Seyler-Str. 4, 72076 Tübingen, Germany

Stanka Stoeva — Abteilung für Physikalische Biochemie des Physiologisch-chemischen Instituts der Universität Tübingen, Hoppe-Seyler-Str. 4, 72076 Tübingen, Germany

| Rania Tsitsilonis | Abteilung für Physikalische Biochemie des Physiologisch-chemischen Instituts der Universität Tübingen, Hoppe-Seyler-Str. 4, 72076 Tübingen, Germany |
|---|---|
| Christian Betzel | Abteilung für Physikalische Biochemie des Physiologisch-chemischen Instituts der Universität Tübingen, Hoppe-Seyler-Str. 4, 72076 Tübingen, Germany |
| M.-Ch. Song | Graduate School of Biotechnology & Plant Metabolism Research Center, KyungHee University, Suwon, 449-701, Korea |
| D.-H. Kim | Graduate School of Biotechnology & Plant Metabolism Research Center, KyungHee University, Suwon, 449-701, Korea |
| Y.-H. Hong | Graduate School of Biotechnology & Plant Metabolism Research Center, KyungHee University, Suwon, 449-701, Korea |
| H.-J. Yang | Graduate School of Biotechnology & Plant Metabolism Research Center, KyungHee University, Suwon, 449-701, Korea |
| I.-S. Chung | Graduate School of Biotechnology & Plant Metabolism Research Center, KyungHee University, Suwon, 449-701, Korea |
| S.-H. Kim | Department of Pharmacy, Woosuk University, Jeunbuk, 565-701, Korea |
| B.-M. Kwon | Graduate School of East-West Medical Science, KungHee University, Suwon, 449-701, Korea |
| D.-K. Kim | Erom Life Co. Ltd., Seoul, 135-825, Korea |
| M.-H. Park | Korea Research Institute of Bioscience and Biotechnology, K/S1, Taejon, 305-333, Korea |
| N.-I. Baek | Graduate School of Biotechnology & Plant Metabolism Research Center, KyungHee University, Suwon, 449-701, Korea |
| Metin Balci | Department of Chemistry, Middle East Technical University, 06531, Ankara-Turkey |
| Murat Çelik | Department of Chemistry, Middle East Technical University, 06531, Ankara-Turkey<br>Department of Chemistry, Ataturk University, 25240 Erzurum-Turkey |

| | |
|---|---|
| Emine Demir | Department of Chemistry, Middle East Technical University, 06531, Ankara-Turkey |
| Murat Ertas | Department of Chemistry, Middle East Technical University, 06531, Ankara-Turkey |
| Serdar M. Gultekin | Department of Chemistry, Middle East Technical University, 06531, Ankara-Turkey<br>Department of Chemistry, Ataturk University, 25240 Erzurum-Turkey |
| Nihal Ozturk | Department of Chemistry, Middle East Technical University, 06531, Ankara-Turkey |
| Yunus Kara | Department of Chemistry, Ataturk University, 25240 Erzurum-Turkey |
| Nurhan Horasan-Kishali | Department of Chemistry, Ataturk University, 25240 Erzurum-Turkey |
| Mir Ezharul Hossain | Department of Medicinal Chemistry, BCSIR Laboratories Chittagong, Chittagong-4220, Bangladesh |
| Sreebash Chandra Bhattacharjee | Department of Medicinal Chemistry, BCSIR Laboratories Chittagong, Chittagong-4220, Bangladesh |
| M.D. Enayetul Islam | Department of Medicinal Chemistry, BCSIR Laboratories Chittagong, Chittagong-4220, Bangladesh |
| Evangeline C. Amor | Institute of Chemistry, College of Science, University of the Philippines, Diliman 1101 Quezon City, Philippines |
| U.L.B. Jayasinghe | Institute of Fundamental Studies, Hantana Road, Kandy, Sri Lanka |
| Y. Fujimoto | Department of Chemistry and Materials Science, Tokyo Institute of Technology, Meguro, Tokyo 152-8551, Japan |
| Ih-Sheng Chen | Graduate Institute of Pharmaceutical Sciences, College of Pharmacy, Kaohsiung Medical University, Kaohsiung 807, Taiwan |
| Che-Ming Teng | Pharmacological Institute, College of Medicine, National Taiwan University, Taipei 100, Taiwan |
| J.U. Mollah | Institute of Biological Sciences, University of Rajshahi, Rajshahi 6205, Bangladesh |
| W. Islam | Institute of Biological Sciences, University of Rajshahi, Rajshahi 6205, Bangladesh |

Atta-ur-Rahman/Choudhary/Khan (Eds.) *Frontiers in Natural Product Chemistry, Vol. 1*

# Rhodium-Catalyzed Asymmetric 1,4-Addition of Organometallic Reagents

Tamio Hayashi*

*Department of Chemistry, Graduate School of Science, Kyoto University, Sakyo, Kyoto 606-8502, Japan*

**Abstract**: Asymmetric 1,4-arylation and -alkenylation was achieved by use of organoboronic acids or their derivatives in the presence of a rhodium catalyst coordinated with binap or its related ligands. The scope of this asymmetric addition is very broad, α,β-unsaturated ketones, esters, amides, 1-alkenylphosphonates, and 1-nitroalkenes being efficiently converted into the corresponding 1,4-addition products with over 95% enantioselectivity. The catalytic cycle of the reaction in water is proposed to involve three intermediates (aryl- or alkenyl-rhodium, (oxa-π-allyl)rhodium, and hydroxorhodium) by NMR studies on the rhodium intermediates. The asymmetric addition of $B$-aryl-9BBN and ArTi(OPr-$i$)$_3$ in aprotic solvents proceeded with high enantioselectivity under mild conditions to give the corresponding metal enolates as the 1,4-addition products.

## INTRODUCTION

Catalytic asymmetric synthesis is a field of great interest in its practical usefulness as well as its scientific interest [1]. Although the asymmetric reduction and oxidation have been developed so well that some of the processes are used for industrial production of enantiomerically enriched compounds, the examples of high efficiency in terms of catalytic activity and enantioselectivity are still rare in the catalytic asymmetric carbon-carbon bond forming reactions. Among the asymmetric carbon-carbon bond forming reactions catalyzed by chiral transition metal complexes, the asymmetric 1,4-addition is one of the most promising reactions because its non-asymmetric version is a basic synthetic reaction often used for the carbon-carbon bond formation which allows us to introduce carbon nucleophiles to the β-position of electron deficient olefins such as α,β-unsaturated ketones and esters [2]. Recently there have been reported two types of 1,4-addition reactions where high enantioselectivity is achieved [3]. One is the copper(I)-catalyzed addition of organozinc reagents by use of copper(I) catalysts coordinated with chiral phosphorous ligands represented by phosphoramidite ligand based on the axially chiral 1,1'-binaphthol [4]. The other is the Michael addition to α,β-unsaturated ketones catalyzed by Shibasaki's heterobimetallic catalysts consisting of chiral 1,1'-binaphthol and two kinds of metals [5]. In these two reactions, sp$^3$-alkyl groups and soft carbon nucleophiles, respectively, are introduced at the stereogenic carbon center at the β-position of α,β-unsaturated ketones.

Miyaura's report in 1997 describing the first example of rhodium-catalyzed 1,4-addition of aryl- and alkenyl-boronic acids to α,β-unsaturated ketones [6] stimulated us to modify the reaction conditions of the rhodium-catalyzed reaction for catalytic asymmetric 1,4-addition reactions. We succeeded in obtaining high catalytic activity and high enantioselectivity by carrying out the reaction in dioxane and water at 100 °C in the

---

*Corresponding author: thayashi@kuchem.kyoto-u.ac.jp

presence of a rhodium catalyst coordinated with (S)-binap ligand, which was reported in 1998 [7]. As a typical example, the reaction of 2-cyclohexenone with phenylboronic acid gave (S)-3-phenylcyclohexanone of 97% ee. After this publication, several reports appeared on the use of some other chiral phosphorus ligands for this type of rhodium-catalyzed 1,4-addition of organoboronic acids to α,β-unsaturated ketones under similar conditions to ours [8]. We have successfully applied the rhodium-catalyzed asymmetric reaction to some other organometallic reagents and electron deficient olefins. In this account described is the recent development of the rhodium-catalyzed asymmetric 1,4-addition reactions recently studied in our research group [9].

## CATALYTIC ASYMMETRIC 1,4-ADDITION OF ORGANOBORONIC ACIDS AND ORGANOBOROXINES

In our first communication, we reported that the rhodium-catalyzed asymmetric 1,4-addition of aryl- and alkenylboronic acids proceeded with high enantioselectivity for both cyclic and linear α,β-unsaturated ketones, Fig. (1) [7]. Important points for the high catalytic activity and the high enantioselectivity at this stage are (1) the use of $Rh(acac)(C_2H_4)_2$ as a rhodium catalyst precursor, (2) binap as a chiral bisphosphine ligand, (3) high reaction temperature (100 °C), and (4) the use of a mixture of dioxane and water in a ratio of 10 to 1 as a solvent. The high reaction temperature is essential, almost no reaction taking place at 60 °C or lower. With $Rh(acac)(CO)_2$ as a catalyst precursor, the reaction is slower and the enantioselectivity is much lower. NMR studies showed that the addition of 1 equiv of binap ligand to $Rh(acac)(C_2H_4)_2$ immediately generates $Rh(acac)(binap)$ quantitatively, while $Rh(acac)(CO)_2$ generates two kinds of unidentified rhodium complexes together with a small amount of the $Rh(acac)(binap)$ complex.

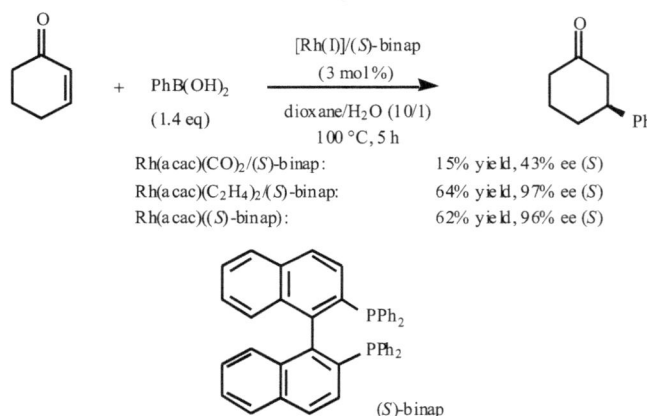

Fig. (1). Rhodium-catalyzed asymmetric 1,4-addition of phenylboronic acid to 2-cyclohexenone.

The scope of this rhodium-catalyzed asymmetric 1,4-addition of organoboronic acids is very broad [7]. Some of the results obtained for the addition to α,β-unsaturated ketones are summarized in Fig. (2). Under standard conditions, that is, 3 mol % of $Rh(acac)(C_2H_4)_2$ and binap in dioxane/$H_2O$ (10/1) at 100 °C, aryl groups substituted with either electron-donating or -withdrawing groups, $4\text{-MeC}_6H_4$, $4\text{-CF}_3C_6H_4$, $3\text{-MeOC}_6H_4$, and $3\text{-ClC}_6H_4$, were introduced onto 2-cyclohexenone with high enantioselectivity by the reaction with the corresponding boronic acids. Asymmetric addition of 1-alkenylboronic acids was as successful as that of arylboronic acids, the alkenylation product with 1-heptenylboronic acid

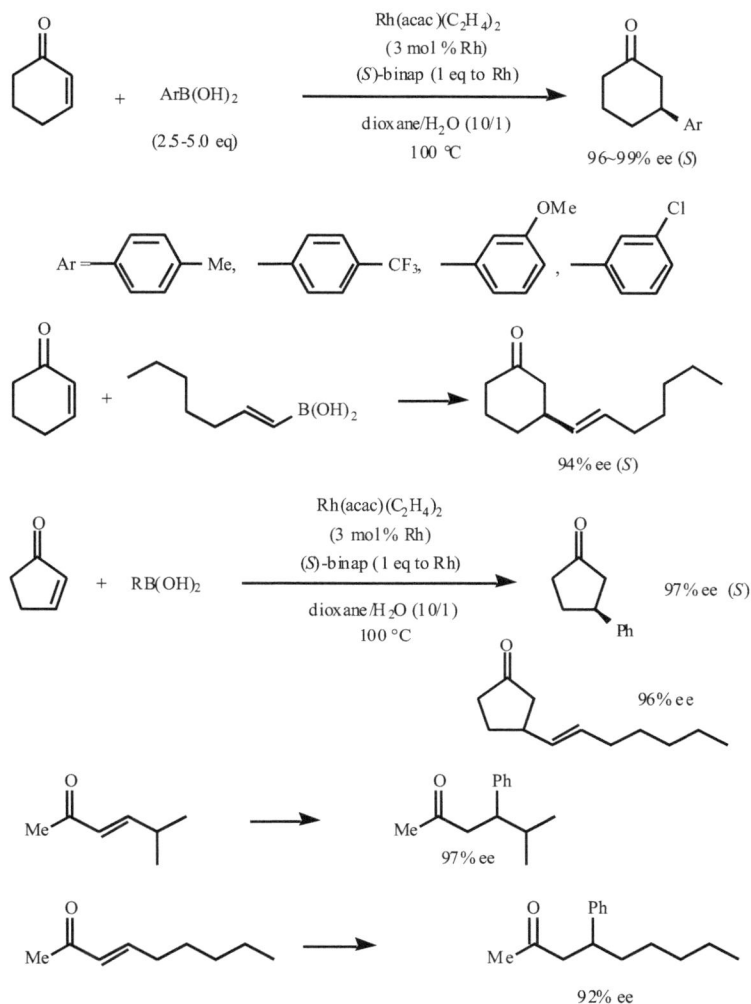

**Fig. (2).** Asymmetric 1,4-addition of organoboronic acids to α,β-unsaturated ketones.

being obtained with 94% enantioselectivity. Cyclopentenone underwent the asymmetric addition of phenyl- and 1-heptenylboronic acids with high enantioselectivity under the same reaction conditions to give 3-substituted cyclopentanones with over 96% ee in high yields. High enantioselectivity was also observed in the reaction of linear enones, 5-methyl-3-hexen-2-one and 3-nonen-2-one, which have *trans* olefin geometry. Thus, the rhodium-catalyzed asymmetric 1,4-addition proceeds with high enantioselectivity for both cyclic and linear α,β-unsaturated ketones with a variety of aryl- and alkenylboronic acids. The procedures for the preparation of (S)-3-phenylcyclohexanone on a scale of several grams have been published in *Organic Synthesis* [10].

Alkenylcatecholboranes obtained by the hydroboration of alkynes with catecholborane were found to be good alkenylating reagents for the asymmetric 1,4-addition, which made one-pot synthesis of the optically active β-alkenyl ketones possible from alkynes, catecholborane, and enones [11]. Lithium trimethyl arylborates, readily generated *in situ* by treatment of aryllithiums with trimethoxyborane, can be also used for the asymmetric 1,4-addition [12]. In the addition to α,β-unsaturated ketones, this one-pot reaction is superior to the reaction of arylboronic acids both in higher catalytic activity resulting in higher chemical yield and in easier manipulation avoiding the isolation of arylboronic acids.

α,β-Unsaturated esters are also good substrates for the rhodium-catalyzed asymmetric addition, Fig. (3) [13,14]. The use of an arylborates generated from aryllithiums and trimethoxyborane gave better results than that of the corresponding boronic acids. Interestingly, the enantioselectivity increases as the steric bulkiness of the ester moiety increases. The enantiomeric purities of the phenylation products are 89%, 91%, 95%, and 96% ee for methyl, ethyl, isopropyl, and tert-butyl esters, respectively, in the reaction of (*E*)-hexenoate esters. The sterically more bulky ester shows the higher enantioselectivity. Aryl groups, $4\text{-}ClC_6H_4$, $4\text{-}MeC_6H_4$, $4\text{-}CF_3C_6H_4$, $3\text{-}MeOC_6H_4$, and 2-naphthyl, were also introduced at the β position of isopropyl ester with enantioselectivity ranging between 93% and 97% ee in high yields in the reactions with the corresponding lithium arylborates. Highest enantioselectivity (98% ee) was observed in the phenylation of isopropyl 4-methyl-2-pentenoate with the phenylborate, though the yield was not high enough.

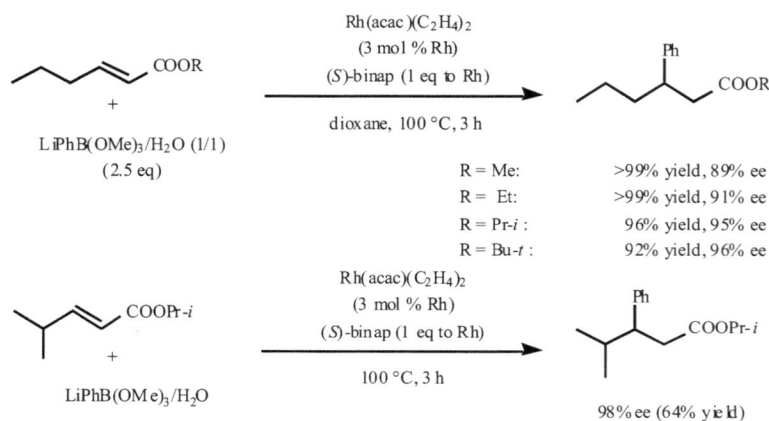

**Fig. (3).** Rhodium-catalyzed asymmetric 1,4-addition to α,β-unsaturated esters.

Asymmetric 1,4-addition to cyclic α,β-unsaturated amides provides a new efficient route to enantiomerically enriched 4-aryl-2-piperidinones, Fig. (4) [15]. For the 1,4-addition of 4-$FC_6H_4B(OH)_2$, which is related to asymmetric synthesis of (−)-Paroxetine, slightly modified conditions were required to obtain a high yield of the arylation product. The main side reaction, that is, hydrolysis of the boronic acid giving fluorobenzene, was suppressed by use of a minimum amount of the water. Thus, the reaction with 4-fluorophenylboroxine and 1 equiv (to boron) of water in the presence of $Rh(acac)(C_2H_4)_2/(R)$-binap catalyst in dioxane at 40 °C gave 63% yield of (*R*)-lactam with 97% enantioselectivity.

Alkenylphosphonates are less reactive toward 1,4-addition compared to α,β-unsaturated carbonyl compounds. Under the reaction conditions used for α,β-unsaturated ketones (phenylboronic acid in dioxane/$H_2O$ (10/1)), the yield of 1,4-addition was very low (44%) for diethyl (*E*)-propenylphosphonate. The asymmetric 1,4-addition was greatly improved (94% yield with 96% ee) by carrying out the reaction using phenylboroxine $(PhBO)_3$ and 1

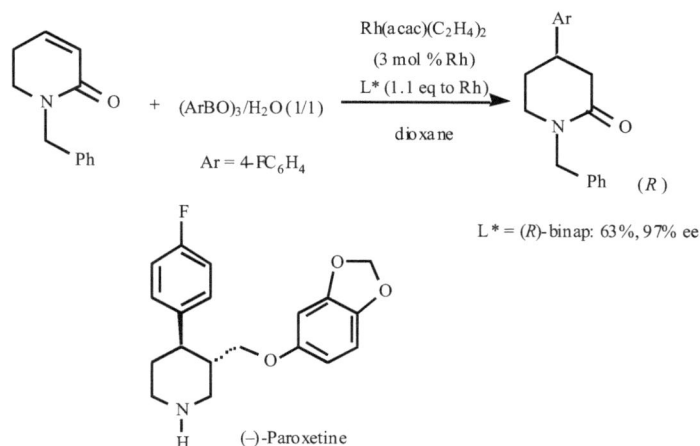

**Fig. (4).** Rhodium-catalyzed asymmetric 1,4-addition to cyclic $\alpha,\beta$-unsaturated amide.

equiv of water, Fig. (5) [16]. The addition of 1 equiv of water is essential for the high yield, almost no reaction taking place in the absence of water. A boroxine and water should be in equilibration with a boronic acid under the reaction conditions [17], and hence the use of arylboroxine in combination with 1 equiv of water for the asymmetric 1,4-addition should result in the same outcome as using the corresponding arylboronic acid with no water added. Nevertheless, the results of the catalytic reactions are better with the combination of boroxine and water. The enantioselectivities and chemical yields were slightly higher with the rhodium catalyst coordinated with unsymmetrically substituted binap ligand, (S)-u-binap, which has diphenylphosphino and bis(3,5-dimethyl-4-methoxyphenyl)phosphino groups at the 2 and 2' positions on the 1,1'-binaphthyl skeleton. In the reaction of diphenyl (E)-propenylphosphonate with phenylboroxine, (S)-u-binap ligand gave 99% yield of the 1,4-addition product with 94% ee while the standard (S)-binap gave 95% yield with 91% ee. It is remarkable that the asymmetric phenylation of (Z) isomer of diethyl 1-propenylphosphonate with phenylboroxine gave R isomer.

Nitroalkenes are good substrates for the rhodium-catalyzed asymmetric 1,4-addition of organoboronic acids [18]. The reaction of 1-nitrocyclohexene with phenylboronic acid in the presence of the rhodium/(S)-binap catalyst at 100 °C for 3 h gave 89% yield of 2-phenyl-1-nitrocyclohexane, Fig. (6). The main phenylation product is a cis isomer (cis/trans = 87/13) and both of the cis and trans isomers are 98% enantiomerically pure. Treatment of the cis-rich mixture with sodium bicarbonate in refluxing ethanol caused cis-trans equilibration giving thermodynamically more stable trans isomer (trans/cis = 97/3). It should be noted that this rhodium-catalyzed asymmetric phenylation produced thermodynamically less stable cis isomer of high enantiomeric purity and it can be isomerized, if one wishes, into trans isomer without loss of its enantiomeric purity. Under similar reaction conditions, 1-nitrocyclohexene underwent asymmetric addition of some other arylboronic acids in good yields with high enantioselectivity. The corresponding cis-2-aryl-1-nitrocyclohexanes were produced with over 85% cis selectivity and with the enantioselectivity ranging between 97.6% and 99.0% ee. The optically active nitroalkanes obtained here are useful chiral building blocks which can be readily converted into a wide variety of optically active compounds by taking advantages of the versatile reactivity of nitro compounds.

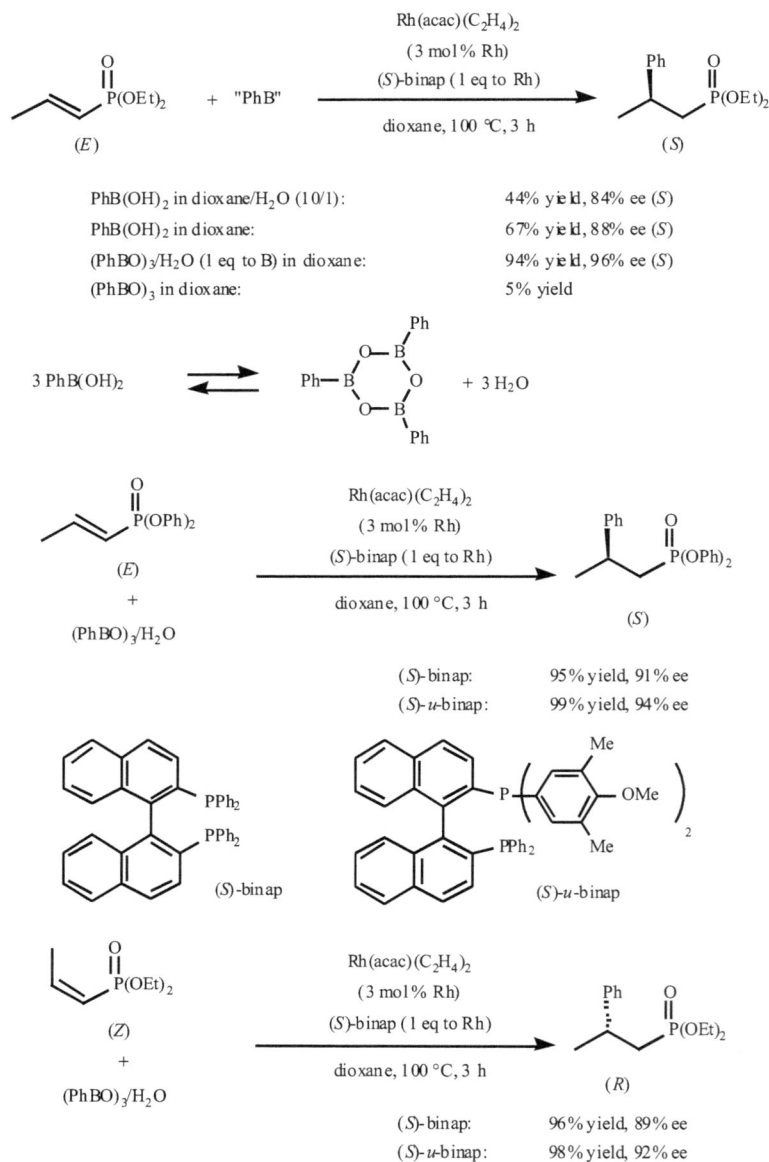

**Fig. (5).** Rhodium-catalyzed asymmetric 1,4-addition to alkenylphosphonates.

## CATALYTIC CYCLE FOR THE RHODIUM-CATALYZED 1,4-ADDITION OF ORGANOBORONIC ACIDS

We succeeded in characterizing the important intermediates involved in the catalytic cycle of the rhodium-catalyzed 1,4-addition by use of RhPh(PPh₃)(binap) as a key intermediate [19]. The catalytic cycle illustrated for the reaction of phenylboronic acid with 2-cyclohexenone is shown in Fig. (7). The reaction proceeds by way of three intermediates,

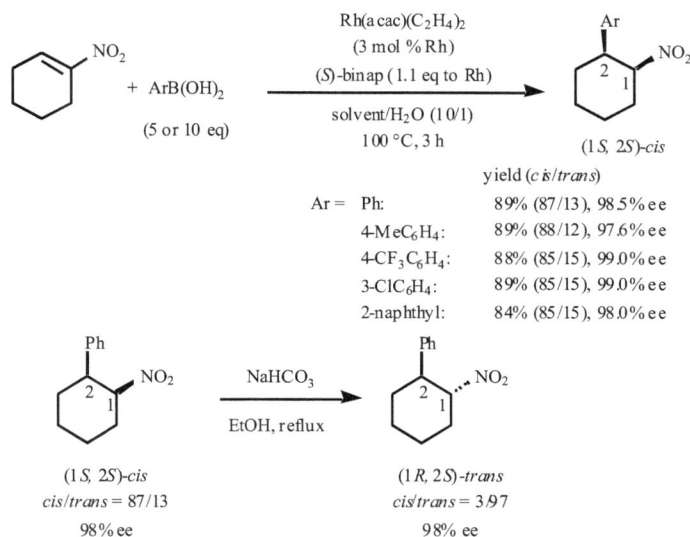

Ar =
Ph:               89% (87/13), 98.5% ee
4-MeC$_6$H$_4$:   89% (88/12), 97.6% ee
4-CF$_3$C$_6$H$_4$:  88% (85/15), 99.0% ee
3-ClC$_6$H$_4$:   89% (85/15), 99.0% ee
2-naphthyl:       84% (85/15), 98.0% ee

(1S, 2S)-cis
cis/trans = 87/13
98% ee

(1R, 2S)-trans
cis/trans = 3/97
98% ee

**Fig. (6).** Rhodium-catalyzed asymmetric 1,4-addition to a nitroalkene.

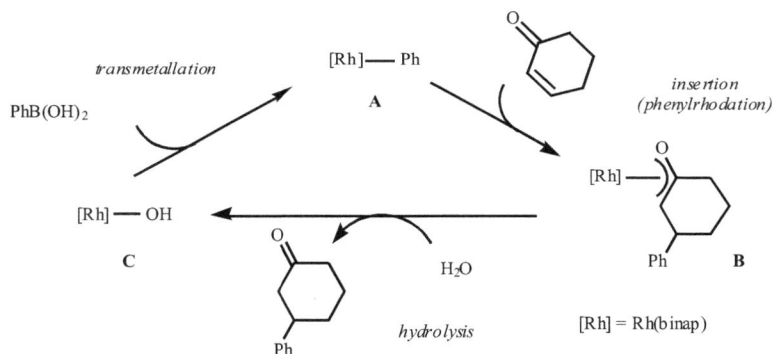

**Fig. (7).** Catalytic cycle for the rhodium-catalyzed 1,4-addition.

phenylrhodium **A**, oxa-π-allylrhodium **B**, and hydroxorhodium **C** complexes. All of the intermediates and transformations between the three complexes were observed in NMR spectroscopic studies, Fig. (**8**). The reaction of phenylrhodium complex RhPh(PPh$_3$)(binap) with 2-cyclohexenone gave oxa-π-allylrhodium which is formed by insertion of the carbon-carbon double bond of enone into the phenyl-rhodium bond followed by isomerization into the thermodynamically stable complex. The oxa-π-allylrhodium complex was converted immediately into hydroxorhodium complex [Rh(OH)(binap)]$_2$ on addition of water, liberating the phenylation product. Transmetallation of phenyl group from boron to rhodium takes place by addition of phenylboronic acid in the presence of triphenylphosphine to regenerate the phenylrhodium RhPh(PPh$_3$)(binap).

All the three transformations in Fig. (**8**) was found to proceed at 25 °C, but the catalytic reaction in the presence of a rhodium catalyst generated from Rh(acac)(C$_2$H$_4$)$_2$ does not proceed at 60 °C or lower. It turned out that the acetylacetonato ligand retards the transmetallation step because of the high stability of the rhodium-acac moiety. Use of the

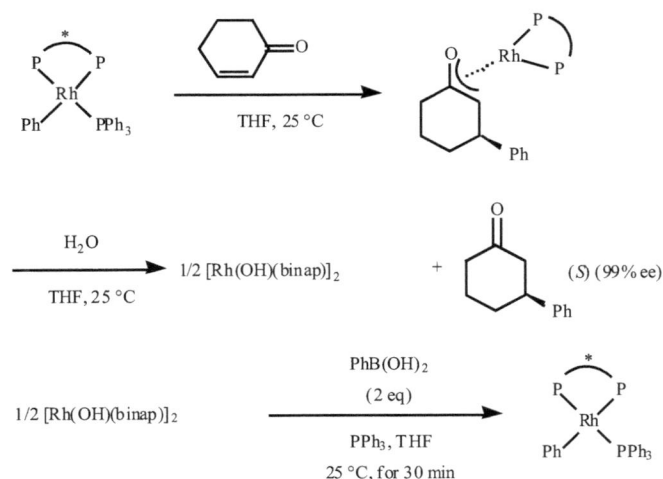

**Fig. (8).** Supporting experiments for the catalytic cycle.

hydroxo complex [Rh(OH)(binap)]₂ as a catalyst made it possible to run the reaction at lower temperature, Fig. (9) [19]. Thus, the addition of phenylboronic acid or phenylboroxine to 2-cyclohexenone is catalyzed by [Rh(OH)(binap)]₂ at 35 °C to give a quantitative yield of 3-phenylcyclohexanone which is over 99% enantiomerically pure. This catalyst system is also applicable to the reaction of other enones and organoboron reagents. The enantioselectivity is always higher than that in the reaction catalyzed by the rhodium-acac complex at 100 °C because the reaction temperature is lower. The chemical yields are higher and less boron reagent is used because the hydrolysis of the boronic acids, which is the main side reaction, is suppressed at the lower temperature.

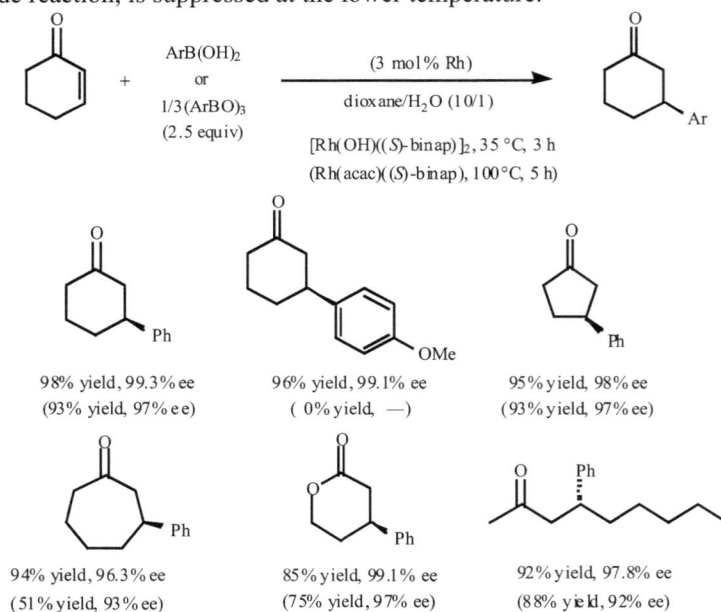

**Fig. (9).** Asymmetric 1,4-addition catalyzed by [Rh(OH)((S)-binap)]2.

Fig. (**10**) shows the stereochemical pathway in the reaction catalyzed by the rhodium complex coordinated with (*S*)-binap [7]. According to the highly skewed structure known for transition metal complexes coordinated with a binap ligand [20], (*S*)-binap–rhodium intermediate **D** should have an open space at the lower part of the vacant coordination site, the upper part being blocked by one of the phenyl rings of the binap ligand. The olefinic double bond of 2-cyclohexenone coordinates to rhodium with its α*si* face forming **E** rather than with its α*re* face, which undergoes migratory insertion to form a stereogenic carbon center in **F** whose absolute configuration is *S*. The absolute configurations of all the 1,4-addition products can be predicted by this type of stereocontrol model, (*S*)-binap–rhodium intermediate attacking the α*si* face of α,β-unsaturated ketones, both cyclic and linear ones, and other electron deficient olefins including α,β-unsaturated esters and alkenylphosphonates.

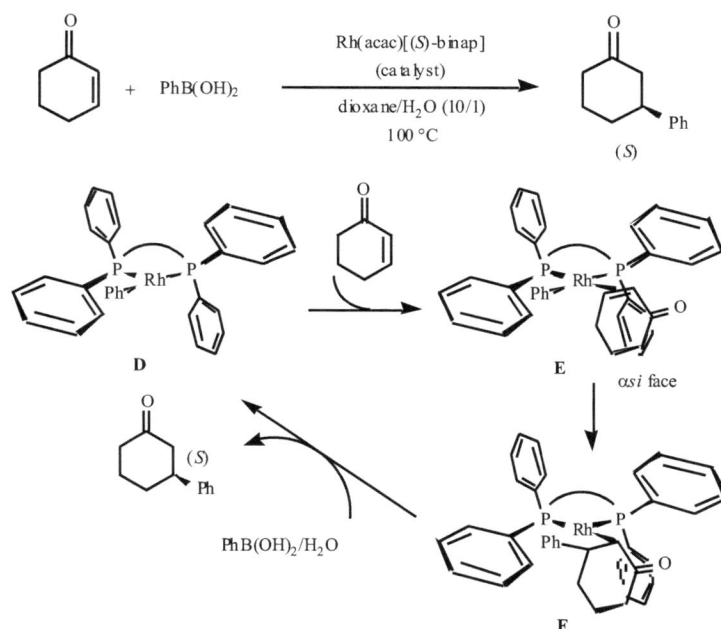

**Fig. (10).** Stereochemical pathway in the rhodium-catalyzed asymmetric 1,4-addition.

## ASYMMETRIC 1,4-ADDITION OF ORGANOBORON AND -TITANIUM REAGENTS FORMING METAL ENOLATES

In the rhodium-catalyzed 1,4-addition of organoboron reagents to electron deficient alkenes described above, protic solvents represented by water play a key role in the catalytic cycle which involves hydrolysis of oxo-π-allylrhodium giving hydroxorhodium species and the hydrolyzed 1,4-addition product, *cf.* Fig. (**7**). The use of water as a cosolvent is one of the advantages of this reaction over other 1,4-addition reactions, but one major drawback is that the 1,4-addition product is obtained as the hydrolyzed product. A catalytic asymmetric 1,4-addition giving boron enolates as the products would be more useful. Recently it was found that the use of *B*-Ar-9BBN realizes the catalytic asymmetric 1,4-addition forming chiral boron enolates, Fig. (**11**) [21]. As a typical example, the reaction of 2-cyclohexenone with 1.1 equiv of *B*-Ph-9BBN in the presence of 3 mol % of a rhodium catalyst generated from [Rh(OMe)(cod)]₂ and (*S*)-binap in toluene at 80 °C for 1 h gave a high yield of the boron enolate which is an *S* isomer of 98% ee. Unfortunately, this reaction forming chiral boron enolate is observed only for 2-cyclohexenone and 2-cycloheptenone. The reaction of boron enolate with electrophiles provides us with a chance for the further transformation as expected.

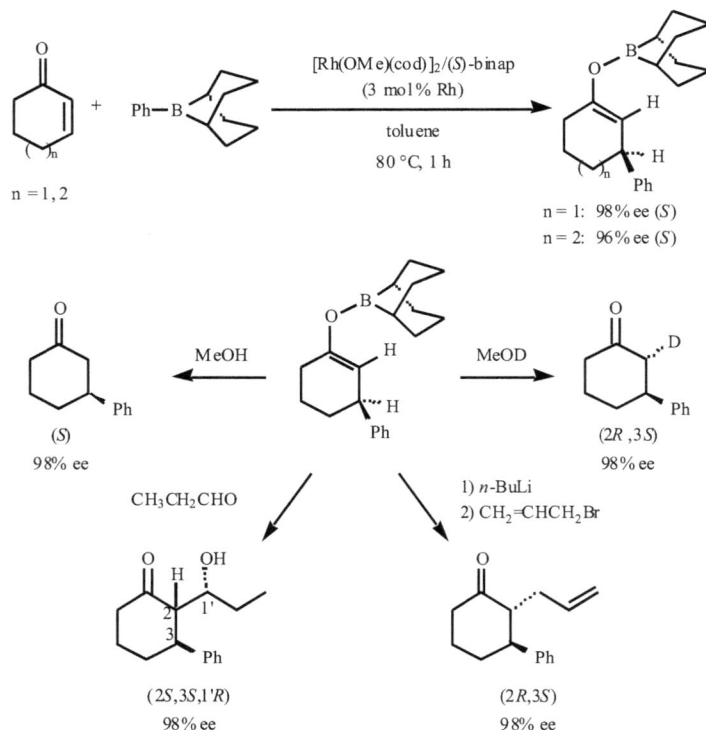

**Fig. (11).** Rhodium-catalyzed asymmetric 1,4-addition of *B*-Ar-9BBN.

A new type of catalytic tandem 1,4-addition–aldol reaction has been also found by use of *B*-Ar-9BBN [22]. The reaction of *B*-Ar-9BBN, vinyl ketone, and aldehyde catalyzed by [Rh(OMe)(cod)]$_2$ proceeded in toluene at 20 °C to give high yield of the aldol-type product with high syn selectivity, Fig. (**12**). Asymmetric reaction using [Rh(OH)((*S*)-binap)]$_2$ as a catalyst gave optically active products, *syn*-(4*S*,5*R*)-aldol of 41% ee and *anti*-(4*R*,5*R*)-**46** of 94% ee, though the *syn/anti* selectivity is low.

Recently we found that a rhodium catalyst and aryltitanium triisopropoxide (ArTi(OPr-*i*)$_3$) is a good combination for the asymmetric 1,4-addition to α,β-unsaturated ketones in an aprotic solvent, Fig. (**13**) [23]. The addition of ArTi(OPr-*i*)$_3$ to 2-cyclohexenone was completed within 1 h in the presence of 3 mol % of [Rh(OH)((*S*)-binap)]$_2$ in THF at 20 °C to give high yields of the titanium enolates as 1,4-addition products. The enantioselectivity is very high, 99.5%, 99.0%, and 99.8% ee, for Ar = Ph, 4-FC$_6$H$_4$, and 4-MeOC$_6$H$_4$, respectively. The titanium enolates were converted into silyl enol ethers by treatment with chlorotrimethylsilane and lithium isopropoxide. Other cyclic enones, 2-cyclopentenone and 2-cycloheptenone, and some linear enones are also good substrates for the asymmetric 1,4-addition of phenyltitanium triisopropoxide giving the corresponding arylation products with over 97% enantioselectivity. The catalytic cycle was demonstrated by NMR studies to

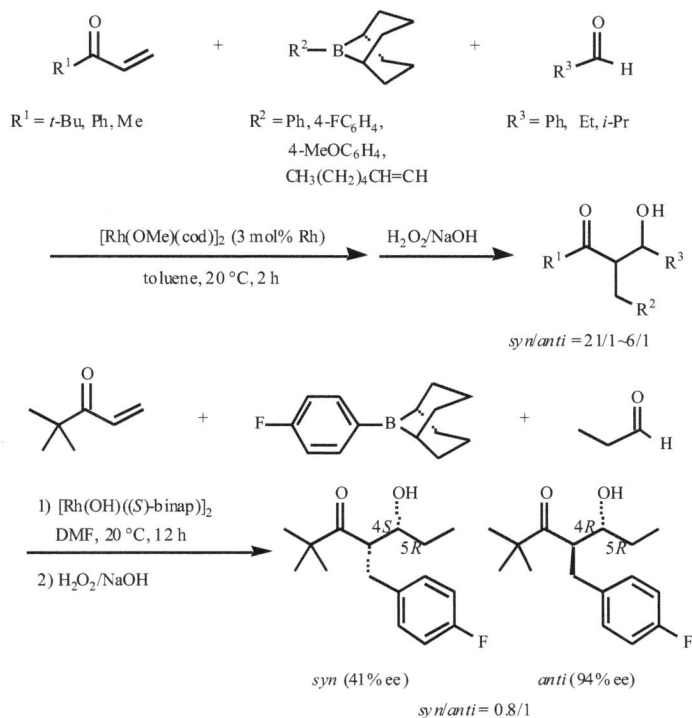

**Fig. (12).** Rhodium-catalyzed tandem 1,4-addition–aldol reaction.

involve the transmetallation of the aryl group from titanium to rhodium of the (oxa-π-allyl)rhodium intermediate leaving an arylrhodium species and the titanium enolate.

The use of alkenyl sulfones for the rhodium-catalyzed addition of aryltitanium reagents (ArTi(OPr-$i$)$_3$) was found to give us an interesting result, Fig. (**14**) [24]. The addition to linear alkenyl sulfones, 1-phenylsulfonyl-1-octene and 2-phenylsulfonyl-1-octene, resulted in a *cine* substitution reaction, where the sulfonyl group is substituted with the phenyl group on the next carbon of the double bond took place regioselectively. The catalytic cycle was established by deuterium labeling studies to proceed through *anti*-elimination of rhodium and sulfonyl group from an alkyl-rhodium intermediate. In the addition reaction to cyclic alkenyl sulfone, 1-phenylsulfonylcyclohexene, the asymmetric carbon center created at the carbo-rhodation step is retained in the substitution product. Thus, the reaction of with aryltitanium triisopropoxides (ArTi(OPr-$i$)$_3$) in the presence of 3 mol % of [Rh(OH)((S)-binap)]$_2$ in THF at 40 °C gave a quantitative yield of 1-arylcyclohexenes with over 99% enantioselectivity.

## CONCLUSION

The rhodium-catalyzed reaction shown here involves a rhodium-aryl or -alkenyl species as an intermediate in the catalytic cycle. Considering the reactivity of the transition metal-carbon bond toward carbon-carbon or carbon-hetero atom multiple bonds, the rhodium intermediate is expected to add to some unsaturated bonds other than the electron deficient olefins. Actually, the addition of organoboron reagents to aldehydes [25] and imines [26]

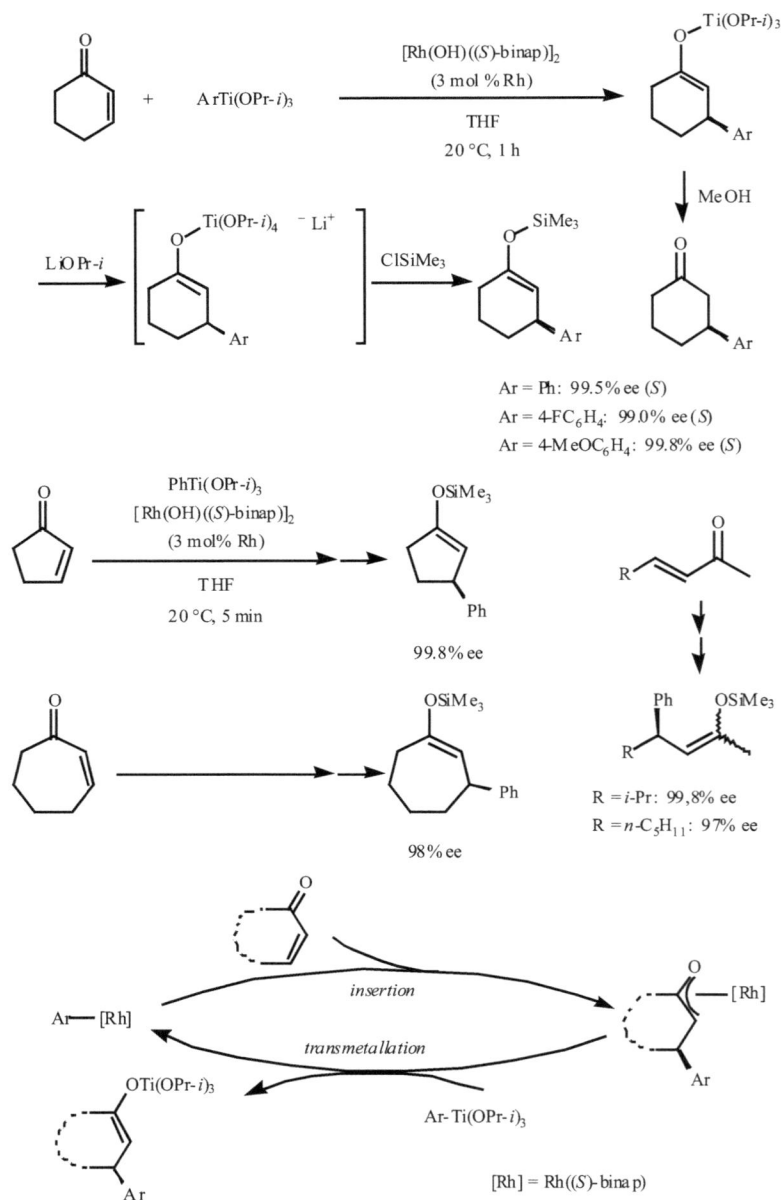

**Fig. (13).** Rhodium-catalyzed asymmetric 1,4-addition of aryltitanium reagents.

has been reported to be catalyzed by a rhodium complex. The addition to aldehydes is applied to asymmetric synthesis of diarylmethanols, though the enantioselectivity is not high enough [25a]. An interesting reactions of arylboronic acids with norbornene and oxanorbornene derivatives have been reported by Miura [27] and Lautens [28], respectively, which involve the addition of rhodium-aryl bond to the norbornene double bond. In the reaction of oxanorbornene derivatives forming chiral functionalized cyclohexenes as ring-opening products, over 90% enantioselectivity has been achieved [28]. The arylrhodium species can be also generated by transmetallation from some other organometallic reagents. The addition of aryltin [29], -silicon [30], and –bismuth [31] reagents to α,β-unsaturated carbonyl compounds catalyzed by a rhodium complex is thought to proceed through a similar catalytic cycle. The addition of arylsilanes has recently been applied to the catalytic asymmetric synthesis [32]. High enantioselectivity has been achieved in the arylation of imines with arylstannanes, which is catalyzed by a rhodium complex coordinated with an axially chiral monodentate phosphine ligand (MOP). Many new catalytic reactions of synthetic value will be developed by combination of various types of organometallic reagents and unsaturated molecules, and some of them will be extended to catalytic asymmetric reactions of high enantioselectivity by proper tuning of the chiral catalyst.

**Fig. (14).** Rhodium-catalyzed asymmetric arylation of alkenylsulfones with aryltitaniums.

## ACKNOWLEDGMENTS

The author is indebted to his co-workers for their experimental and intellectual contribution to this work. Much of the work at the initial stage has been supported by

"Research for the Future" Program, the Japan Society for the Promotion of Science and a Grant-in-Aid for Scientific Research, the Ministry of Education, Japan.

## REFERENCES

[1]     a) Ojima, I. Catalytic Asymmetric Synthesis, 2nd Ed., Wiley-VCH: New York, 2000. b) Jacobsen, E. N.; Pfaltz, A.; Yamamoto, H. Comprehensive Asymmetric Catalysis, Springer: Berlin, 1999; Vols. *1-3.* c) Noyori, R. *Asymmetric Catalysis in Organic Synthesis*, Wiley: New York, 1994.

[2]     For reviews on 1,4-addition reactions: a) Perlmutter, P. Conjugate Addition Reactions in Organic Synthesis, Pergamon Press: Oxford, 1992. b) Schmalz, H.-G. In *Comprehensive Organic Synthesis*, Trost, B. M.; Fleming, I. Eds.; Pergamon: Oxford, 1991; Vol. *4*, Chapter 1.5. c) Rossiter, B. E.; Swingle, N. M. *Chem. Rev.*, 1992, *92*, 771.

[3]     For recent reviews on catalytic asymmetric 1,4-addition: a) Krause, N.; Hoffmann-Röder, A. *Synthesis*, 2001, 171. b) Sibi, M. P.; Manyem, S. *Tetrahedron*, 2000, *56*, 8033. c) Tomioka, K.; Nagaoka, Y. In *Comprehensive Asymmetric Catalysis*; Jacobsen, E. N.; Pfaltz, A.; Yamamoto, H. Eds.; Springer: Berlin, 1999, Vol. *3*, Chapter 31.1. d) Kanai, M.; Shibasaki, M. In *Catalytic Asymmetric Synthesis*, 2nd Ed., Ojima, I. Ed.; Wiley: New York, 2000, pp. 569-592.

[4]     For examples of the copper-catalyzed asymmetric 1,4-addition of organozinc reagents: a) Mizutani, H.; Degrado, S. J.; Hoveyda, A. H. *J. Am. Chem. Soc.,* 2002, *124*, 779. b) Alexakis, A.; Benhaim, C.; Rosset, S.; Humam, M. *J. Am. Chem. Soc.*, 2002, *124*, 5262. c) Arnold, L. A.; Naasz, R.; Minnaard, A. J.; Feringa, B. L. *J. Am. Chem. Soc.*, 2001, *123*, 5841. d) Alexakis, A.; Trevitt, G. P.; Bernardinelli, G. *J. Am. Chem. Soc.*, 2001, *123*, 4358. e) Degrado, S. J.; Mizutani, H.; Hoveyda, A. H. *J. Am. Chem. Soc.*, 2001, *123*, 755. f) Escher I. H.; Pfaltz, A. *Tetrahedron*, 2000, *56*, 2879. g) Yan, M.; Chan, A. S. C. *Tetrahedron Lett.*, 1999, *40*, 6645.

[5]     For examples for catalytic asymmetric Michael addition of malonate esters: a) Yamaguchi, M.; Shiraishi, T.; Hirama, M. *J. Org. Chem.*, 1996, *61*, 3520. b) Arai, T.; Sasai, H.; Aoe, K.; Okamura, K.; Date, T.; Shibasaki, M. *Angew. Chem. Int. Ed.*, 1996, *35*, 104. c) Shibasaki, M.; Sasai, H.; Arai, T. *Angew. Chem. Int. Ed.*, 1997, *36*, 1236. d) Kim, Y. S.; Matsunaga, S.; Das, J.; Sekine, A.; Ohshima, T.; Shibasaki, M. *J. Am. Chem. Soc.*, 2000, *122*, 6506, and references cited therein.

[6]     Sakai, M.; Hayashi, H.; Miyaura, N. *Organometallics*, 1997, *16*, 4229.

[7]     Takaya, Y.; Ogasawara, M.; Hayashi, T.; Sakai, M.; Miyaura, N. *J. Am. Chem. Soc.*, 1998, *120*, 5579.

[8]     a) Kuriyama, M.; Nagai, K.; Yamada, K.; Miwa, Y.; Taga, T.; Tomioka, K. *J. Am. Chem. Soc.*, 2002, *124*, 8932. b) Reetz, M. T.; Moulin, D.; Gosberg, A. *Org. Lett.*, 2001, *3*, 4083. c) Amengual, R.; Michelet, V.; Genêt, J.-P. *Synlett.*, 2002, 1791. d) Boiteau, J.-G.; Imbos, R.; Minnaard, A. J.; Feringa, B. L. *Org. Lett.*, 2003, *5*, 681.

[9]     For reviews concerned with the rhodium-catalyzed asymmetric addition: a) Fagnou K.; Lautens, M. *Chem. Rev.*, 2003, *103*, 169. b) Hayashi, T.; Yamasaki, K. *Chem. Rev.*, 2003, *103*, 2829. c) Bolm, C.; Hildebrand, J. P.; Muniz, K.; Hermanns, N. *Angew. Chem. Int. Ed.*, 2001, *40*, 3284. d) Hayashi, T. *Synlett.*, 2001, 879.

[10]    Hayashi, T.; Takahashi, M.; Takaya, Y.; Ogasawara, M. *Org. Synth.*, 2002, *79*, 84.

[11]    Takaya, Y.; Ogasawara, M.; Hayashi, T. *Tetrahedron Lett.*, 1998, *39*, 8479.

[12]    Takaya, Y.; Ogasawara, M.; Hayashi, T. *Tetrahedron Lett.*, 1999, *40*, 6957.

[13]    Takaya, Y.; Senda, T.; Kurushima, H.; Ogasawara, M.; Hayashi, T. *Tetrahedron: Asymmetry*, 1999, *10*, 4047.

[14]    Similar results for the asymmetric 1,4-addition of arylboronic acids to α,β-unsaturated esters and amides has been independently reported by Miyaura: a) Sakuma, S.; Sakai, M.; Itooka, R.; Miyaura, N. *J. Org. Chem.*, 2000, *65*, 5951. b) Sakuma, S.; Miyaura, N. *J. Org. Chem.*, 2001, *66*, 8944.

[15]    Senda, T.; Ogasawara, M.; Hayashi, T. *J. Org. Chem.*, 2001, *66*, 6852.

[16]    Hayashi, T.; Senda, T.; Takaya, Y.; Ogasawara, M. *J. Am. Chem. Soc.*, 1999, *121*, 11591.

[17]    Tokunaga, Y.; Ueno, H.; Shimomura, Y.; Seo, T. *Heterocycles*, 2002, *57*, 787.

[18]    Hayashi, T.; Senda, T.; Ogasawara, M. *J. Am. Chem. Soc.*, 2000, *122*, 10716.

[19]    Hayashi, T.; Takahashi, M.; Takaya, Y.; Ogasawara, M. *J. Am. Chem. Soc.*, 2002, *124*, 5052.

[20]    Ozawa, F.; Kubo, A.; Matsumoto, Y.; Hayashi, T.; Nishioka, E.; Yanagi, K.; Moriguchi, K. *Organometallics*, 1993, *12*, 4188, and references cited therein.

[21]    Yoshida, K.; Ogasawara, M.; Hayashi, T. *J. Org. Chem.*, 2003, *68*, 1901.

[22]    Yoshida, K.; Ogasawara, M.; Hayashi, T. *J. Am. Chem. Soc.*, 2002, *124*, 10984.

[23]    Hayashi, T.; Tokunaga, N.; Yoshida, K.; Han, J. W. *J. Am. Chem. Soc.*, 2002, *124*, 12102.

[24]    Yoshida, K.; Hayashi, T. *J. Am. Chem. Soc.*, 2003, *125*, 2872.

[25]    Sakai, M.; Ueda, M.; Miyaura, N. *Angew. Chem. Int. Ed.*, 1998, *37*, 3279. b) Ueda, M.; Miyaura, N. *J. Org. Chem.*, 2000, *65*, 4450.

[26]    Ueda, M.; Miyaura, N. *J. Organomet. Chem.*, 2000, *595*, 31.

[27]    Oguma, K.; Miura, M.; Satoh, T.; Nomura, M. *J. Am. Chem. Soc.*, 2000, *122*, 10464.

[28]    Lautens, M.; Dockendorff, C.; Fagnou, K.; Malicki, A. *Org. Lett.*, **2002**, *4*, 1311. b) Lautens, M.; Fagnou, K.; Hiebert, S. *Acc. Chem. Res.*, **2003**, *36*, 48.

[29]    a) Oi, S.; Moro, M.; Ono, S.; Inoue, Y. *Chem. Lett.*, **1998**, 83. b) Oi, S.; Moro, M.; Ito, H.; Honma, Y.; Miyano, S.; Inoue, Y. *Tetrahedron*, **2002**, *58*, 91. c) Huang, T.-S.; Li, C.-J. *Org. Lett.*, **2001**, *3,* 2037. d) Venkatraman, S.; Meng, Y.; Li, C.-J. *Tetrahedron Lett.*, **2001**, *42*, 4459.

[30]    a) Oi, S.; Honma, Y.; Inoue, Y. *Org. Lett.*, **2002**, *4*, 667. b) Oi, S.; Moro, M.; Inoue, Y. *Organometallics*, **2001**, *20*, 1036. c) Mori, A.; Danda, Y.; Fujii, T.; Hirabayashi, K.; Osakada, K. *J. Am. Chem. Soc.*, **2001**, *123*, 10774. d) Koike, T.; Du, X.; Mori, A.; Osakada, K. *Synlett*, **2002**, 301. e) Mori A.; Kato, T. *Synlett*, **2002**, 1167.

[31]    Venkatraman, S.; Li, C.-J. *Tetrahedron Lett.*, **2001**, *42*, 781.

[32]    Oi, S.; Taira, A.; Honma, Y.; Inoue, Y. *Org. Lett.*, **2003**, *5*, 97.

# Tandem Stereospecific Radical Cation-Mediated Syntheses of Oligostilbenoid Dimers

Atta-ur-Rahman/Choudhary/Khan (Eds.) *Frontiers in Natural Product Chemistry, Vol. 1*

# Tandem Stereospecific Radical Cation-Mediated Syntheses of Oligostilbenoid Dimers

Noel F. Thomas[a]*, Kiew C. Lee[b], Jean-Frédéric F. Weber[c], Ibtisam Abdul Wahab[c], Khalijah Awang[a], A. Hamid A. Hadi[a] and Pascal Richomme[d]

[a] *Department of Chemistry, Faculty of Sciences, Universiti Malaya, 59100 Kuala Lumpur, Malaysia,* [b] *Department of Chemistry, Faculty of Sciences, National University of Singapore, 117543 Singapore,* [c] *Faculty of Pharmacy, Universiti Teknologi MARA, 40450 Shah Alam, Malaysia,* [d] *Faculté des Sciences, Université d'Angers, 2, boulevard Lavoisier, 49045 Angers, France*

**Abstract:** Protected trihydroxystilbenes have been synthesized by Heck coupling methodology in three steps. Treatment of 3,4-dimethoxy-12-benzyloxymethyl stilbene with ferric chloride in dichloromethane (room temperature), gave catechol analogues of ampelopsin F and of restrytisol C, while 3,4-dimethoxy-12-acetoxymethyl stilbene treated in the same conditions yielded two other analogues of restrytisol C (but no trace of ampelopsin F analogues). All the structures were unambiguously confirmed by 1D- and 2D- homo- and heteronuclear nmr experiments. All transformations were stereospecific. The ampelopsin F-type compounds are the result of radical cation pathways. By contrast, the restrytisol C-type compounds are the products of pericyclic pathways.

## INTRODUCTION

Resveratrol **1** and piceatannol **2** are natural building blocks for oligostilbenoids from dipterocarpaceous timber trees, such as heimiol A **3**, distichol **4**, hopeaphenol **5**, or cassigarol D **6** [1, 2].Oligostilbenoids have shown *in vitro* numerous biological activities (antimicrobial, antifungal, antioxidant, antiulcer, anti-HIV, cytotoxic, antiplatelet, anti-inflammatory, protein kinase C inhibitor, etc.), but their real potential as drug candidate remains to be determined [1].

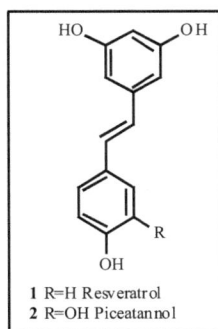

**1** R=H Resveratrol
**2** R=OH Piceatannol

*Corresponding author: E-mail: noelfthomas@um.edu.my

THOMAS *et al.*

The majority of oligostilbenoid polymers possess the substitution pattern of resveratrol **1**, from which they are biosynthesised. Potential stilbene monomer building blocks that have the less often encountered catechol arrangement do exist, but seem to be relatively infrequently used in oligostilbenoid biosynthesis. One of the few exceptions to the above, is cassigarol D **5** which is an oligostilbenoid dimer possessing the catechol arrangement and also the phenanthrene ring system. The biosynthetic building block for this synthesis is not resveratrol **1** but piceatannol **2**.

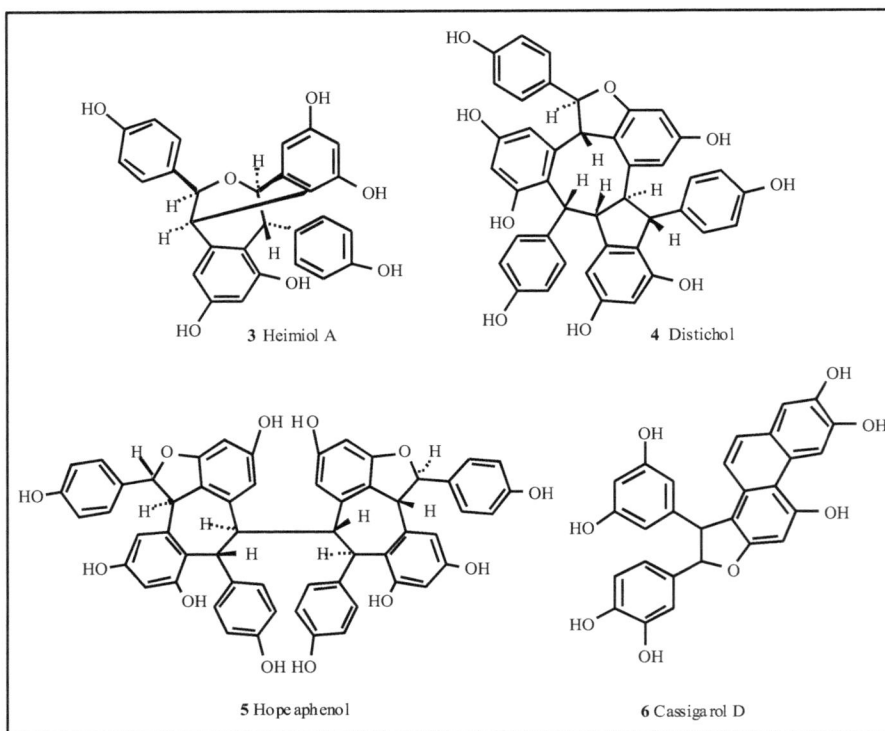

For these reasons, we are investigating biomimetic syntheses of these compounds so that, eventually, various analogues can be produced on demand for studies on structure-activity relationships. In this first phase of our investigations and consistent with the biomimetic principle, the synthetic strategy was based on oxidative phenolic coupling. Protected trihydroxystilbenes were treated with one-electron oxidants. In a previous communication, we have described the regioselective oxidative lactonization of stilbenes with Mn(OAc)₃ [3]. We have also described FeCl₃-promoted synthesis of catechol analogues of restrytisol C [4]. Some aspects of this chemistry are described in this paper, together with new ones.

## DISCUSSION

We have synthesized stilbenes using standard Heck coupling conditions [3] (PdCl₂, Ph₃P, K⁺OAc⁻, AgNO₃, DMF, 120°C), Fig. (**1**). The protected iodophenols **9a** and **9b** and protected styrene **10** were generated by standard benzylation [4] and Wittig [5] methodologies. When stilbenes **11a** and **11b** were treated with ferric chloride in dichloromethane, Fig. (**1**), several stilbene dimers were isolated whose nmr spectra indicated

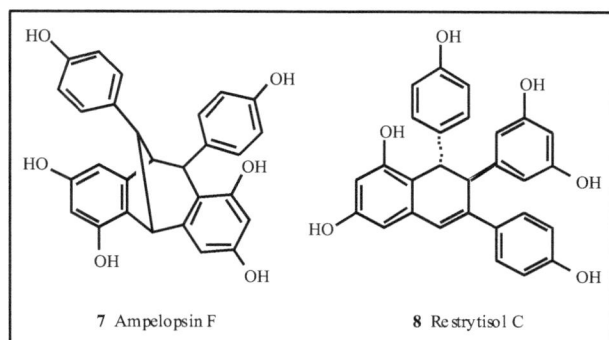

four methoxymethyl singlets. Two types of skeletons were generated, that of ampelopsin F **7** and that of restrytisol C **8**. We will now discuss the mechanistic aspects of the transformation leading to these novel dimers.

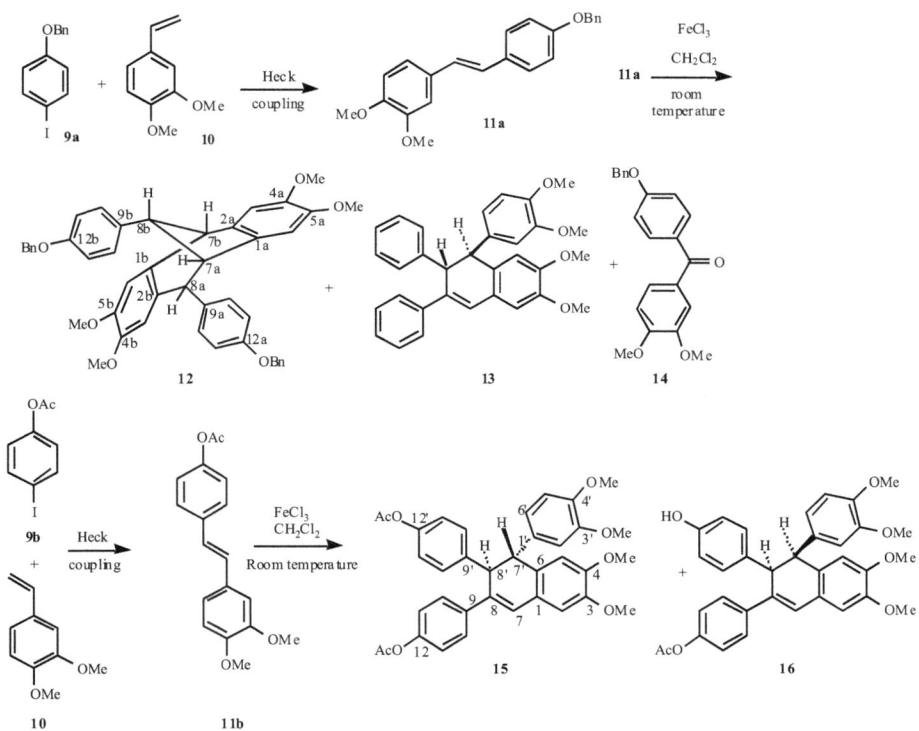

**Fig. (1).** Syntheses of stilbene monomers and dimers.

## Synthesis of the Ampelopsin F Analogue 12

Complete structural elucidation of **12** was possible by exploiting [1]H NMR (400 MHz), [13]C (DEPT), COSY, TOCSY, HMQC, HMBC, NOESY, and high resolution mass spectra.

The mechanism for the formation of **12** is as follows, Fig. (**2**). Radical cation dimerization of **17**, which could also involve the resonance-stabilised form **18**, followed by attack on the benzylic carbocation of one component by the electron-rich catechol ring of the other component would give rise to **19**. Intramolecular nucleophilic attack involving the *para* position of one catechol ring on the electrophilic quinone methyl completes the installation of the bicyclo[3,2,1] system present in **20**. Further oxidation of the radical cation in **20** followed by rapid deprotonation/aromatisation would produce **12**.

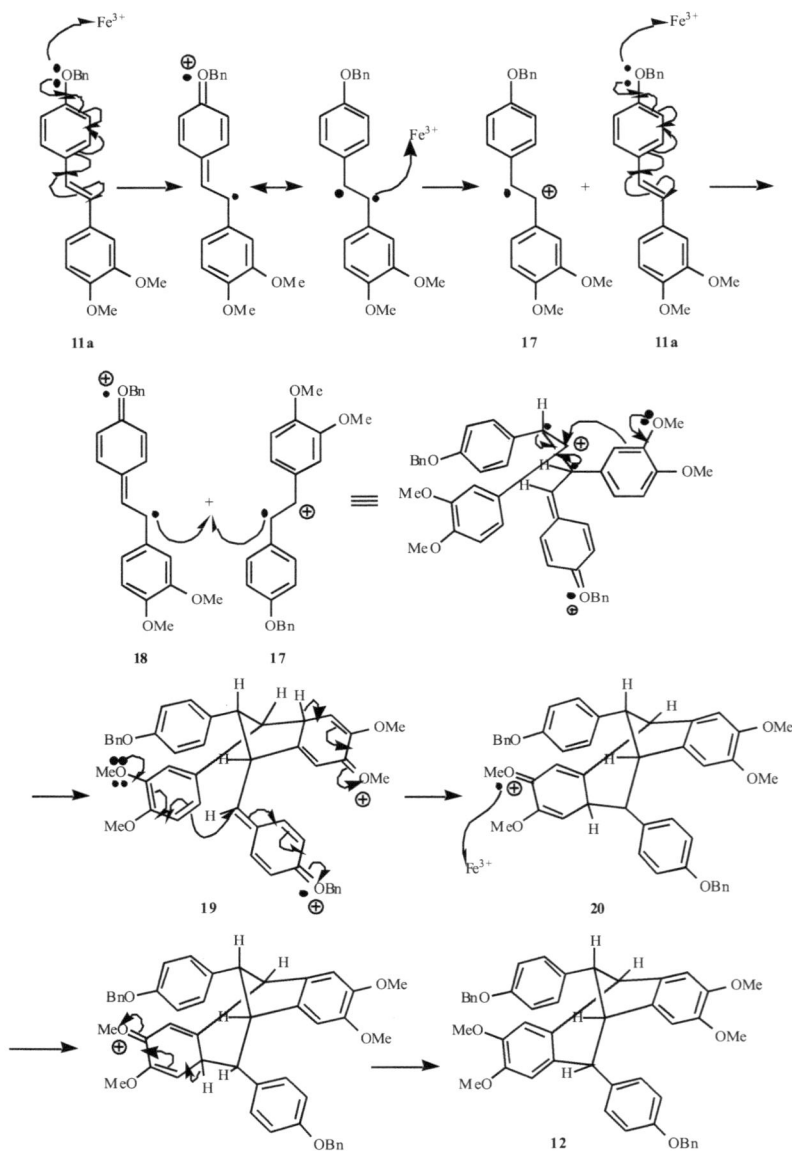

**Fig. (2).** Proposed mechanism formation of **12**.

### Synthesis of Restrytisol C Analogue 13

**13** was obtained as a yellowish oil, exhibiting a strong blue fluorescence under UV-254 nm light which revealed the presence of a strong conjugated structure. The structure of **11** was fully elucidated from HRMS and 2D NMR.

The mechanism for the pericyclic transformation of compound **13** can be explained by application of the Woodward-Hoffmann rules [6]. The mechanism is initiated by the formation of radical cation **21** followed by coupling of the two radical and rapid deprotonation leading to the diene **22**, Fig. (**3**).

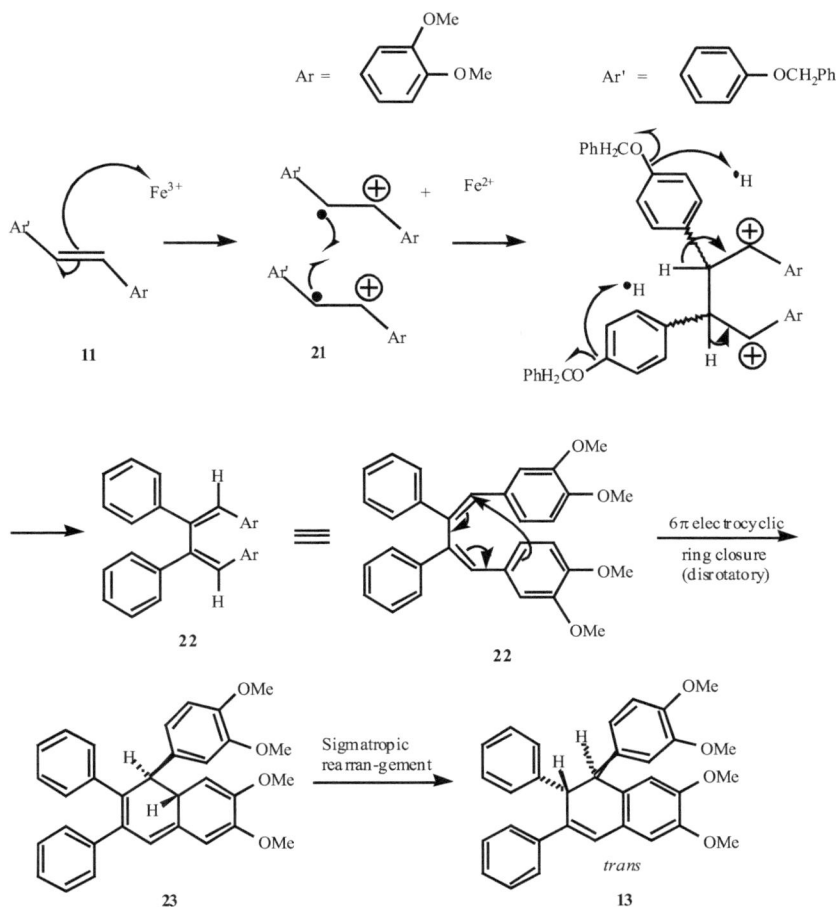

**Fig. (3).** Proposed mechanism from **11** to **13**.

There is a competition between $4\pi$ and $6\pi$ electrocyclic closure. However in this case only $6\pi$ electrocyclic ring closure is involved in the formation of **23**, followed by a sigmatropic rearrangement ([1,5]-hydride shift) to provide **13**. The cleavage of the both benzyloxy groups also occur in this step. The steric effect of the two benzyl groups might be the driving force of their cleavage. There are two possible pathways for the bisbenzyloxy cleavage, Fig. (**4**). In pathway A, homolytic cleavage of **24** would give rise to the aryl radical **25** and benzaldehyde. This radical can be quenched by a hydrogen radical, which is in turn obtained by $Fe^{3+}$ oxidation of hydride ion. For pathway B, loss of a hydride ion would generate the oxocarbenium **26**, which then undergoes hydrolysis in the work-up to give aryl cation, which is then reduced by a hydride ion. It should be observed that pathway B is the source of hydride both for reduction of $Ar^+$ and for generation of hydrogen radical as previously described. Logically pathways A and B are concurrent.

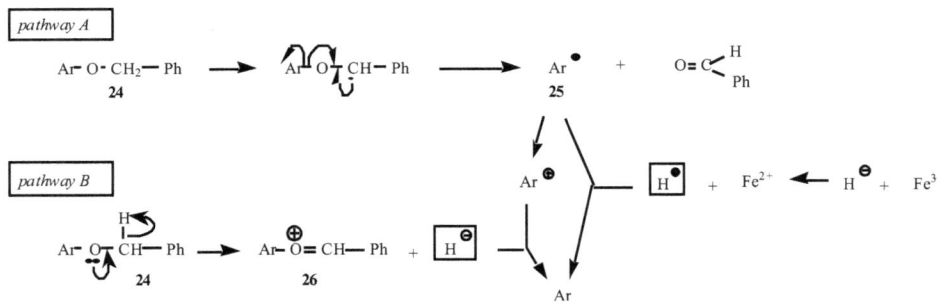

**Fig. (4).** Formation of the hydride ion and hydrogen radical.

The transformation of **22** to **13** can be explained by frontier orbital considerations, as shown in **scheme 5**. By considering the highest occupied molecular orbital (HOMO) for the $6\pi$ system (hexatriene) **22**, disrotatory ring closure leading to 27 culminating in the *trans* disposed hydrogens at the two new stereogenic centres is to be expected. This is then followed by symmetry-allowed [1,5] suprafacial hydride shifts. This pericyclic transformation is thermally allowed based on the Woodward Hoffmann rules, [6].

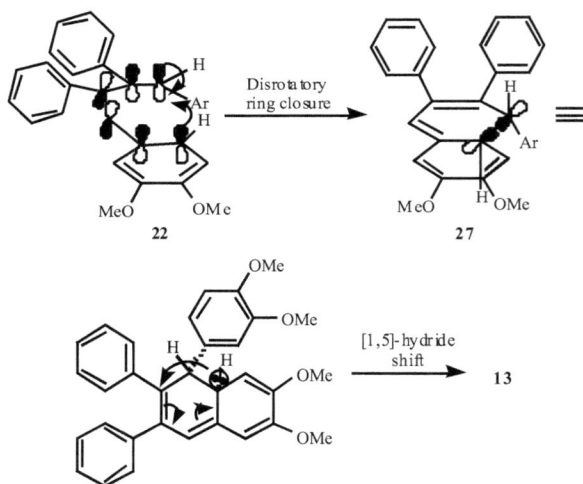

**Fig. (5).** Thermally allowed $6\pi$-electron electrocyclizations leading to *trans*-configuration (Woodward-Hoffmann rules).

## Synthesis of (4-Benzyloxyphenyl)-(3,4-Dimethoxyphenyl)-Methanone 14

**14** was obtained as colourless crystals. Our mechanistic hypothesis begins with formation of the radical cation **28** and followed by oxidation and addition of water to produce the diol

**29**. Further oxidation to produce the hydroxyketone **30** was followed by a Wagner-Meerwein-type rearrangement to produce the aldehyde **31**. $C\equiv O$ extrusion from **32**, probably assisted the presence of $Fe^{3+}$, completes the rearrangement leading to **14**, Fig. (**6**).

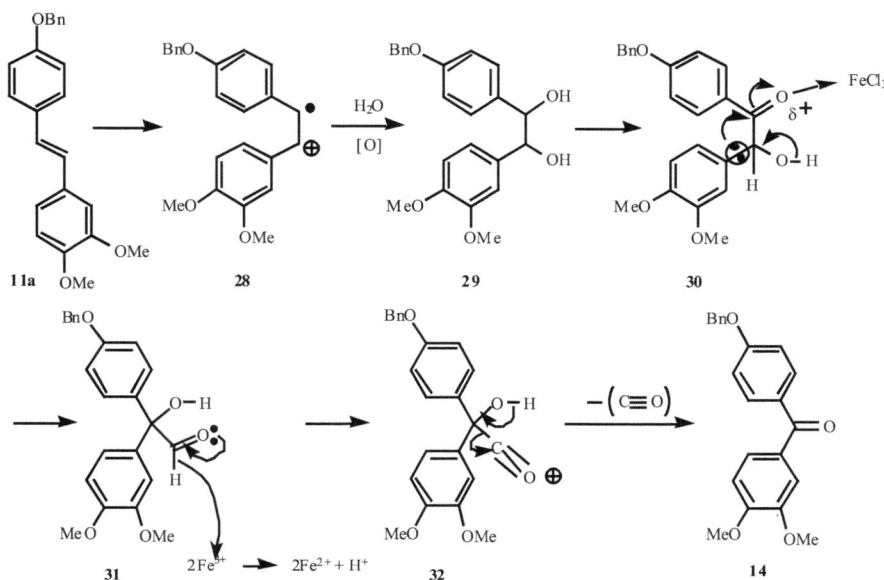

**Fig. (6).** Proposed mechanism to (4-benzyloxy-phenyl)-(3,4-dimethoxy-phenyl)-methanone **14**.

## Synthesis of Restrytisol C Analogues 15 and 16

Compounds **15** and **16** were both obtained as a yellowish oils, strongly blue fluorescent under UV-254 nm light. The formation of **15** and **16** also can be explained by thermally-allowed pericyclic transformations. The mechanism is initiated by $Fe^{3+}$ reduction to $Fe^{2+}$ with removal of one electron from the olefinic system **11b** to form a radical cation **33**, Fig. (**7**). This is followed by coupling of two radical cationic species to **34**. Rapid deprotonation of **34** would yield the dienes **35a** and **35b** with Z,Z-isomer and Z,E-isomer respectively. $6\pi$ electrocyclic ring closure of **35a** and **35b** would give **36a** and **36b** respectively. This would be followed by sigmatropic rearrangements to provide **15** and **16**. Both *cis* and *trans* isomers were isolated from the reaction mixture. The *trans* isomer was isolated as the major compound. This may be due to its greater thermodynamic stability. Its predominance probably also reflects the fact that it is formed from the more abundant diene **35a**. The transformation of **35a** to **15** and **35b** to **16** can be explained by frontier orbital considerations, as shown in **scheme 8**. Considering the highest occupied molecular orbital (HOMO) for both $6\pi$ system (hexatriene) **35a** and **35b**, disrotatory ring closure of **35a** would provide the *trans*-disposed hydrogen at the two new stereogenic centres **36a** and then followed by [1,5]-suprafacial hydride shifts to **15**. By contrast disrotatory ring closure of **35b** would produce the *cis* configuration shown in **36b**. This is then followed by symmetry allowed [1,5]-suprafacial hydride shifts and deprotection of the acetate leading to **15**.

Radical cation dimerization were observed previously in the work of R.T. Bushby *et al.* [9] (promoted by $FeCl_3$) and K.C. Nicolaou et al. [10] (promoted by cerium ammonium nitrate). Our studies have confirmed the synthetic and versatility of such reactions.

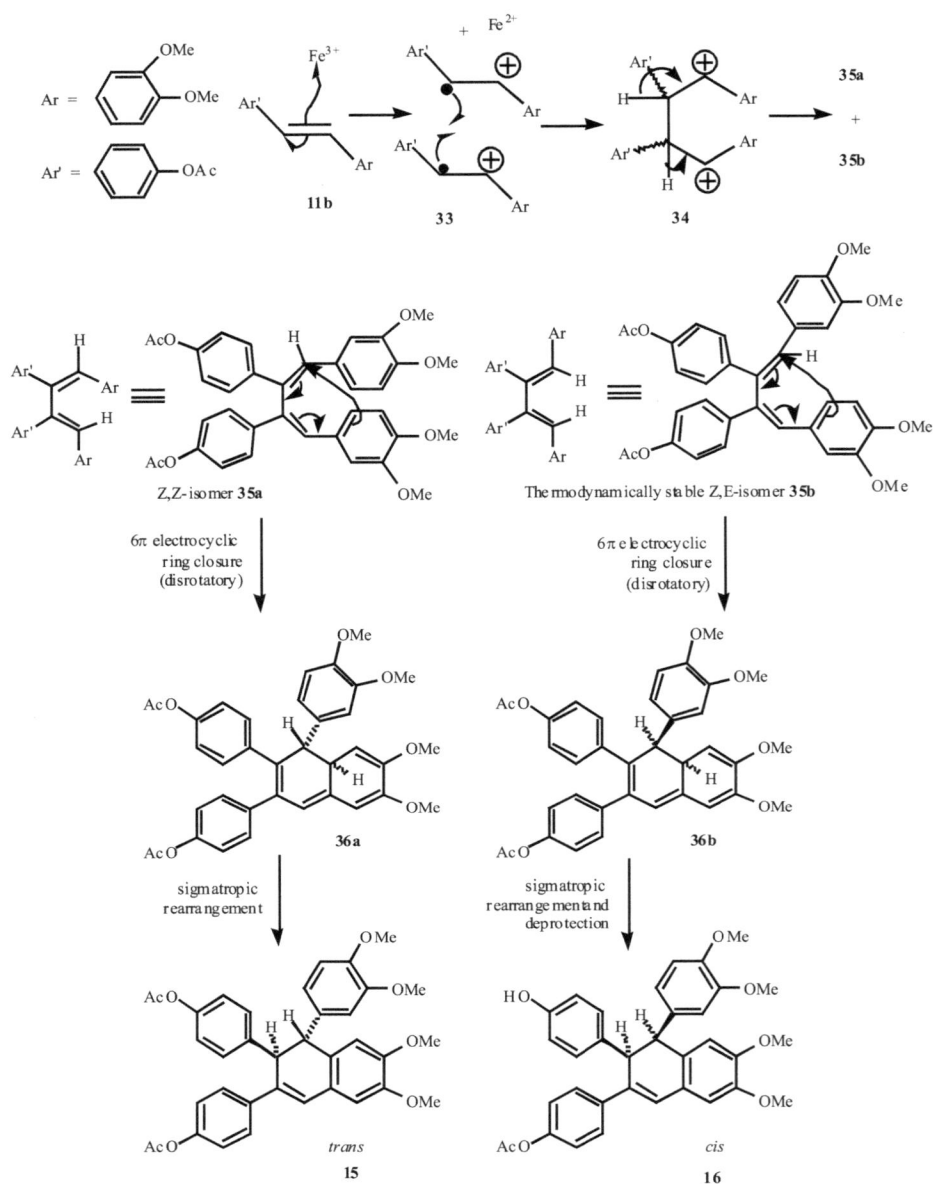

**Fig. (7).** Pericyclic mechanism leading to **15** and **16**.

## EXPERIMENTAL

### Synthesis of 3,4-dimethoxy-12-benzyloxy Stilbene 11a

The starting material, iodophenylbenzylether **9a** (5.13 g, 0.017 mol) dissolved in dry DMF (50 ml). The solution was allowed to stir under nitrogen for a few minutes. Palladium

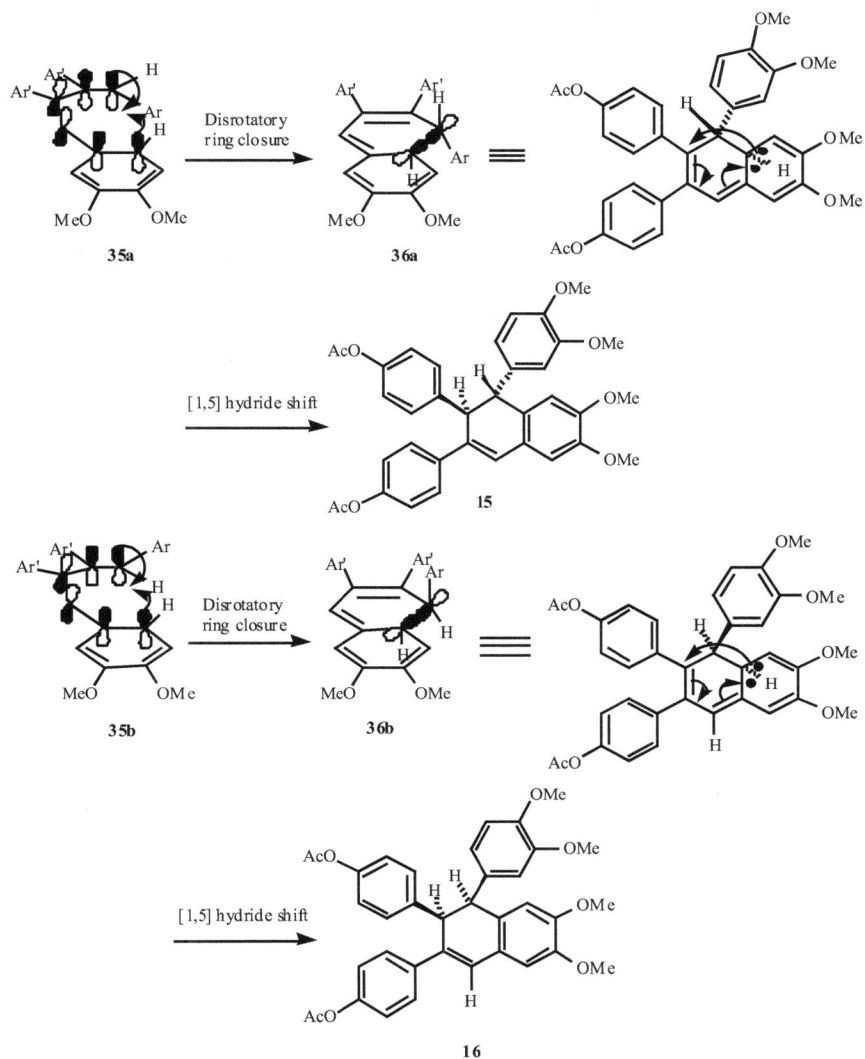

**Fig. (8).** Orbital symmetry consideration relating to the mechanism leading to **15** and **16**.

(II) chloride (0.30 g, 1.7 mmol) was then added, followed by addition of triphenylphosphine (1.28 g, 4.8 mmol), silver nitrate (3.0g, 0.018 mol), potassium acetate (2.1 g, 0.022 mol) and 3,4-dimethoxy styrene **10** (2.95 g, 0.018 mol). The mixture was refluxed under nitrogen for 3 days. The reaction mixture was filtered and quenched by saturated sodium chloride and extracted by ethyl acetate. The combined ethyl acetate extracts were dried over anhydrous Na$_2$SO$_4$. The crude will be purified by column chromatography to yield 63 % crystals.

### 3,4-Dimethoxy-12-benzyloxy Stilbene 11a

Colourless crystals. $^1$H NMR (400 MHz, CDCl$_3$) 7.05 (d; J = 2 Hz; 1H), 7.02 (d; J = 8.0,2.0 Hz; 1H), 6.82 (d; J = 8.0 Hz; 1H), 6.92 (s; 1H), 6.92 (s; 1H), 7.43 (d; J = 8.8 Hz;

1H), 7.43 (d; J = 8.8 Hz; 1H), 6.96 (d; J = 8.8 Hz; 1H), 6.96 (d; 8.8 Hz; 1H), 5.08 (s; 1H), 3.89 (d; 6H). $^{13}$C NMR (100.4 MHz, CDCl$_3$) 130.83 (C-1), 108.67 (C-2), 149.15 (C-3), 148.69 (C-4), 111.31 (C-5), 119.54 (C-6), 126.39 (C-7), 126.57 (C-8), 130.63 (C-9), 127.47 (C-10,14), 115.11 (C-11, 13), 158.30 (C-12), 70.09 (C-15), 136.96 (C-16), 127.47 (C-17, 21), 128.60 (C-18, 20), 127.99 (C-19), 55.96 (C$_3$-OC$\underline{H}_3$), 55.88 (C$_4$-OC$\underline{H}_3$).

### Synthesis of 3,4-dimethoxy, 12-acetoxy Stilbene 11b

4-iodophenylacetate **9b** (3.6 g, 0.013 mol) was dissolved in dry DMF. Palladium (II) chloride (0.24 g, 1.3 mmol), triphenylphosphine (0.70 g, 2.7 mmol), silver nitrate (2.3 g, 0.013 mol), potassium acetate (1.7 g, 0.017 mol) and 3,4-dimethoxy styrene (**9**) (2.2 g, 0.013 mol) were then added. The mixture was refluxed under nitrogen for a week. The reaction mixture was filtered and extracted with ethyl acetate. The combined ethyl acetate extracts were dried over anhydrous Na$_2$SO$_4$. The crude was purified by column chromatography to give 32 % yield of crystals.

### 3,4-Dimethoxy, 12-acetoxy Stilbene 11b

Colourless crystals. $^1$H NMR (400 MHz, CDCl$_3$) δ ppm: 7.49 (d; J = 8.6 Hz; 2H; H-10,14), 7.07 (d; J = 8.6 Hz; 2H; H-11,13), 7.06 (d; J = 2.2 Hz; 1H; H-2), 7.04 (dd; J = 8.0, 2.2, 1H; H-6), 7.00 (d; J = 16.4 Hz; 1H; H-7), 6.97 (d; J = 16.4 Hz; 1H; H-8), 6.86 (d; J = 8.0 Hz; 1H; H-5), 3.95 (s; 3H; C$_3$-OMe), 3.90 (s; 3H; C$_4$-OMe), 2.31 (s; 3H; C$_{12}$-OAc). $^{13}$C NMR (100.4 MHz, CDCl$_3$) 130.08 (C-1), 108.57 (C-2), 148.93 (C-3), 148.80 (C-4), 111.04 (C-5), 119.75 (C-6), 128.51 (C-7), 125.53 (C-8), 135.15 (C-9), 126.95 (C-10,14), 121.57 (C-11, 13), 149.61 (C-12), 169.28 (C-15), 55.71 (C$_3$-OC$\underline{H}_3$), 55.65 (C$_4$-OC$\underline{H}_3$), 20.91 (C$_{16}$-CH$_3$).

### Oxidative Coupling with Stilbene 11a

Stilbene **11a** (1.0 g, 2.9 mmol) was dissolved in 100 ml dichloromethane. FeCl$_3$.6H$_2$O (7.3 g, 27 mmol) was added into the flask. After 3 hours reactions, the reaction mixture was worked-up with MeOH. The crude mixture was dried under reduce pressure and its components separated by column and centrifugal chromatography. Three pure compounds were isolated.

### Ampelopsin F Analogue 12

17 % yield. Yellowish oil. $^1$H NMR (400 MHz, CDCl$_3$) 7.27-7.46 (m; 10H), 7.16 (d; J = 8.8 Hz, 2H), 6.94 (d; J = 8.8 Hz, 2H), 6.83 (d; J = 8.8 Hz; 2H), 6.73 (d; J = 8.8 Hz; 2H), 6.724 (s; 1H), 6.720 (s; 1H), 6.97 (s; 1H), 6.40 (s; 1H), 5.06 (s; 2H), 4.94 (s; 2H), 4.21 (s; 1H), 3.89 (s; 1H), 3.77 (s; 1H), 3.37 (s; 1H), 3.93 (s; 3H), 3.87 (s; 3H), 3.81 (s; 3H), 3.64 (s; 3H). $^{13}$C NMR (100.5 MHz, CDCl$_3$) 139.3 (C-1), 127.1 (C-1'), 130.1 (C-2,6), 128.0 (C-2',6'), 114.8 (C-3,5), 114.4 (C-3',5'), 157.4 (C-4), 157.1 (C-4'), 53.3 (C-7), 51.4 (C-7'), 50.8 (C-8), 56.5 (C-8'), 134.9 (C-9), 135.8 (C-9'), 142.2 (C-10), 137.5 (C-10'), 108.6 (C-11), 106.1 (C-11'), 148.2 (C-12), 148.0 (C-12'), 148.1 (C-13), 147.2 (C-13'), 108.1 (C-14), 115.1 (C-14'), 137.2 (C-15,15'), 127.6 (C-16,20), 127.5 (C-16',20'), 128.7 (C-17,17',19,19'), 128.6 (C-18,18'), 56.2 (C$_{12}$-OC$\underline{H}_3$), 56.0 (C$_{12'}$-OC$\underline{H}_3$), 56.1 (C$_{13}$-OC$\underline{H}_3$), 56.0 (C$_{13'}$-OC$\underline{H}_3$), 70.2 (C$_5$-OC$\underline{H}_2$), 70.0 (C$_{5'}$-OC$\underline{H}_2$).

### 1-(3,4-Dimethoxy-phenyl)-6,7-dimethoxy-2,3-diphenyl-1,2-dihydro-naphthalen 13

3 % yield. Yellowish oil. $^1$H NMR (400 MHz, CDCl$_3$) δ ppm: 7.33 (d; J = 7.6 Hz; 2H), 7.28 (d; J = 7.6 Hz; 2H), 7.22 (t; J = 7.3 Hz; 2H), 7.20 (t; J = 7.8 Hz; 2H), 7.16 (t; J = 7.8

Hz; 2H), 7.13 (s; 1H), 6.88 (s; 1H), 6.79 (s; 1H), 6.72 (s; 2H), 6.51 (s; 1H), 4.20 (s; 1H), 4.12 (s; 1H), 3.95 (s; 3H), 3.80 (s; 3H), 3.76 (s; 3H), 3.74 (s; 3H). $^{13}$C NMR (100.5 MHz, CDCl$_3$) 127.02 (C-1), 138.01 (C-1'), 110.04 (C-2), 110.79 (C-2'), 147.58 (C-3), 147.87 (C-3'), 148.67 (C-4), 148.73 (C-4'), 112.52 (C-5), 111.15 (C-5'), 127.42 (C-6), 119.31 (C-6'), 125.07 (C-7), 52.85 (C-7'), 135.99 (C-8), 51.68 (C-8'), 140.63 (C-9), 142.71 (C-9'), 127.48 (C-10,14), 125.45 (C-10',14'), 128.64 (C-11,13), 128.28 (C-11',13'), 126.60 (C-12), 127.06 (C-12'), 55.71 (C$_3$-OCH$_3$)*, 55.74 (C$_3$'-OCH$_3$)*, 55.76 (C$_4$-OCH$_3$)*, 55.89 (C$_4$'-OCH$_3$)*.

### (4-Benzyloxy-phenyl)-(3,4-dimethoxy-phenyl)-methanone 14

8 % yield. Colourless crystals. $^1$H NMR (400 MHz, CDCl$_3$) δ ppm: 7.79 (d; J = 8.5 Hz, 2H), 7.38-7.46 (m; 5H), 7.36 (dd; J = 8.3, 1.5 Hz; 1H), 7.35 (d; J = 1.5 Hz; 1H), 7.04 (d; J = 8.5 Hz; 2H), 6.89 (d; J = 8.3 Hz; 1H), 5.15 (s; 2H), 3.96 (s; 3H), 3.94 (s; 3H). $^{13}$C NMR (100.5 MHz, CDCl$_3$) 130.95 (C-1), 109.74 (C-2), 148.98 (C-3), 152.49 (C-4), 112.26 (C-5), 124.81 (C-6), 194.57 (C-7), 130.78 (C-8), 132.20 (C-9,13), 114.31 (C-10,12), 161.99 (C-11), 70.15 (C-14), 136.28 (C-15), 127.47 (C-16,20), 128.67 (C-17, 19), 128.20 (C-18), 56.05 (C$_4$-OCH$_3$)*, 56.02 (C$_3$-OCH$_3$)*.

### Oxidative Coupling with Stilbene 11b

Stilbene **11b** (0.4 g, 1.3 mmol) was dissolved in 40 ml dichloromethane. FeCl$_3$.6H$_2$O (3.6g, 13 mmol) was added. The same procedure used for the reaction on **11a** allowed the isolation of two pure compounds.

### Acetic Acid 4-[3-(4-acetoxy-phenyl)-4-(3,4-dimethoxy-phenyl)-6-methoxy-3,4-dihydro-naphthalen-2-yl]-phenyl Ester 15

Yellowish oil. 17 % yield. $^1$H NMR (400 MHz, CDCl$_3$) δ ppm: 7.30 (d; J = 8.6 Hz; 2H; H-10,14), 7.25 (d; J = 8.4 Hz; 2H; H-10',14'), 7.08 (s; 1H; H-7), 6.93 (d; J = 8.6; 2H; H-11',13'), 6.91 (d; J = 8.4 Hz; 2H; H-11,13), 6.85 (s; 1H; H-2), 6.73 (s; 1H; H-2'), 6.68 (m; 2H; H-5',6'), 6.50 (s; 1H; H-5), 4.14 (s; 1H;H-8'), 4.02 (s; 1H; H-7'), 3.87 (s; 3H; C$_3$-OMe)*, 3.73 (s; 3H; C$_4$-OMe)*, 3.69 (s; 6H; C$_{3',4'}$-OMe)*, 2.22 (s; 6H; C$_{12,12'}$-OAc). $^{13}$C NMR (100.5 MHz, CDCl$_3$) 126.77 (C-1), 137.69 (C-1'), 110.14 (C-2), 110.81 (C-2'), 147.70 (C-3)*, 147.97 (C-3')*, 148.80 (C-4)*, 148.89 (C-4')*, 112.62 (C-5), 111.29 (C-5'), 127.20 (C-6), 119.31 (C-6'), 125.35 (C-7), 52.74 (C-7'), 134.95 (C-8), 51.17 (C-8'), 138.23 (C-9), 139.94 (C-9'), 126.45 (C-10,14), 128.48 (C-10',14'), 121.66 (C-11,13), 121.42 (C-11',13'), 149.42 (C-12)*, 149.74 (C-12')*, 55.94 (C$_3$-OCH$_3$)*, 55.81 (C$_3$'-OCH$_3$,C$_4$'-OCH$_3$)*, 55.74 (C$_4$-OCH$_3$)*, 21.05 (C$_{12}$-COCH$_3$)*, 21.00 (C$_{12'}$-COCH$_3$)*, 169.40 (C=O).

### Acetic Acid 4-[4-(3,4-dimethoxy-phenyl)-3-(4-hydroxy-phenyl)-6,7-dimethoxy-3,4-dihydro-naphthalen-2-yl]-phenyl Ester 16

Yellowish oil. 7 % yield. $^1$H NMR (400 MHz, CDCl$_3$) δ ppm: 7.32 (d; J = 8.8 Hz; 2H; H-10,14), 7.10 (d; J = 8.5 Hz; 2H; H-10',14'), 7.06 (s; 1H; H-7), 6.91 (d; J = 8.8; 2H; H-11,13), 6.64 (d; J = 8.5 Hz; 2H; H-11',13'), 6.86 (s; 1H; H-2), 6.74 (d; J = 1.7; 1H; H-2'), 6.70 (m; 2H; H-5',6'), 6.51 (s; 1H; H-5), 4.08 (s; 1H; H-8'), 4.06(s; 1H; H-7'), 3.93 (s; 3H; C$_3$-OMe)*, 3.79 (s; 3H; C$_3$'-OMe)*, 3.75 (s; 3H; C$_4$-OMe)*, 3.74 (s; 3H; C$_4$'-OMe)*, 2.24 (s; 3H; C$_{12}$-OAc). $^{13}$C NMR (100.5 MHz, CDCl$_3$) 126.96 (C-1), 137.90 (C-1'), 110.03 (C-2), 110.84 (C-2'), 147.81 (C-3)*, 147.50 (C-3')*, 148.66 (C-4,4'), 112.59 (C-5), 111.24 (C-5'), 127.47 (C-6), 119.33 (C-6'), 125.00 (C-7), 53.05 (C-7'), 135.46 (C-8), 51.02 (C-8'), 138.49 (C-9), 134.32 (C-9'), 126.45 (C-10,14), 128.61 (C-10',14'), 121.30 (C-11,13), 115.54 (C-11',13'), 149.53 (C-12), 154.77 (C-12'), 55.91 (C$_3$-OCH$_3$)*, 55.73 (C$_3$'-OCH$_3$)*, 55.79 (C$_4$-OCH$_3$, C$_4$'-OCH$_3$)*, 21.04 (C$_{12}$-COCH$_3$), 169.61 (C=O).

## REFERENCES

[1]    Gorham, J. *The Biochemistry of Stilbenoids*, TJ Press Padstow, Cornwall, **1995**.

[2]    Weber, J.F.F.; Abd. Wahab, I.; Marzuki, A.; Thomas, N.F.; Abd. Kadir, A.; A. Hadi, A.H.; Awang, K.; Abd. Latiff, A.; Rashwan, H.; Richomme P.; Delaunay, J. *Tetrahedron Lett.*, **2001**, *42*, 4895-4897.

[3]    Thomas, N.F.; Lee, K.C.; Paraidathathu, T.; Weber, J.F.F.; Awang, K. *Tetrahedron Lett.*, **2002**, *43*, 3151-3155.

[4]    Thomas, N.F.; Lee, K.C.; Paraidathathu, T.; Weber, J.F.F.; Awang, K.; D. Rondeau, D.; Richomme, P. *Tetrahedron*, **2002**, *58*, 7201–7206.

[5]    Grigg, R.; Dorrity, M.J.; Malone, J.F.; Sridharan, V.; Sukirthalingam, S. *Tetrahedron Lett.* **1990**, *31*, 1343-1346.

[6]    Greene, T.W.; Wuts, P.G.M. *Protecting Groups in Organic Synthesis* 2nd edn, John Wiley, New York, **1991**.

[7]    Larock, R.C. *Comprehensive Organic Transformations*, 2nd edn, John Wiley, New York, **1999**.

[8]    Woodward, R.B.; Hoffmann, R. *Angew. Chem. Int. Ed.*, **1969**, *8*, 781-932.

[9]    Boden, N.; Bushby, R.J.; Lu, Z.; Headdock, G. *Tetrahedron Lett.*, **2000**, *41*, 10117-10120.

[10]   Nicolaou, K.C.; Gray, D. *Angew. Chem. Int. Ed.*, **2001**, *40*, 761.

# Structure and Biological Activity - Diversity Orientated Synthesis

## E. Winterfeldt*

*Organic Chemistry Department, Hannover University, Schneiderberg, 1B, D-30167, Hannover, Germany*

**Abstract:** The cephalostatins ( *Cephalodicus gilchristi* ) and the agelorins (*Agelas oroides* ) represent two groups of marine natural products showing high biological activity. The total synthesis of enantiopure analogues reveals for the cephalostatins and the decisive role of molecular dissymmetry and of a chiral curvature, while the agelorins were shown to be prodrugs, which under stress conditions are undergoing an enzymatically induced fragmentation, generating the highly active cyclohexadiene aeroplysinin. Finally a simple diversity oriented enantioselective synthesis of wistarin precursor is reported.

## INTRODUCTION

Although natural sources have been providing biologically active compounds of various types of structures for more than 3000 years by now, nature continues to offer every year hundreds of new and exciting structures to natural products chemists and pharmacologists.

As extraction and separation methods have been developed to very high standards and since they are accompanied today by extremely powerful and highly redundant spectroscopic techniques, more or less every habitat –may it be at the edge of volcanoes or at the bottom of the ocean- can nowadays be explored and every type of substance –may it be very sensitive or unstable, volatile or of high molecular weight- can be purified and their structure elucidated.

These efforts have revealed the constitution and the relative as well as the absolute configuration of dozens of highly active compounds, which could be good candidates for drug development themselves, but will more likely serve as a lead-structure in medicinal chemistry.

The reason for this is quite simple. One has to realize that the compound in question was evolutionary developed in a worm or fish or a plant to protect it against hostile invaders or to send messages to friends and spouses.

Having been optimized for this particular biological system, the chances are very low that it can at the same time operate also highly satisfactorily in human therapy or any application in general.

Nevertheless the overall structure is representing a very promising invitation to structural diversifications aiming at an optimized drug.

These circumstances lead us directly to todays, main motivations for synthetic exercises in this field.

*Corresponding author: Fax: 0049-511-762-3011; E-mail: winterfeldt@mbox.oci.uni-hannover.de

Thirty years ago the main driving force for endeavours of this type originated from the desire to prepare the compound itself and to consider its complicated structure an interesting test-ground for the established synthetic methodology. In many cases it even called for improvements or extensions of the existing techniques.

The unequivocal structural proof resulting additionally from these efforts has lost its splendour to quite an extent, since nowadays we generally have high confidence in the overall structure elucidation and a questionmark may only show up with the absolute configuration or the proper assignments in diastereomers.

Additionally there is a well filled arsenal of very reliable and highly chemoselective as well as stereoselective or enantioselective transformations, which results in a shift of motivation into the following areas.

As the highly potent compounds are of course the most interesting ones, one can safely predict they will be available in small amounts only, with the additional complication that particularly with marine sources the corresponding organisms will not be easily accessible and may also in an unpredictable way migrate to various locations.

One of the tasks of synthetic chemistry therefore, could be to provide material for biological evaluation and since the structure at this stage will be well established it should be very attractive to locate the pharmacologically important substructures, to melt the compound down to these essentials for biological activity and to devise efficient and reliable routes to these entities.

Pursuing these aims diversity emerges of course as the second important task for synthetic chemistry. Intermediates prepared in the process as well as the reactions employed for their further elaboration should show high synthetic flexibility. This means that the reactive functional groups present in key-intermediates should guarantee a maximum of structural and configurational variations in subsequent transformations and that they should be susceptible to quite a variety of broadly applicable reactions. Starting in this case from a structure or substructure of a proved and well defined biological activity, the success rate of molecular ensembles, generated with this background, will be much higher than with arbitrarily devised ad hoc libraries.

Since this opens the road to a wide variety of related compounds of comparable biological activity, one may additionally gain informations on the mechanism of their biological activity from these investigations and I shall give an example for this at a later stage.

Finally, having secured high flexibility as far as structures and transformations are concerned, one should be in a position to reach high sustainability, in case large scale production of any drug developed this way, would be considered. From quite a set of reactions applicable for the preparation one could in these cases exclusively select those employing easily available or regrowing starting materials and mild or benign reaction conditions.

My research group in Hannover was in the late nineties also very much guided by the motivations described above in various synthetic endeavours with marine natural products. A particularly hopeless case as far as reisolation was concerned became known with the tumorinhibitor cephalostatin (1) [1] which had been isolated by Petit and his colleagues in 1988 [2] and they had needed large amounts of the worm.

*Cephalodiscus Gilchristii* to lay hands on only a few hundred milligrams of this material. Since one had additionally many difficulties to relocate this source some time

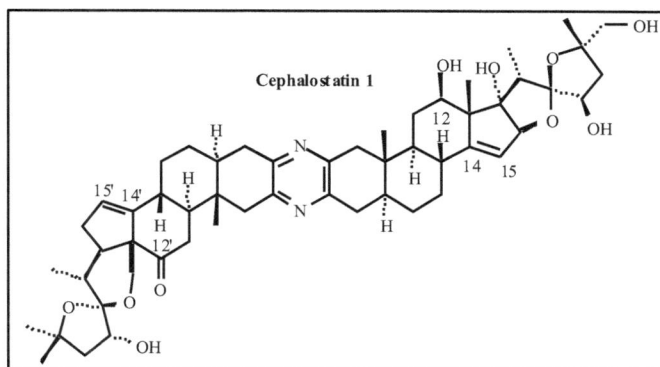

Cephalostatin 1

later, the outlook for further supply was quite disappointing. As Petits structure elucidation, however, had proven the highly active cephalostatines to be novel non-symmetric bis-steroidal pyrazines, this was clearly the hour of synthetic chemistry and compounds of this type quickly became an important synthetic target worldwide.

The very obvious first question of course was: would any steroidderivative of this type do, or is the generally observed dissymmetry essential for high biological activity. This problem was most simply addressed easily to make symmetric diketone (2) [3], which on the one hand documents that multigram amounts of bis-steroidal pyrazines are readily available, but on the other hand being at least one power of ten less active than even the weakest non-symmetric compound derived from it, it also proves the importance of dissymmetry.

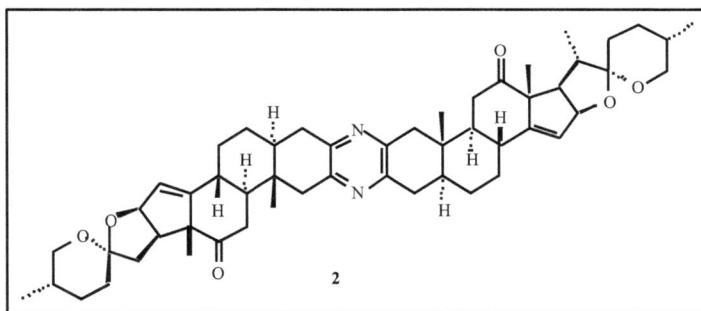

2

Wile selective and diastereoselective reductions are of course the most obvious way of desymmetrisation Dr. Mansour Nawasreh from Jordania in his dissertation at the university of Hannover [4] also investigated selective Wittig-olefination and demonstrated the nonsymmetric main hydroboration stereoisomer (3), resulting after monoolefination, to strongly inhibit renal cancer cells.

The most remarkable result in this case is that the substitution pattern generated here, does not show any natural product. The compound being nonsymmetric, however, it nevertheless showed a highly selective biological activity.

This proves diketone 2 to be a highly flexible master-key intermediate, which may give rise to natural as well as non-natural dissymmetric cephalostatin analogues. While these

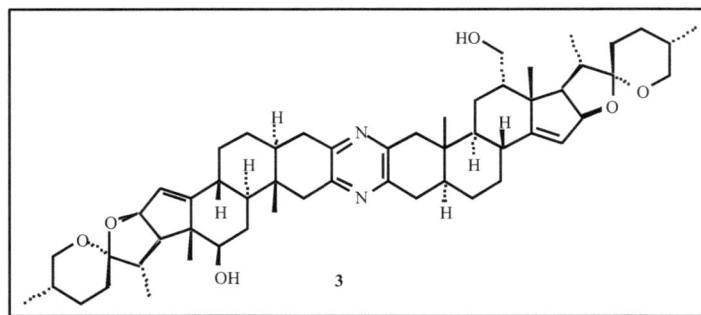

observations clearly proved the decisive role of dissymmetry one also had to investigate the contribution of characteristic functional groups. It should be noted in this context that the 14/15-double bond, which is present in all highly active cephalostatins, is by no means a common functional group in the steroid field.

Its decisive role can indeed easily be proven in a comparison of these diolefins to corresponding tetrahydro counterparts. Luckily these structures are easily accessible by standard procedures and while their extremely low solubility was a clear warning already, activity studies proved them to be inactive indeed.

Looking for an explanation for this remarkable difference in solubility a clue can be found in the very characteristic molecular shape of all 14/15 unsaturated compounds.

In contrast to their more or less flat, saturated analogues, these molecules, according to their x-ray data, are bent into a very characteristic chiral curvature. Due to the presence two sp-2-centres in the five-membered rings these entities are pointing downward thus bending the molecule like a bow.

The relationship between the solubility of pure enantiomers and their molecular shape has been noticed with various types of molecules already [5] and was recently described in detail by J.M. Lehn and his colleagues [6].

They demonstrated that with racemic mixtures the two complementing mirror-images fit very nicely into a densely packed crystal lattice, while one single enantiomer is missing this chiral partner. This leads to a widened crystal lattice, which results in higher solubility. As good solubility is a prerequisite for high biological activity, this proves the crucial role of the 14/15 double bonds.

The important take-home message from this investigation can be summarized in the recommendation to make sure for a chiral curvature if polycyclic compounds create solubility problems, as they very often do.

Now we shift from the bottom of the Indian Ocean to the shallow warm waters of the Barrier Reef where G. König found the sponge *Agelas Oroides* and isolated the agelorins and fistularins [7] Fig. (**1**). These compounds show moderate antibiotic activity and they are characterized by two spiro-isoxazoline-systems linked to a diamine *via* amide bonds.

An off-hand structure-activity-analysis indicated very clearly that the spiro-substructures should represent the essential pharmacophoric group of these compounds.

However, the result from the first synthetic investigations turned out to be quite confusing.

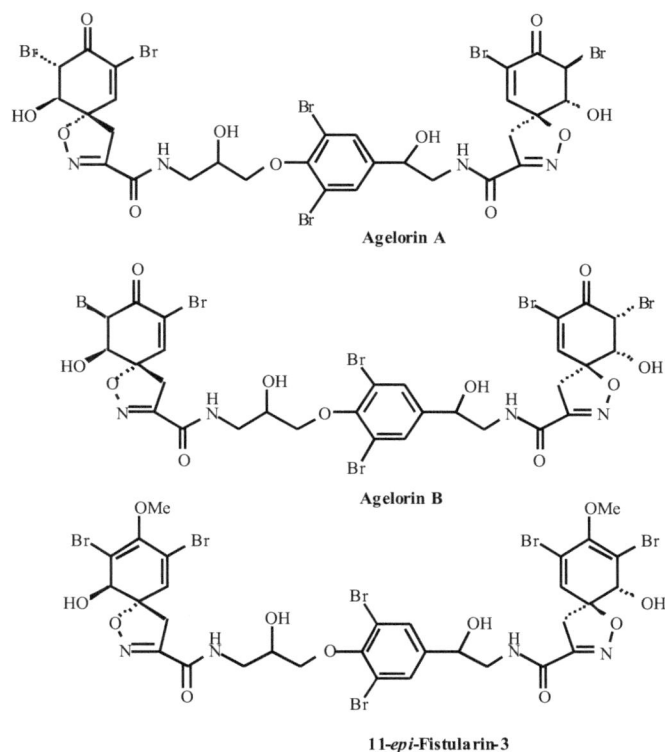

Agelorin A

Agelorin B

11-epi-Fistularin-3

**Fig. (1).**

When various enantiopure spiro-isoxazolines were prepared via enantiopic double bond differentiation of the corresponding spirocyclohexadienones with a homochiral cyclopentadiene, all of them showed moderate antibiotic activity and some of these were even superior to the natural products themselves.

An explanation for these unexpected, curious results came from an investigation aiming at the defence mechanism of *Agelas Oroides*.

Prof. P. Proksch and his students observed that the sponge when injured releases an enzyme at this spot, which catalyzes the fragmentation of all these spiroamides into a hydroxynitrile, which turned out to be a strong antibiotic [8]. (Fig. **2**) This proves the spirocompounds to be prodrugs, which are converted into a powerful antibiotic if an enemy attacks.

In contrast to the quiet deep sea-ambiente where a constant shield of defence substances could easily be maintained, this strategy will of course fail in shallow waters, since strong agitations and constant streaming would immediately strongly dilute any defence material in this case.

So the sponge keeps his powder dry and just waits till an intruder attacks. Any damage will immediately release the stress-enzyme, which triggers the fragmentation of the prodrug into a highly active antibiotic. Obviously one deals with a highly economical strategy here, as owing to the structure of the agelorins the enzyme will release two molecules of antibiotic in every case.

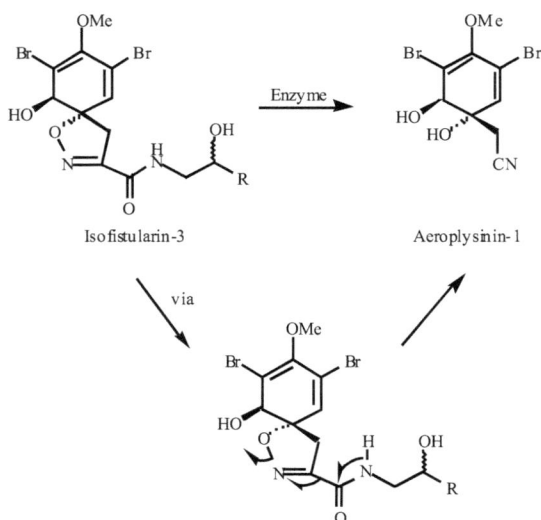

**Fig. (2).**

This makes the defence system operate like a double barreled shotgun.

A comparison of the various spirocompounds prepared in our laboratory [8] demonstrated the enzyme to be quite substrate specific. While different substitution patterns in the cyclohexenone moiety just led to different reaction rates, a change from secondary amides to tertiary ones, lacking the decisive N-H-bond, as expected led to a complete failure of the fragmentation process.

## REFERENCES

[1]    Pettit, G.R.; Inoue,M.; Kamano, Y.; Heraldt, D.L.; Arm, C.; Dufresne, C.; Christie, N.D.; Schmidt, J.M.; Doubek, D.L.; Krupa, T.S. *J. Am. Chem. Soc.,* **1988**, *110*, 2006.
[2]    Pettit, G.R.; Tan, R.; Yu, J.P.; Ichihara, Y.; Williams, M.D.; Boyd, M.R. *J. Nat.,* **1998**, *61*, 955.
[3]    Drögemüller, M.; Flessner, T.; Jautelat, R.; Scholz, U.; Winterfeldt, E. *Eur. J. Org. Chem.,* **1998**, *1*, 2811.
[4]    Dissertation Mansour Nawasre, University Hannover, **2000**.
[5]    Hakam, K.; Thielmann, M.; Thielmann, T.; Winterfeldt, E. *Tetrahed.,* **1987**, *43*, 2035.
[6]    Brienne, M.J.; Gabard, J.; Leclerq, M.; Lehn, J.M.; Cesario, M.; Pascard, C.; Cheve, M.; Dutruc-Rosset, G. *Tetrahed. Lett.,* **1994**, *35*, 8157.
[7]    König, G.M.; Wright, A.D. *Heterocycles,* **1993**, *36*, 1351.
[8]    Goldenstein, K.; Fendert, T.; Proksch, P.; Winterfeldt, E. *Tetrahed.,* **2000**, *56*, 4173.

# The Nitroaldol (Henry) Reaction as the Key Step for the Synthesis of Some Natural Products

Roberto Ballini*, Giovanna Bosica, Dennis Fiorini and Alessandro Palmieri

*Dipartimento di Scienze Chimiche dell'Università di Camerino, 62032 Camerino, Italy*

**Abstract:** The nitroaldol (Henry) reaction although has been discovered more than one century ago is still largely employed as the key step for the synthesis of many targets. The reaction is performed under basic condition by mixing primary or secondary nitroalkanes (and nitromethane) with a carbonyl, allowing the formation of a β-nitroalkanol. The latter shows an high versatility since it can be converted into a lot of different functionalities and many natural products have been prepared using the Henry reaction as the key step. Some of these synthesis will be reported.

## INTRODUCTION

Aliphatic nitro compound have been proved to be valuable intermediates and chemical literature continuously reports progress in their utilization for a variety of target molecules [1]. Different conversions can be performed by nitroalkanes and the Henry reaction is one of the most important. The Henry reaction, an aldol-type reaction, represents one of the classical C-C bond-forming processes that allows the synthesis of β-nitroalkanols A (Scheme **1**) [2,3].

The classical nitroaldol reaction is performed in a homogeneous solution by dissolving an aliphatic nitroderivative and an aldehyde, in the presence of an appropriate base, in an organic solvent. However, the use of water as solvent or the use of heterogeneous catalysis have been extensively studied. Stronger conditions could give the nitroaldolic "condensation" allowing the direct formation of conjugated nitroalkenes B [1].

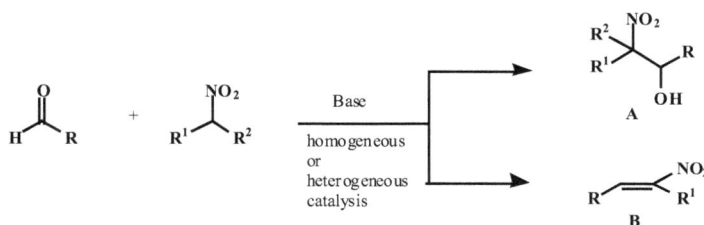

**Scheme 1.**

Some years ago we reported the use of nitroalkanes in the synthesis of different natural products [4], while here we'll present the preparation of some of the above targets in which the nitroalkanols, obtained through the Henry reaction, are the key building blocks.

---

*Corresponding author: Fax: +39-0737-402297; E-mail: roberto.ballini@unicam.it

## RESULTS

Then, *(Z)*-heneicos-6-en-11-one 4, the Douglas Fir Tussok Moth (*Orgya pseudotsugata*) sex pheromone, can be prepared in good yield starting from the nitroaldol reaction of 1-nitro-dec-4-ene 1 with undecanal 2 (Scheme **2**) [5]. The reaction allows, after oxidation, the α-nitro ketone 3, that after further elaboration produces 4.

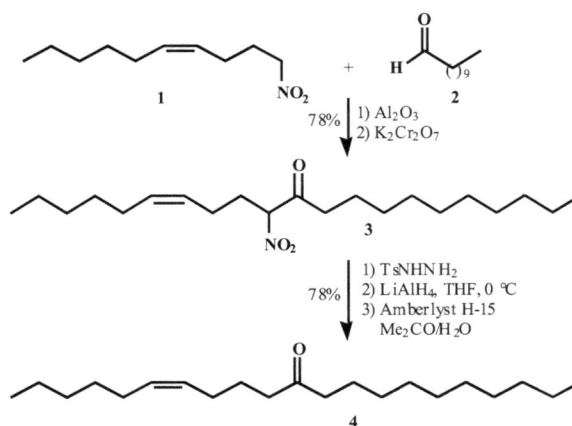

**Scheme 2.**

The Scheme **3** shows a new synthesis of the *trans*-2-methyl-1,7-dioxaspiro[5.5] undecane 8, a component of cephalic secretions of the female of *Epeolus cruciger* [6]. The starting step is the nitroaldol condensation of the nitro ketone 5 with the hydroxy-protected aldehyde 6. Then, the polyfunctionalized nitroalkene 7 converts, one-pot, to 8 in good yield.

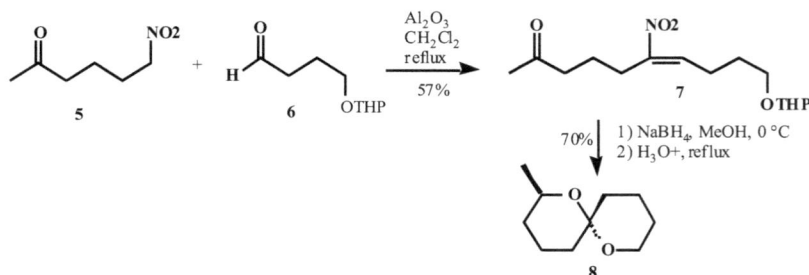

**Scheme 3.**

The roots of *Chiococca alba*, of Rubinaceae family, are used in folk medicine as a tonic for ganglion inflammation, a diuretic, an antivirus, an antioedema and an aphrodisiac. The main components of the leaf-extract have been found to be two hydroxyketones: 4-hydroxyheptadecan-7-one 10 and 14-hydroxyoctadecan-8-one 13. Few years ago we reported the first synthesis of both the hydroxyketones 10 and 13, starting from the nitroaldolic condensation of a nitroalkanol with an aldehyde (Scheme **4** and **5**) [7].

An elegant synthesis of the A ring of Taxol (Scheme **6**) has been published through a nitroaldol cyclisation (16 to 17) [8].

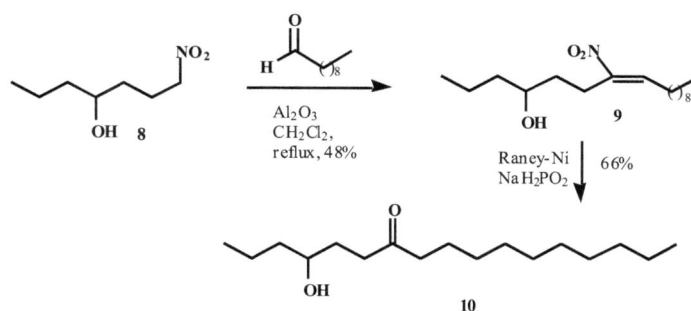

**Scheme 4.**

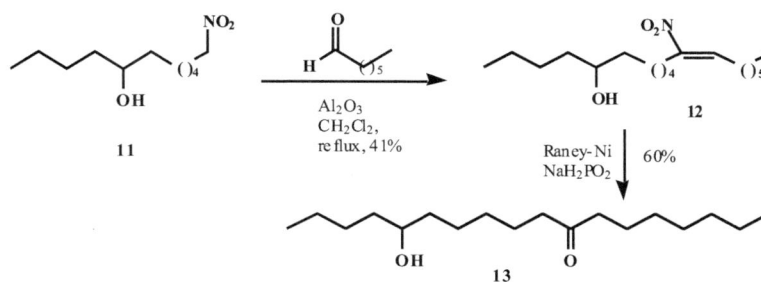

**Scheme 5.**

Then, the nitroalkanol 17 is dehydrated to 18 that, after Nef conversion and reduction (DIBAL) yields the A ring 19.

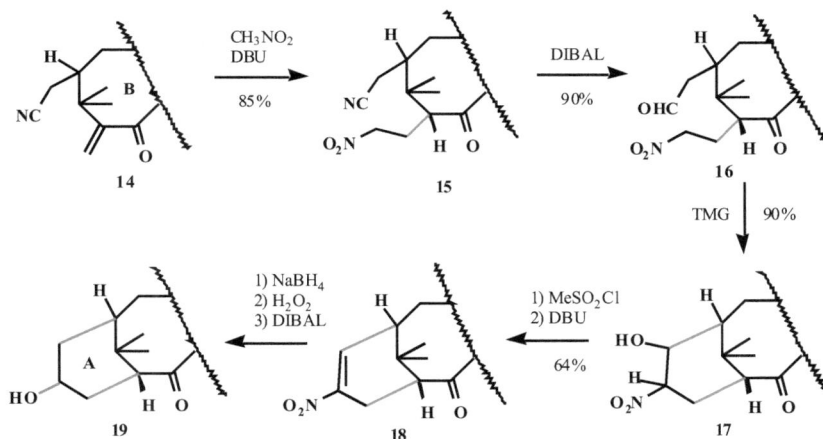

**Scheme 6.**

Stingless bees in the genus *Trigona tataira* and their relatives are particularly noteworthy because of the unusual properties of their mandibular gland secretion. This aphid successfully plunders the food reserves from the nests of other species of stingless bees. Because of the vescicatory properties of its exudates, it is frequently referred to as the fire bee. Analysis of the volatile compounds derived from cephalic secretion of workers of *T. tataira* revealed the presence, as the main component, of *(E)*-non-3-ene-2,5-dione 24 (Scheme **7**). We reported the first synthesis of the enedione 24 starting by the Henry reaction (20 to 21), followed by nitrous acid elimination of the nitro-dione 23, obtained after oxidation of the diol 22 [9].

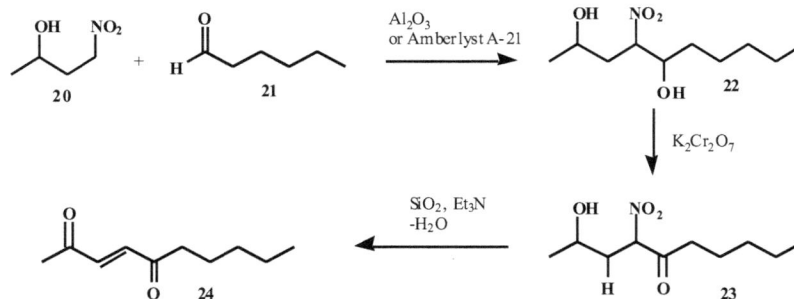

**Scheme 7.**

The extracts of *Artabotrys odoratissima* are largely employed in traditional medical treatment. A decoction of the leaves is given in cholera, extracts of leaves of this plant have shown irregular oestrus cycle in albino rats, the essential oil obtained from flowers is used in perfumery industries. Due to the importance of the *Artabotrys o.*, recently some authors characterized the main chemical components in the leaves of the above plant and they found a new interesting hydroxyester that was identified as the pentadecyl 6-hydroxydodecanoate 29. Then, we planned the first synthesis of 29 starting from a cyclic α-

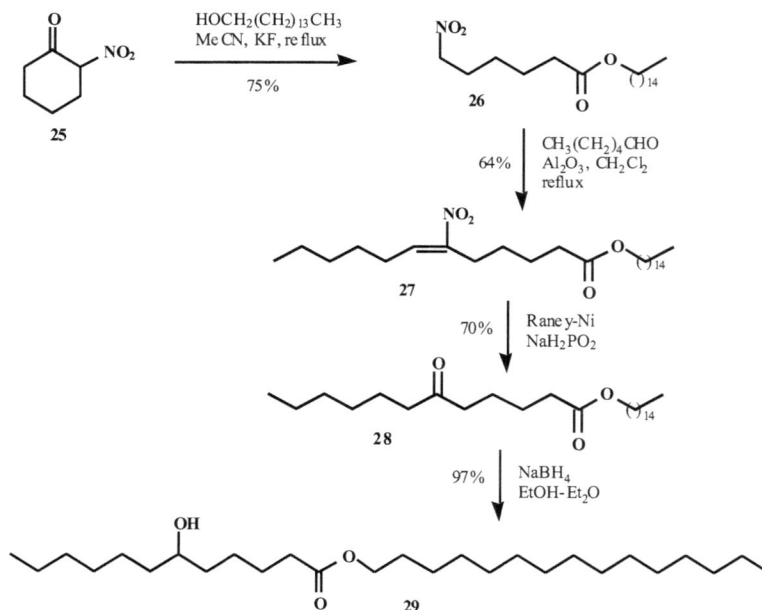

**Scheme 8.**

nitro ketone, such as $\alpha$-nitrocyclohexanone. It is well known that the above nitro ketones are prone to nucleophilic ring cleavage [10], so by action of 1-pentadecanol, 25 converts to the nitro ester 26. This nitro ester is the appropriate nitroalkane for the Henry reaction with hexanal. Further steps (Nef reaction and $NaBH_4$ reduction) produces the natural product 29 [11].

## CONCLUSIONS

In conclusion, we have reported some representative examples in which the Henry reaction has been employed as the key step for the synthesis of several natural products.

## ACKNOWLEDGEMENTS

The authors thank the University of Camerino-Italy and Fondazione della Cassa di Risparmio della Provincia di Macerata-Italy for financial support.

## REFERENCES

[1]     Rosini, G.; Ballini, R. *Synthesis*, **1998**, 833-847.
[2]     Ballini, R.; Bosica, G. *J. Org. Chem.,* **1997**, *62*, 425-427.
[3]     Ballini, R.; Bosica, G.; Livi, D.; Palmieri, A.; Maggi, R.; Sartori, G. *Tetrahedron Lett.,* **2003**, *44*, 2271-2273 and references cited therein.
[4]     Ballini, R. In *Studies in Natural Products Chemistry*; Atta-ur-Rahman, Ed.; Elsevier Science B. V: Amsterdam, **1997**, Vol. *19*, pp.117-184.
[5]     Ballini, R. *J. Chem. Soc., Perkin Trans 1*, **1991**, 1419-1421.
[6]     Ballini, R.; Bosica, G.; Schaafstra, R. *Liebigs Ann. Chem.*, **1994**, 1235-1237.
[7]     Ballini, R.; Bosica, G.; Rafaiani, G. *Helv. Chim. Acta*, **1995**, *78*, 879-882.
[8]     Magnus, L. *J. Chem. Soc., Chem. Commun.*, **1995**, 1933-1935.
[9]     Ballini, R.; Astolfi, P. *Liebigs Ann. Chem.*, **1996**, 1879-1880.
[10]    Ballini, R. *Synlett*, **1999**, 1009-1018.
[11]    Ballini, R.; Gil, M. V.; Fiorini, D.; Palmieri, A. *Synthesis*, **2003**, 665-667.

Atta-ur-Rahman/Choudhary/Khan (Eds.) *Frontiers in Natural Product Chemistry, Vol. 1*

# Synthesis of Vinblastine Derivatives

Hedvig Bölcskei[1,*], Lajos Szabó[2] and Csaba Szántay[2]

[1]*Gedeon Richter Ltd. H-1475 Budapest, P.O.B. 27 Hungary,* [2]*Institute of Organic Chemistry, Budapest University of Technology and Economics, H-1111 Budapest, Gellért tér 4, Hungary*

**Abstract:** The bisindole alkaloids of the Madagascan periwinkle *Catharanthus Roseus* vincristine **1** and vinblastine **2** are widely used clinically in the chemotherapy of cancer. Many efforts were made to synthesize more efficient new derivatives having less side effects than vinblastine **2**. New anhydrovinblastine derivatives were obtained by the ferric chloride mediated coupling reaction of catharanthine and vindoline and their derivatives. The nitro- dinitro-, amino- and hydroxymethyl analogues of the alkaloids **1, 2** and **3** showed promising antitumor activity.

## INTRODUCTION

The evergreen *Catharanthus roseus* is known Madagascan periwinkle. The plant contains about 90-100 alkaloids. The most valuable of them vincristine **1** and vinblastine **2** are antineoplastic agents. They are used in the treatment of leukaemia, Hodgkin's disease and other lymphomas. They are also of use in the treatment of some inoperable malignant neoplasms too [1]. Besides the naturally occuring **1** and **2** synthetic derivatives are also used in the chemotherapy of cancer e.g. vindesine **4** (Eli Lilly) or vinorelbine **5** (Pierre Fabre).

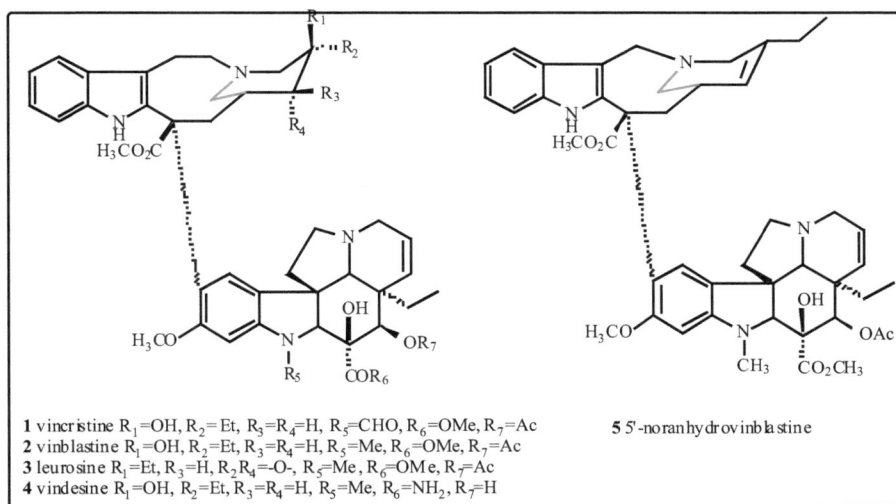

**1** vincristine $R_1$=OH, $R_2$=Et, $R_3$=$R_4$=H, $R_5$=CHO, $R_6$=OMe, $R_7$=Ac
**2** vinblastine $R_1$=OH, $R_2$=Et, $R_3$=$R_4$=H, $R_5$=Me, $R_6$=OMe, $R_7$=Ac
**3** leurosine $R_1$=Et, $R_3$=H, $R_2$$R_4$=-O-, $R_5$=Me, $R_6$=OMe, $R_7$=Ac
**4** vindesine $R_1$=OH, $R_2$=Et, $R_3$=$R_4$=H, $R_5$=Me, $R_6$=NH$_2$, $R_7$=H

**5** 5'-noranhydrovinblastine

Worldwide many efforts have been made to synthesize new efficient and less toxic vinblastine analogues [2]. There are two possibilities to synthesize new indole-indoline

*Corresponding author: E-mail: h.bolcskei@richter.hu

derivatives: either by the coupling reaction of the corresponding monomer indole alkaloids, catharanthine and vindoline and their derivatives or by transformation of the VLB-type dimer itself isolated from the plant.

## AVLB DERIVATIVES BY COUPLING OF THE MONOMERS

After many attempts [3] the modified Polonovski reaction of catharanthine **6a** and vindoline **7a** resulted in anhydrovinblastine **8a** AVLB having the right stereochemistry [4]. In 1988 Vukovic *et al.* [5] published a more efficient and simple coupling method in the presence of ferric chloride in aqueous medium. Using extreme excess of $NaBH_4$ the borane complex of AVLB **9a** could be isolated as main product which seemed to be extremely stable allowing the detailed NMR study of it [6]. We have employed the above mentioned coupling method in case of deethylcatharanthine **6b** with vindoline **7a** and N-demethyl-vindoline **7b**. N-demethyl-AVLB **8c** was synthesized too in similar way [7].

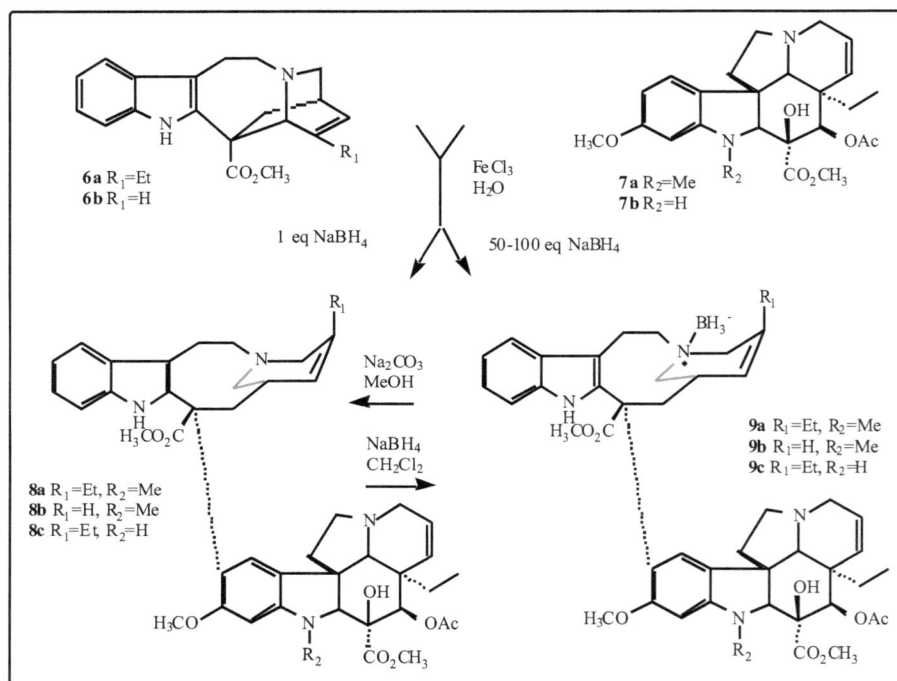

Studying chemical behaviour of catharanthine a rearranged 5-nor-catharanthine **10** was obtained. The ferric ion mediated coupling reaction of **10** with vindoline **7a** produced three dimer compounds **11**, **12** and **13** having unusual structure[8].

The above mentioned N-demethyl-vindoline **7b** was prepared by removal of the formyl group of N-formyl-vindoline (**7c** $R_2$=CHO) gained by the $MnO_2$ oxidation of vindoline **7a** [9]. Studying this reaction new other vindoline derivatives among them the N-formyl-derivative **14** were obtained. Usually N-formyl-vindoline derivatives aren't suitable for a coupling reaction neither by the Polonovski-Potier reaction nor the ferric ion method. The $NaBH_4$ reduction of **14** led to two new hydroxymethyl derivatives of vindoline **15a** and **15b** [10].

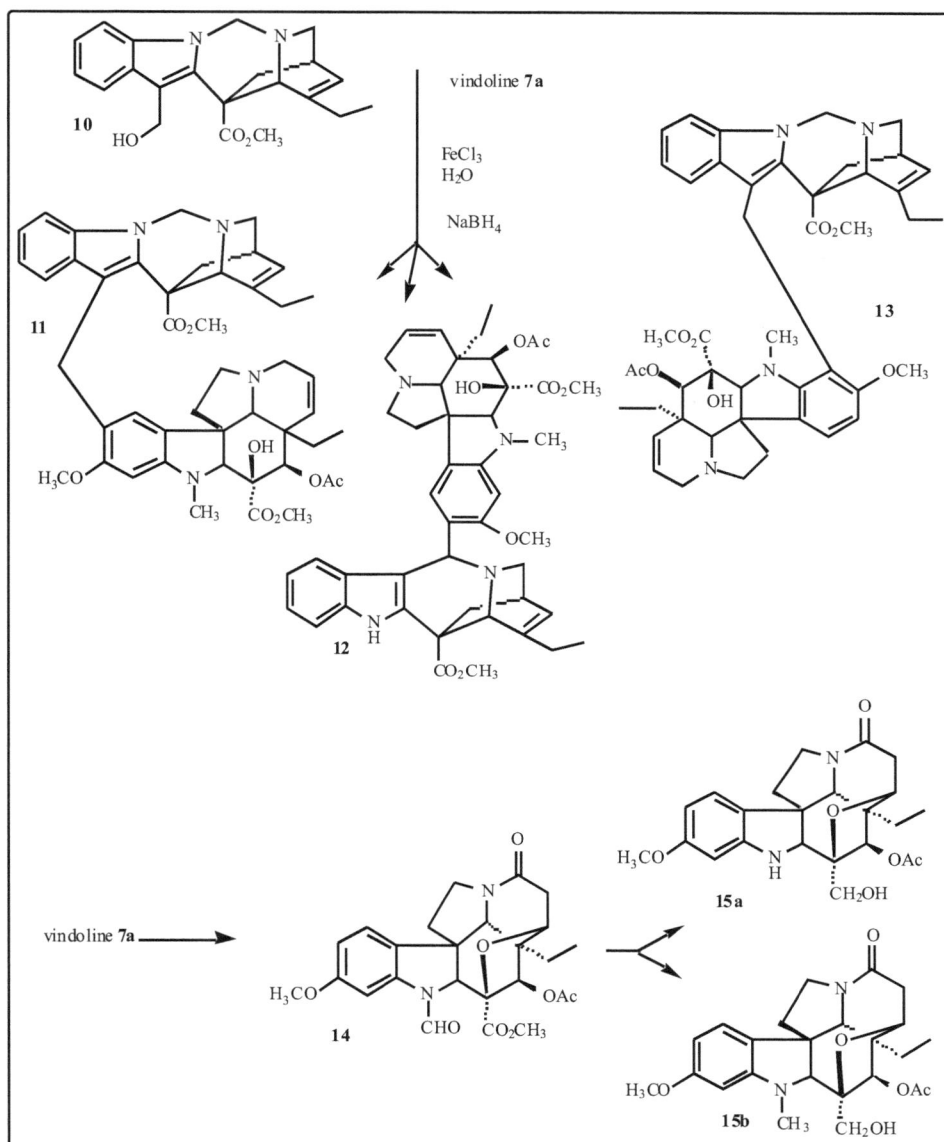

The ferric ion mediated coupling reaction of **15a** with catharanthine resulted in the desired new hydroxymethyl-AVLB derivatives **16a**, but in case of **15b** the AVLB derivative of the corresponding N-methyl derivative **16b** was obtained in quite small amount and new vindoline dimer **17** seemed to be the main product [10].

## TRANSFORMATION OF THE VLB-TYPE DIMERS

### Reduction of Leurosine 3 and Vinblastine 2

Besides the main alkaloids VLB **2** and VCR **1** leurosine **3** can be isolated in relative large amount from the plant. The reduction of leurosine **3** was studied using several

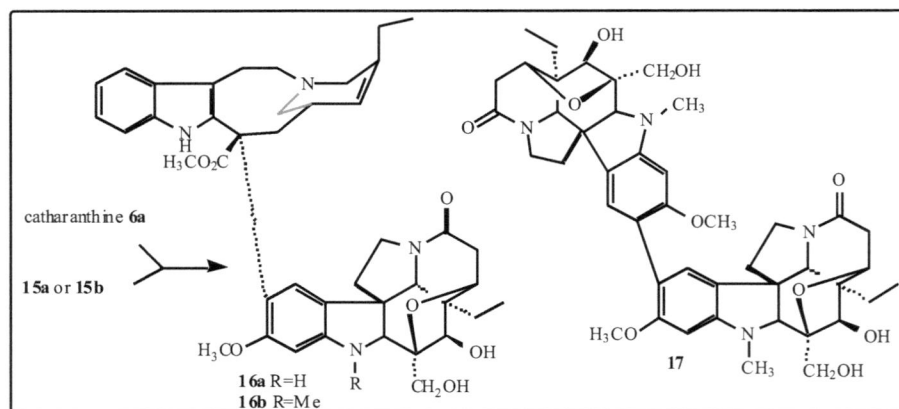

reducing agents e.g. Zn(BH$_4$)$_2$ supported on silicagel which led two main products **18** and **19** depending on the reaction conditions [10]. After 0.5 h at 40°C **18** was the main product, where the methoxycarbonyl group of th vindoline moiety was reduced only. Under thermodynamicallly controlled conditions (1 hours reflux) mainly compound **19** was obtained where the acetyl group was hydrolyzed too.

The analogous hydroxymethyl derivative of VLB **20** could be prepared in good yield by the NaBH$_4$ reduction of **2** in boiling t-butanol dropping methanol to the reaction mixture [10]. Deacetylvinblastine **21** the byproduct of this reduction could be transformed into **20** under the above mentioned reaction conditions. Deacetoxyvinblastine **22** gave a similar reaction resulting in **23**.

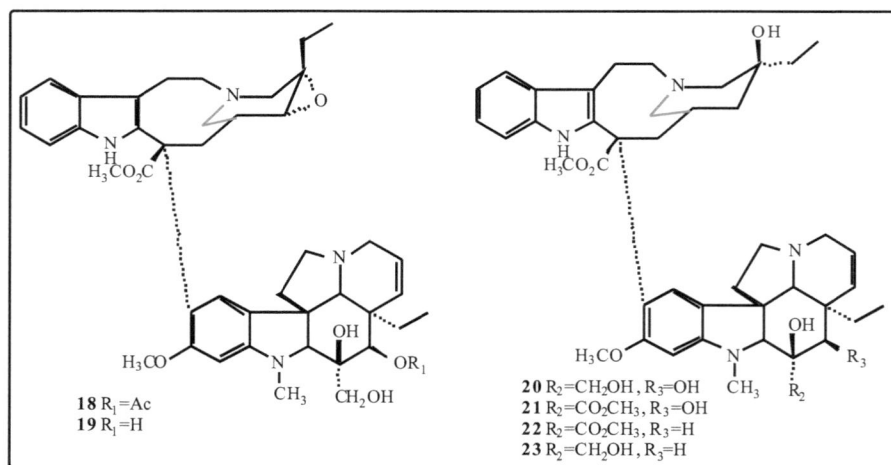

## Nitration of the VLB-type Indole-indoline Alkaloids

Earlier we published the nitration of VCR **1** with fuming nitric acid in a mixture of acetic acid and CHCl$_3$ resulting in **24** 11'-nitro-VCR (60 %), 9'-nitro-VCR **25** (5 %) and 7'-nitro-derivative **26** (31 %) [11]. Due to the deactivating effect of the formyl group  the nitration took place on the cleavamine moiety of the compound only.

Starting from N-formyl-leurosine **27** the corresponding 11'-nitro-derivative **28** and 7'-nitro-derivative **29** could be isolated in a similar manner. The vindoline moiety remained intact in this case too [12].

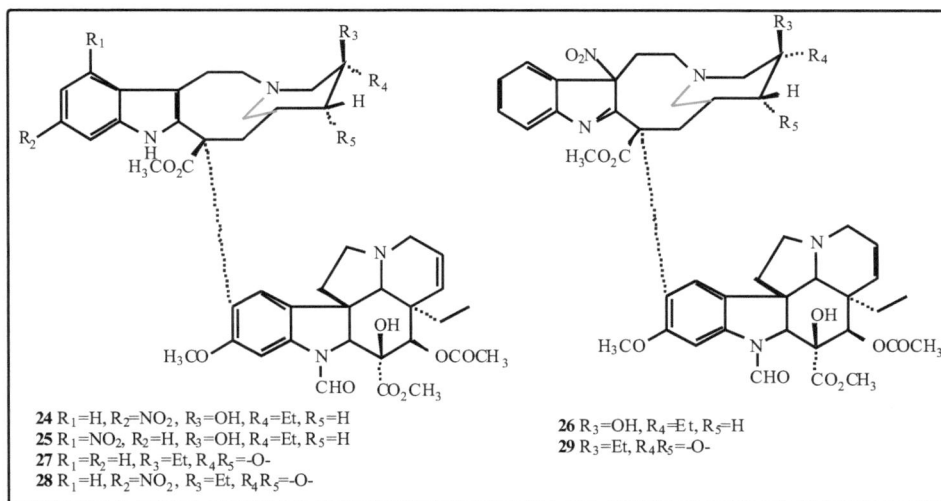

**24** R₁=H, R₂=NO₂, R₃=OH, R₄=Et, R₅=H
**25** R₁=NO₂, R₂=H, R₃=OH, R₄=Et, R₅=H
**27** R₁=R₂=H, R₃=Et, R₄R₅=-O-
**28** R₁=H, R₂=NO₂, R₃=Et, R₄R₅=-O-

**26** R₃=OH, R₄=Et, R₅=H
**29** R₃=Et, R₄R₅=-O-

The nitration of VLB **2** led to the 12-nitro-VLB **30** as main product and in small amount to dinitro-VLB-derivatives **31** and **32** too. Due to the activating effect of the tertiary amine group every product had nitro group on the vindoline moiety.

Similarly to VLB the nitration of leurosine **3** resulted in 12-nitro-LEU **33** and dinitro-LEU-derivatives **34-36** [13].

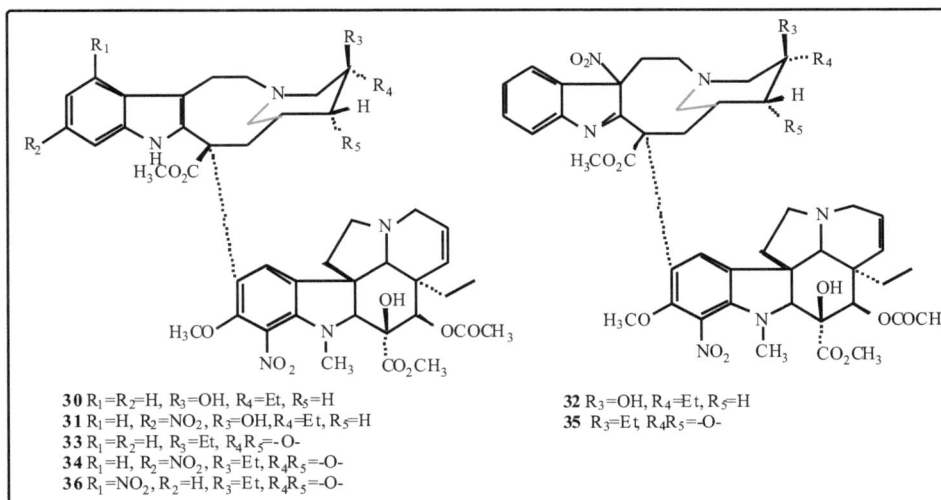

**30** R₁=R₂=H, R₃=OH, R₄=Et, R₅=H
**31** R₁=H, R₂=NO₂, R₃=OH, R₄=Et, R₅=H
**33** R₁=R₂=H, R₃=Et, R₄R₅=-O-
**34** R₁=H, R₂=NO₂, R₃=Et, R₄R₅=-O-
**36** R₁=NO₂, R₂=H, R₃=Et, R₄R₅=-O-

**32** R₃=OH, R₄=Et, R₅=H
**35** R₃=Et, R₄R₅=-O-

After previous biological results 15',20'-anhydro-VCR **37** showed promising antitumour activity. Thus treating 11'-nitro-VCR **24** as well as 12-nitro-VLB **30** with thionyl-chloride the corresponding anhydro-derivatives **38** and **39** were prepared [12].

Several methods were checked for the reduction of the nitro group. 12-nitro-VLB **30** was reduced to 12-amino-VLB **40** either with sodium borohydride in presence of Pd/C or sodium dithionite in water/ethanol. This reducing agent was applied in case of 11'-nitro-VCR **24** and 11',12-dinitro-VLB **31** resulting in the desired 11'-amino-VCR **41** and the 11',12-diamino-VLB **42** respectively. Interestingly after the reduction of 7'-nitro-VCR **26** with sodium-borohydride in presence of Pd/C the original VCR **1** was recovered [11]. Similarly to this 7',12-dinitro-VLB with sodium dithionite led to 12-amino-VLB **40** instead of the diamino-derivative [12].

Further promising new amino-derivative 12-formylamino-VLB **43** could be obtained by formylation of 12-amino-VLB **40**. 12-Amino-17-deacetyl-VLB **44** was obtained by Zemplén deacetylation (NaOCH₃/CH₃OH) of **40** [12].

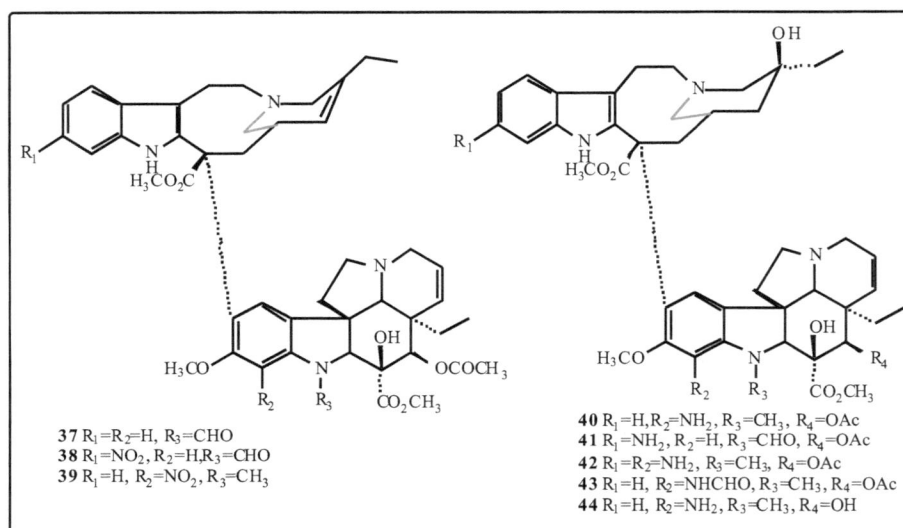

37 $R_1$=$R_2$=H, $R_3$=CHO
38 $R_1$=NO₂, $R_2$=H,$R_3$=CHO
39 $R_1$=H, $R_2$=NO₂, $R_3$=CH₃

40 $R_1$=H,$R_2$=NH₂, $R_3$=CH₃, $R_4$=OAc
41 $R_1$=NH₂, $R_2$=H, $R_3$=CHO, $R_4$=OAc
42 $R_1$=$R_2$=NH₂, $R_3$=CH₃, $R_4$=OAc
43 $R_1$=H, $R_2$=NHCHO, $R_3$=CH₃, $R_4$=OAc
44 $R_1$=H, $R_2$=NH₂, $R_3$=CH₃, $R_4$=OH

## Pharmacology

The biological experiments were performed at the European Organization for Research and Treatment of Cancer (EORTC) and at the National Cancer Institute (NCI). The antitumour activity of a compound was measured for 64 human tumor cell lines. In the case of compounds **20**, **40** and **44** cytotoxic activity was found for non-small cell lung cancer in the concentration range tested ($10^{-5}$-$10^{-9}$). Compound **20** showed activity against small cell lung cancer and ovarian cancer too. 12-Amino-VLB **40** and its 17-deacetyl-derivative **44** also had potency in the screen for colon cancer, breast cancer and leukemia [12, 13].

## REFERENCES

[1]     Jong-Keun Son, Rosazza, J. P. N.; Duffel, M. W.: *J. Med. Chem.* **1990**, *33*, 1845-1848
[2]     *The Alkaloids*. Ed. By Brossi, A. Academic Press. New York **1990** Vol.*37*.
[3]     a) Harley-Mason, J.; Atta-ur-Rahman: *J. Chem. Soc. Chem. Comm.* **1967**, 1048-1049. b) Kutney, J. P.; Beck, J.; Bylsman, F.; Cook, J.; Cretney, W. J.; Fuji, K.; Inhof, R.; Treasurywala, A. M.; *Helv. Chim. Acta* **1975**, *58*, 1690-1719
[4]     Langlois, N.; Guéritte, F.; Langlois, Y.; Potier, P. *J. Am. Chem. Soc.* **1976**, *98*, 7017-7024.
[5]     Vukovic, J.; Goodbody, A. E.; Kutney, J .; Misawa, M. *Tetrahedron*, **1988**, *44*, 325-331.
[6]     Szántay, Cs. Jr.; Balázs, M.; Bölcskei, H.; Szántay, Cs. *Tetrahedron*, **1991**, *47*, 1265-74.
[7]     Balázs, M. ; Szántay, Cs. Jr.; Bölcskei, H.; Szántay, Cs. *Tetrahedron Lett.*, **1993**, *34*, 4397-4398.

[8]　　Balázs, M.; Szántay, Cs. Jr.; Bölcskei, H.; Szántay, Cs. *Nat. Prod. Lett.* **1994**, *4* 189-193

[9]　　Bölcskei, H.; Gács-Baitz, E.; Szántay, Cs.; *Tetrahedron Letters* **1989**, *30,* 7245-48

[10]　　Bölcskei, H.; Szántay Cs. Jr;.; Mák, M.; Balázs, M.; Szántay, Cs. *J. Ind. Chem. Soc.* **1997**, *74*, 904-907.

[11]　　Szabó, L.; Szántay, Cs.; Gács-Baitz, E.; Mák, M, *Tetrahedron Lett.* **1995**, 5265-5266.

[12]　　Szabó, L.; Bölcskei, H.; Gács-Baitz, E.; Mák, M.; Szántay, Cs. *Arch. Pharm. Pharm. Med.Chem.* **2001**, *334*, 399-405.

[13]　　Bölcskei, H.; Szántay, Cs. Jr.; Mák, M.; Balázs, M.; Szántay, Cs. *Acta Pharm. Hung.* **1998** *68,* 87-93.

Atta-ur-Rahman/Choudhary/Khan (Eds.) *Frontiers in Natural Product Chemistry, Vol. 1*  51

# Nature as Source and Inspiration for the Synthesis of New Anticancer Drugs

Daniele Passarella*, Alessandra Giardini, Giordano Lesma,
Alessandra Silvani and Bruno Danieli*

*Dipartimento di Chimica Organica e Industriale, Università degli Studi di Milano, Via Venezian, 21 - 20133 Milano, Italy*

**Abstract:** The bifunctional taxoid-colchicinoid hybrids were synthesised and evaluated in assays of cytotoxicity and tubulin assembly/disassembly. All compounds showed a high degree of cytotoxicity.

## INTRODUCTION

Nature was a generous provider of a great number of compounds displaying fascinating structural diversity with different biological activity. For anticancer treatment a considerable number of approved drugs are of natural origin. Humankind appreciates this gift from Nature but the treatment with these drugs often results in a number of undesired side effects as well as multi-drug resistance. Therefore, it remains essential to develop new anticancer agents with fewer side effects and improved activity against various classes of tumors. In an inspiring seminar at Berkely, François Jacobs once remarked that "natural selection works like a tinker who does not know exactly what he is going to produce but uses whatever he finds around him to produce some kind of workable object. None of the material at the tinker's disposal has a precise and definite function. Each can be used in different ways. ... *Novelty comes from previously unseen association of old material. To create is to recombine*" [1]. Although originally referring to genes, this observation holds true also for secondary metabolites, their ultimate plant and microbial products. Compounds like indole alkaloids, flavonoids, cannabinoids, tocopherols and furanocoumarins cogently testify how different metabolic pathways can be combined by Nature to generate a bewildering range of molecular diversity [2]. Nature has also deftly exploited various coupling strategies to assemble homo- and heterodimeric molecules whose activity can dramatically transcend that of their monomeric units. The bis-indole alkaloid vincristine (**1**) [3], the bis-steroid pyrazine cephalostatine 1 (**2**) [4] and the dimeric sesquiterpene lactone absinthine (**3**) [5] are remarkable examples of how Nature has harnessed coupling strategies based, respectively, on oxidative-, condensative- and pericyclic chemistry to induce bioactivity.

The idea of combining different anticancer agents into a single, biologically multivalent molecule is not new and dual drugs obtained by coupling spindle poisons to various DNA-damaging agents have been prepared in the hope of simultaneously targeting crucial end-points of cell division [9]. The inherent weakness of these approaches is the different cellular localization of tubulin and DNA, who critically interact only during mitosis, and therefore the need of a precise spatio-temporal coordination for the dual activity [6]. Furthermore, ligand affinity of DNA and tubulin differ substantially, making it difficult to simultaneously optimise both individual drug concentrations. By focusing on distinct and functionally different binding sites of the same target, we hoped to overcome these

---

*Corresponding author: E-mail: Daniele.Passarella@unimi.it

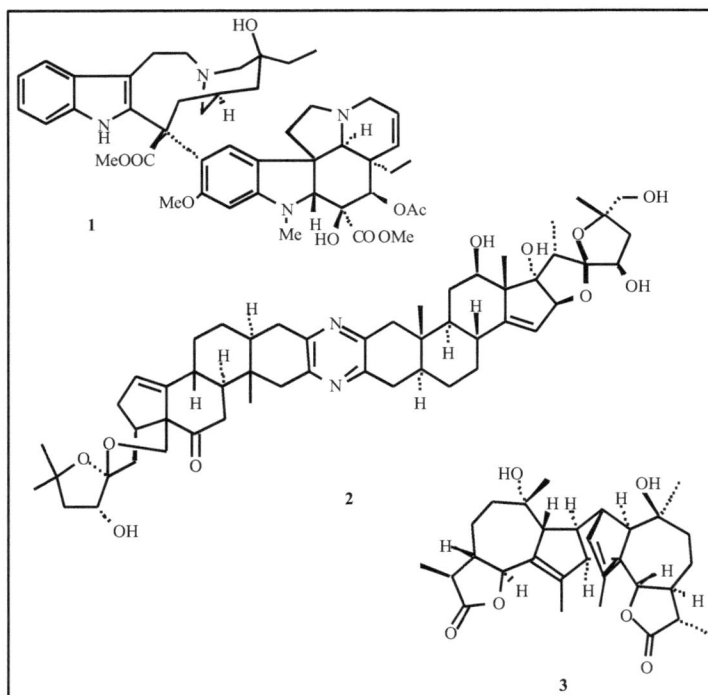

limitations, exploiting the potentially synergistic effect resulting from the presence in the same molecule of two mechanistically distinct inhibitor moieties of comparable affinity.

In this light, we have synthesised and investigated in cytotoxicity and tubulin binding assays the taxoid-colchicinoid hybrids **4-6**. In these compounds, a taxoid moiety is bound to an *N*-deacetylcolchicinoid by a succinate spacer linking the 10-, 7- or 2'-hydroxyl of the taxoid unit with the basic amino group of the colchicinoid moiety. Chalcogenic modification of the enolic oxygen of colchicine [10] and benzoyl- to Boc swap of the amide moiety of Taxol [7] are known to increase the biological activity of the natural products. We planned to incorporate this simple molecular editing into our final targets, using thiocolchicine (**7**) [10a] and 10-deacetylbaccatin III (**8**), a taxane devoid of the aminoacidic side chain, as starting materials. The chemistry of taxoids and baccatines is relatively well known, but several unexpected difficulties surfaced *en route* to the targets, requiring extensive remodelling of the original synthetic sequences.

The Taxoid-cholchicinoid hybrids **4-6** were assayed for cytotoxicity in MCF7 breast cancer cells. The results showed that compounds **4** and **5** are mechanistically multifunctional tubulin inhibitors, behaving as interesting probes to investigate not only tubulin biology, but also the complex and so far poorly understood relationship between tubulin binding and cytotoxicity of taxoids. On the other hand, the biological profile of **6** is quite surprisingly and might well involve a target different from tubulin [11].

We moved our attention toward the incorporation of other anticancer agents that present a functional group available for the construction of different hybrids. Preliminary biological evaluation suggested the not trivial importance of the spacer. For this reason the preparation

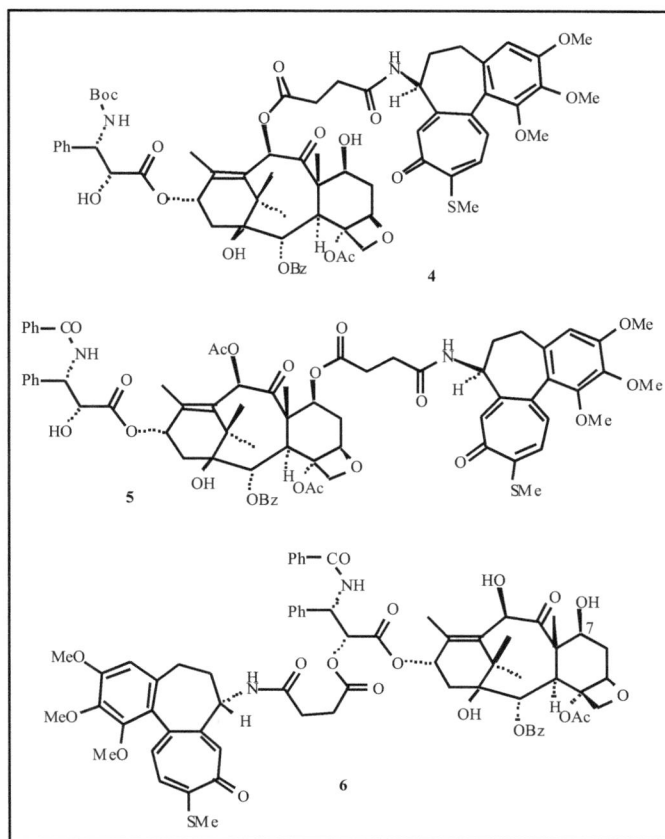

of such kind of compounds is a problem with three variables: the two anticancer agents and the spacer to be merged in a single hybrid product. We then decided to introduce a combinatorial approach for the preparation of new hybrids and this research is going on in our laboratory.

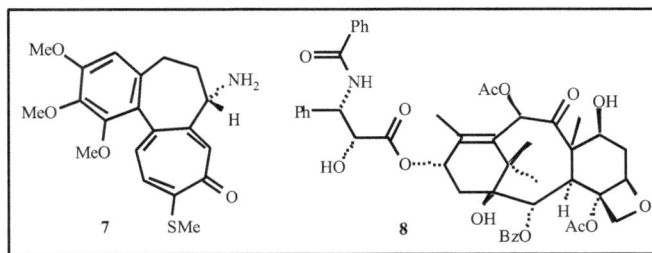

# REFERENCES

[1]    Jacob, F. *Science* **1977**, *196*, 1161.
[2]    Mann, J. In *Secondary Metabolism*, Oxford University Press, Oxford **1980**, pp. 237-278.

[3]      for a comprehensive review on isolation, chemistry and structure-activity relationships of vincristine and related compounds see: *The Alkaloids, Antitumor Bisindole Alkaloids from Catharanthus raseus (L.)* Brossi A. and Suffness M. Eds., Accademic Press: New York, **1990**, Vol. *37*.

[4]      Pettit, G. R., Inoue, M., Kamano, Y., Herald, D. L., Arm, C., Dufresne, C., Christie, N. D., Schmidt, J. M., Doubek, D. L., Krupa, T. S. *J. Am. Chem. Soc.* **1988**, *110*, 2006.

[5]      Novotny, L., Herout, V., Sorm, F. *Coll. Czech. Chem. Commun.* **1960**, *25*, 1492.

[6]      For a review on tubulin binders, see: Jordan, A., Hadfield, J. A., Lawrence, N. J., McGown, A. T. *Med. Res. Rev.* **1998**, *18*, 259.

[7]      For a recent and comprehensive review on the structure-activity relationships of paclitaxel, see: Kingston, D. G. I., Jagtap, P. G., Yuan, H., Samala, L., in *Progress in the Chemistry of Organic Natural Products*; Herz, W., Falk, H., Kirby, G. W. Eds.; Springer: New York, **2002**; Vol. *84*, pp 53-225.

[8]      Boyè, O., Brossi, A. Tropolonic Colchicum Alkaloids and Allo Congeners. In *The Alkaloids,* Brossi, A., Ed., Accademic Press: New York, **1992**, Vol. *41*, pp.125

[9]      a) Taxol-calichemicin hybrid: Py, S., Harwig, C. W., Banerjee, S., Brown, D. L., Fallis, A. G. *Tetrahedron Lett.* **1998**, *39*, 6139; b) Taxol-daunorubicin dimers: Kar, A. K., Braun, P. D., Wandless, T. J. *Bioorg. Med. Chem. Lett.* **2000**, *10*, 261; c) Taxol-chlorambucil hybrid: Wittman, M. D., Kadow, J. F., Vyas, D. M., Lee, F. L., Rose, W. C., Long, B. H., Fairchild, C., Johnston, K. *Bioorg. Med. Chem. Lett.* **2001**, *11*, 811; d) Taxol-epipodophyllotoxin conjugates: Shi, Q., Wang, H.-K., Bastow, K. F., Tachibana, Y., Chen, K., Lee, F.-Y., Lee, K.-H.*Bioorg. Med. Chem.* **2001**, *9*, 2999-3004. (e) Taxol-camptothecin coniugates: Ohtsu, H., Nakanishi, Y., Bastow, K. F., Lee, F.-Y., Lee, K.-H. *Bioorg. Med. Chem.* **2003**, *11*, 1851.

[10]     a) Velluz, L., Muller, G. *Bull. Soc. Chim. Fr.* **1954**, 755; b) Brossi, A., Yeh, H. J. C., Chrzanowska, M., Wulff, J., Hamel, E., Lin, C. M., Quinn, F., Suffness, M., Silverton, J. *Med. Res. Rev.* **1988**, *8*, 77.

[11]     Danieli, B., Giardini, A., Lesma, G., Passarella, D., Silvani, A., Appendino, G., Noncovich, A., Fontana, G., Bombardelli, E., Sterner, O. *Chemistry and Biodiversity* **2004**, *1*, 327.

Atta-ur-Rahman/Choudhary/Khan (Eds.) *Frontiers in Natural Product Chemistry, Vol. 1*

# Stereocontrol in Organic Synthesis Using Silicon Compounds

Ian Fleming*

*Department of Chemistry, Lensfield Road, Cambridge CB2 1EW, UK*

**Abstract:** Electronic control of diastereoselectivity is discussed; only electrophilic attack adjacent to a stereogenic centre carrying an electropositive element **3** makes a coherent story.

## INTRODUCTION

Substituent effects on *reactivity* are well established, as is the language with which to explain them. An electronegative element X is a $\sigma$-acceptor and a $\pi$-donor, and the balance between these effects changes from the dominance of the former to the dominance of the latter, as we go from right to left along the periodic table. Carbon substituents have less dramatic and more various effects, ranging from the $\sigma$-neutral but $\pi$-donor alkyl groups, through the $\pi$-donor or acceptor alkenyl and aryl groups, to the $\sigma$- and $\pi$-withdrawing carbonyl and C-X groups. Electropositive elements M are the opposite of electronegative elements, being $\sigma$-donors and $\pi$-acceptors, but they are less familiar perhaps when they are not themselves the site of reaction. When they are simply substituents modifying the reactivity, only the least electropositive elements can survive, and foremost among these is silicon. The $\beta$-effect of a silyl group, stabilising cations, is a consequence of its $\sigma$-donor character, and the ability to stabilise an $\alpha$-anion is a consequence of its $\pi$-acceptor character.

Substituent effects on *stereoselectivity* are much less well established, and there is no consistent language with which to discuss them, except perhaps for straightforward steric effects, where one can often say, in the absence of any electronic effects that a reagent will attack from the less hindered side. But it is precisely the electronic effects that I want to discuss today, hoping, but largely failing as we shall see, to tease out a simple way of understanding their influence. We shall concentrate on the four fundamental cases: nucleophilic attack **1** and **4** and electrophilic attack **2** and **3** on a double bond adjacent to a stereogenic centre carrying either an electronegative atom X or an electropositive atom M.

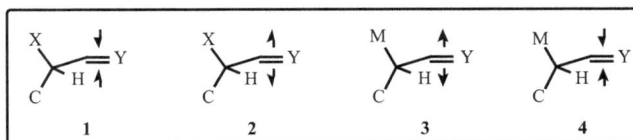

## DISCUSSION

To understand how an electronic effect might be transmitted into the $\pi$-framework in such a way as to make the two sides of the $\pi$-bond different, we would like to apply molecular orbital theory. If we look in Fig. (**1**) at the atomic orbitals that contribute to the C—X bond and the $\pi$-bond, we see that none of the $p_x$, $p_y$ or $p_z$ orbitals can have any effect

*Corresponding author: E-mail: if10000@cam.ac.uk

that would differentiate the top and bottom of the π-bond—the p-orbitals are either orthogonal ($p_x$ and $p_y$) or equally placed ($p_z$) with respect to the top and bottom surfaces. Only the s-orbital on the carbon atom of the π-bond can have any effect, illustrated in Fig. 1 for a hybrid ψ between the π orbital and the s-orbital on the first carbon atom of the double bond, where the s orbital is arbitrarily given the same sign (shaded) as the s-orbital on the neighbouring carbon and the top surface of the p orbital. In this case the upper lobe is increased in size, and, since this is a filled orbital, we can expect it to encourage electrophilic attack on that surface. The complication is that there is no easy way to choose the sign of the s atomic orbital for each of the molecular orbitals created from these components, let alone in the appropriate frontier orbital, although an attempt has been made [1].

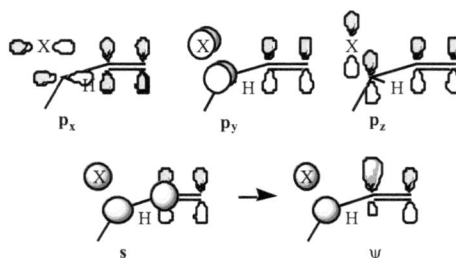

**Fig. (1).** Only mixing in the s atomic orbital can make the two surfaces of a π-bond differ.

Thus we are unable easily to explain the way electronic effects can be transmitted into a π-bond. Many attempts have been made [2], but none yet commands everyone's allegiance. We turn, therefore, to the experimental observations, to see what coherence there is there.

## NUCLEOPHILIC ATTACK ON A CARBONYL GROUP

The longest known reactions in any of these classes are nucleophilic attack on a carbonyl group **1** (Y=O) governed by Cram's rule, and most convincingly explained by Felkin and Anh. The electronic effect, which Anh added to Felkin [3], says that, in the absence of chelation, one counts an electronegative substituent as the large group, whatever its actual size. High level calculations by Frenking [4] agree that the lowest-energy transition structure **5** fits the rule. Furthermore, it is understandable, since both the hydride nucleophile and the electronegative chlorine atom carry an excess of negative charge, and they repel each other.

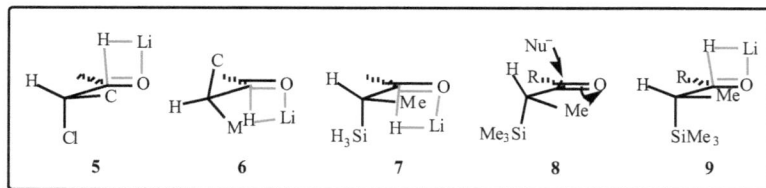

Strict application of this version of Anh's rule when the polar substituent is an electropositive group M places the incoming nucleophile *anti* to the carbon group **6**, since carbon is now the most electronegative element [5]. In support of this analysis, a calculation by Paddon-Row [6] at the same level as Frenking's gave the lowest-energy transition structure **7**, which also has preferred attack from below (if we keep the order of the three substituents on the stereogenic centre constant, as it is throughout this paper). This is understandable too, because the negatively charged nucleophile will be attracted to the positively charged silicon atom. The only problem with this story is that it is not in agreement with observation—almost all examples of this type of reaction take place from above in the sense **8**. We have recently repeated the Paddon-Row calculation using the trimethylsilyl group in place of the unsubstituted silyl group. The lowest-energy transition structure proved to be **9** [7], in agreement with observation. We conclude that the effect is largely steric, and that the electronic effect detected in Paddon-Row's calculation is overridden—the trimethylsilyl group effectively buries its positively charged core.

## NUCLEOPHILIC AND ELECTROPHILIC ATTACK ON A C=C DOUBLE BOND

When we turn to the more complicated story for attack on a C=C double bond (Y=CR$_2$), we have four situations **1-4** to discuss, and we shall take them in that order.

### Nucleophilic Attack on a C=C Double Bond with a Neighbouring Electronegative Substituent 1 (Y=CR$_2$)

At first sight we might expect the rule to be the same as Felkin's and Anh's, and this is what is observed in the representative reaction $Z$-**10**→**11** [8], with attack favoured from above. But the reason is not the same: in the first place the medium-sized group no longer easily fits 'inside', as it is called, more or less eclipsing the C=C double bond in the way that it prefers to eclipse the C=O double bond in all the structures **5-9**, and secondly, attack apparently takes place syn to the electronegative element **12**.

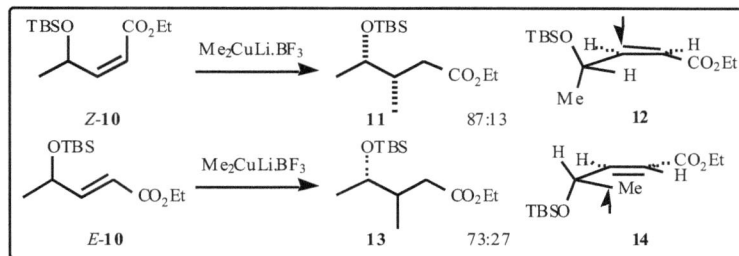

Furthermore, the sense of attack changes from above to below when the double bond geometry is changed, with $E$-**10** giving largely the diastereoisomer **13**. The attack is still apparently from the side carrying the electronegative substituent **14**, but now the methyl group sits 'inside'. We shall often see this 'inside methyl' effect, which complicates the story most tiresomely by not always showing up.

The pattern of attack syn to the electronegative element is not always observed, but seems to be more common than not. It is certainly not restricted to organocuprate reactions, and it is clearly not what might be expected by comparison with the Anh rule. Suggestions have been made that the nucleophile is delivered intramolecularly following coordination to the electronegative element, but this seems unlikely for the conjugate addition of malonates, for example, or for the S$_N$2' reaction **15**→**16** [9], which is stereospecifically syn **17**, like most but not all S$_N$2' reactions.

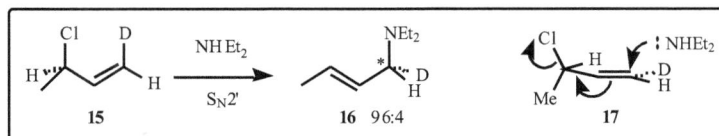

## Electrophilic Attack on a C=C Double Bond with a Neighbouring Electronegative Substituent 2 (Y=CR$_2$)

The reaction of osmium tetroxide on an alkene is electrophilic in character, and typically follows the pattern shown in the reactions of the alkenes Z-**18** and E-**18** [10].

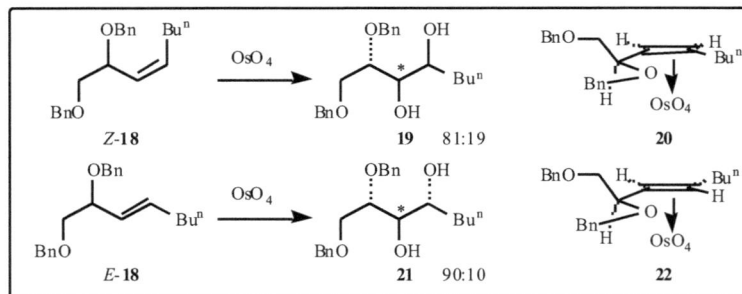

The explanation usually offered (although not in ref. 10) is that the C—O bond, if it were conjugated to the π-bond, would be deactivating. Attack by an electrophile therefore takes place with the C—O bond 'inside' **20** and **22**, out of conjugation, and the stereochemistry is simply attack on the less hindered side.

In contrast, the hydroboration of the alkenes **23** appears to take place with the hydrogen atom inside, and with attack **25** and **27** from the same side as the electronegative atom, which this time is the medium-sized group [11].

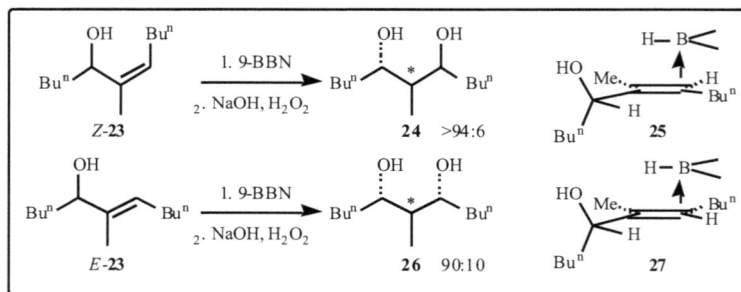

And in another variation, the osmium tetroxide reaction on the sulfones **28** appears to take place with the hydrogen atom inside in the Z-alkene and with the methyl group inside with the E-alkene, and with attack **30** and **32** from the opposite side from the electronegative atom [12]. In this case, Vedejs suggests that the sulfone is too large to sit inside.

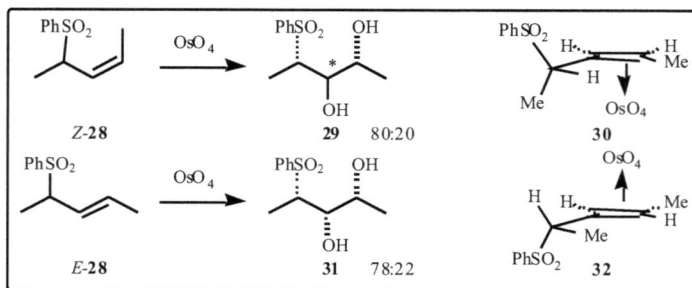

### Electrophilic Attack on a C=C Double Bond with a Neighbouring Electropositive Substituent 3 (Y=CR$_2$)

Vedejs also looked at a similar reaction, replacing the allylsulfones **28** with the corresponding allylsilanes **33**, for which he found that the diastereoselectivities, both in sense and in degree, were essentially the same as for the sulfones [12]. He argued that since the sense of attack is the same whether the substituent is an electronegative element or an electropositive element, the diastereoselectivity in both cases is simply controlled by a steric effect, with the methyl group sitting inside in the *E*-alkenes **32** and **37**, when there is only a small energetic penalty, exposing a relatively very unhindered upper surface.

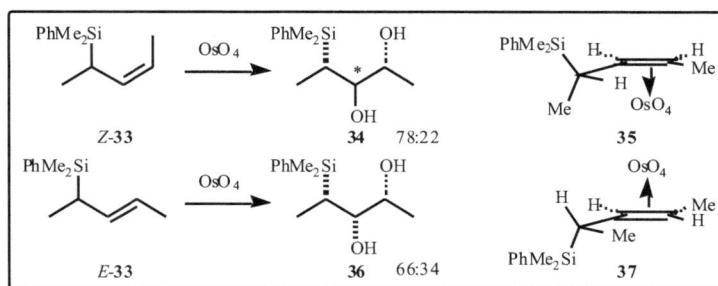

Our own work [13] has shown the same pattern of attack reliably anti to the silyl group in a wide variety of reactions, some showing the 'inside methyl' effect and some not. The best studied of the reactions showing this pattern is the S$_E$2' reaction of allylsilanes **38**, in which the stereochemical information is transferred from C-1 to C-3 [14]. The *E*-isomer *E*-**38** reacts a little over half the time (60:40, as revealed by the double bond geometry in the product) in the 'methyl inside' conformation, but all the reactions are stereospecifically highly anti.

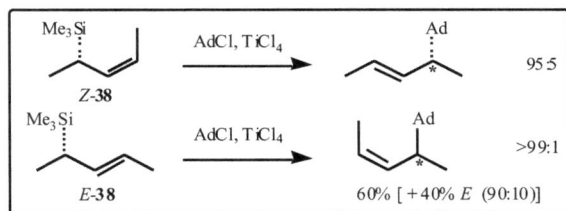

Similarly, hydroboration is highly anti, except that both geometries *Z*-**33** and *E*-**33** react with 9-BBN in the conformation with the hydrogen atom inside [15].

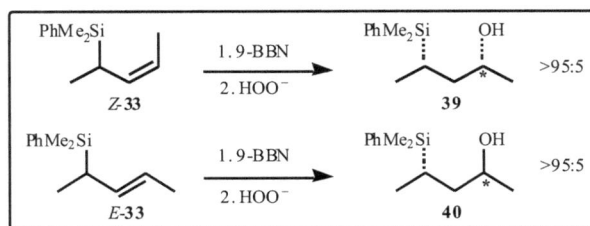

Another reaction with high levels of attack anti to the silyl group is enolate alkylation and protonation, where either diastereoisomer **41** or **42** can be obtained with almost equal ease by exchanging the resident group and the electrophile [16].

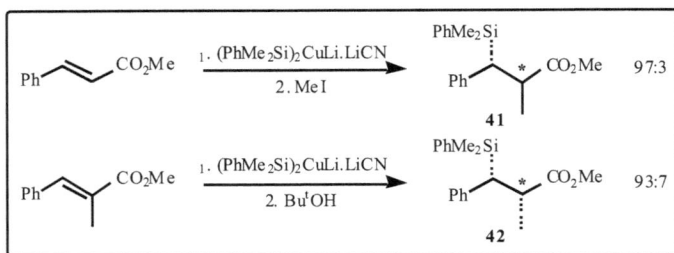

In the last two reactions, the silyl group remains in the molecule, and to use the stereochemical information embedded in it a reaction is needed in which the silyl group is converted into something more generally useful in synthesis.

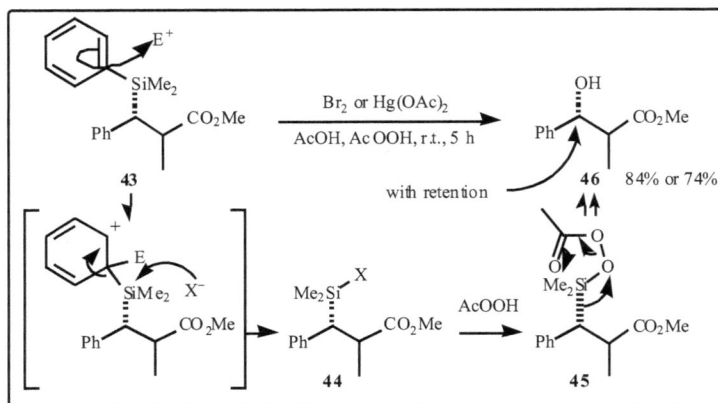

This reaction is the silyl-to-hydroxy conversion 43→46 [17], which takes place in two stages: the removal of the phenyl group by an ipso electrophilic substitution 43→44, using bromine or mercuric ion, and the oxidative rearrangement step, using peracid or a peroxide, in which the carbon groups attached to the silicon atom move to the electrophilic oxygen atom 45 (arrows) with the usual retention of configuration seen in all [1,2]-sigmatropic rearrangements to electrophilic atoms.

Using one or more of the four kinds of reactions seen immediately above, we synthesised ten natural products having one, two, three or four stereogenic centres [18], and have also been working on the synthesis of ebelactone A 47, which has seven stereogenic centres and one double bond to be controlled. The plan was to synthesise the three fragments A, B and C, each enantiomerically enriched, and with *all the relative stereochemistry and the double bond geometry controlled by the presence of the silyl group.*

This was a more substantial target, requiring us to invent solutions to some of the problems, but constraining us so severely that we were not able actually to synthesise this molecule. We did control all the relative stereochemistry by making each of the molecules 48, 49 and 50 as our fragments A, B and C, respectively, and we reported this work in an earlier lecture in this place [19].

Since then, we have joined the pieces together, but an inversion of the stereocentre at C-2 occurred in the step involving the allyllithium intermediate 51. This compound was designed to abstract the silyl group on the C-9 oxygen atom in a reaction (arrows) with good precedent [20]. Had it done so, the allylsilane 52 would have undergone a clean

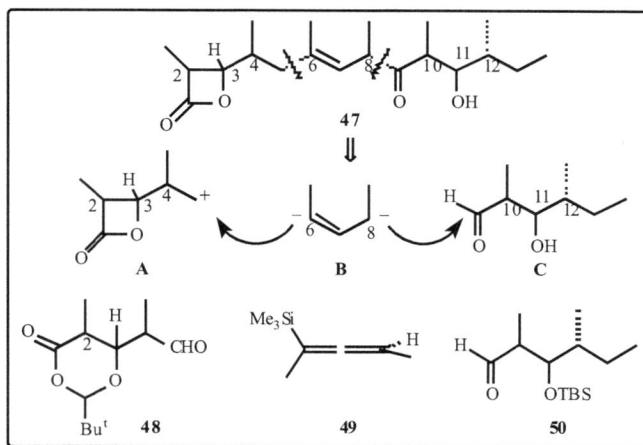

regioselective protodesilylation placing the double bond between C-6 and C-7, and with the right geometry.

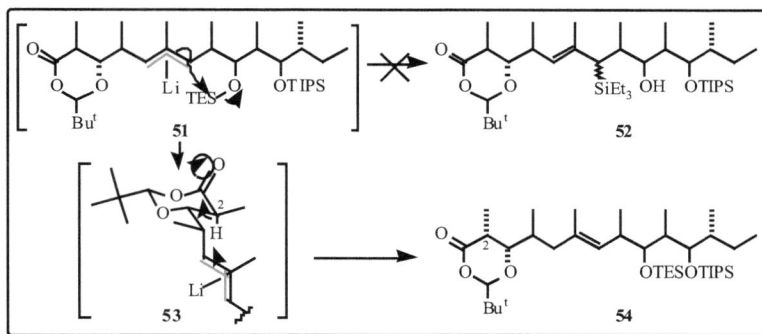

In the event the allyllithium intermediate **51** calamitously took the proton off C-2 **53** (arrows), and the resulting enolate reprotonated on the less hindered side of the dioxanone ring, inverting the configuration at C-2 in the product **54**. As a result, we made 2-epi-ebelactone A, and even that largely as the 11-benzenesulfonate, because the β-lactone was so slow to form, being cis disubstituted, that the C-11 hydroxyl was esterified.

In spite of this setback, we had proved yet again that electrophilic attack on a double bond with a neighbouring electropositive element was a reliable strategy for the control of relative stereochemistry in open-chain systems. In all probability, the stereoselectivity is a consequence only of the steric effect of the large silyl group, but it cannot be unhelpful that any electronic effect is probably in the same direction—encouraging attack anti to the silyl group.

## Nucleophilic Attack on a C=C Double Bond with a Neighbouring Electropositive Substituent 4 (Y=CR₂)

Nucleophilic attack on such systems, where the steric and electronic effects might be opposing each other, has hardly been investigated. The nearest known reaction was on an intermediate in the reaction of the acetal **55** with a silyl enol ether, where the diastereoselectivity followed what might be expected for attack on the less hindered side, anti to the silyl group, in the conformation **57** [21].

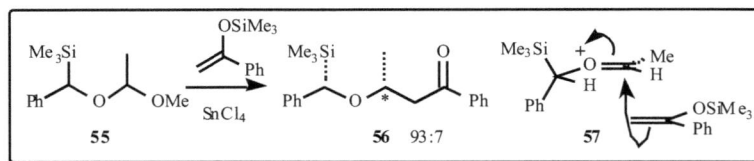

In our first work in this area, we investigated the enone **58**, which also underwent nucleophilic attack anti to the silyl group to give the silyl enol ether **59** (R=Et) with a high degree of diastereoselectivity [22]. The conformation **58** was calculated to have the lowest energy, in spite of the large group's being axial, and it is also the conformation adopted in the solid state, as shown by a low-temperature X-ray structure.

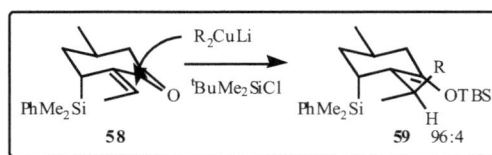

Following this result, we repeated the reaction with the isohexylcuprate to give the silyl enol ether **59** (R=isohexyl), and used this to prepare the ketone **60** in a synthesis of (±)-phytol **63**. The fragmentation **61** → **62** revealed the open-chain 1,5-relationship, and the remaining carbons were attached in a prenylation reaction between a silyl dienol ether and the aldehyde derived from the nitrile **62**.

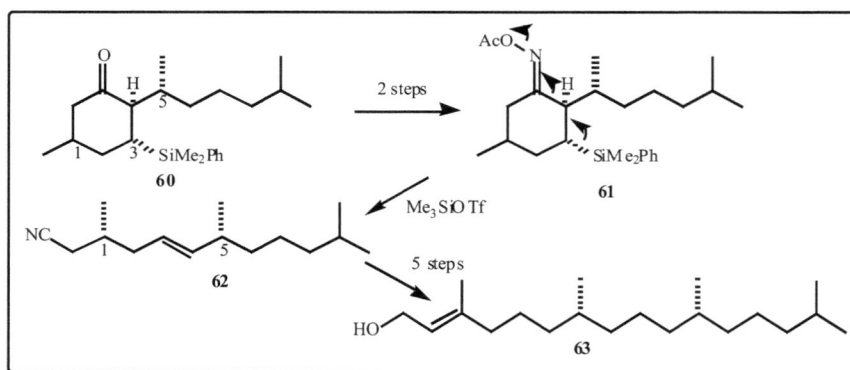

However, these results were in a relatively rigid system **58**, and we wanted to know how well the silyl group controlled the diastereoselectivity directly in an open-chain system. We therefore examined the α,β-unsaturated ester **64**, moderately confident, since we deliberately chose a Z-isomer that attack would take place anti to the silyl group in the conformation with the hydrogen atom inside. Our thinking was prejudiced by the accumulated experience with electrophilic attack, coupled with the results immediately above, that steric effects could explain the diastereoselectivity that we and everyone else had seen—there was no evidence for any difference in nucleophilic attack from that seen so regularly in electrophilic attack. In the event, we were surprised to find that there was little diastereoselectivity (58:42). Insofar as there was any diastereoselectivity, the major product, judging by the coupling constant between the protons on C-3 and C-4 ($J$ 1.1 Hz for the major and 6.7 for the minor), was the isomer **65** we had not expected [23]. A coupling constant argument was fairly reliable in this system, since the values are so different, and they so nearly match those calculated from an assessment of the Boltzmann distribution of the low energy conformations, summarised in the Newman projections **66** and **67**.

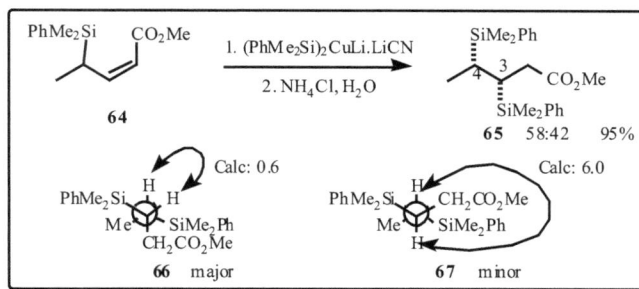

Another $\alpha,\beta$-unsaturated ester **68**, available as $E$- and $Z$-isomers, was more complicated, because there were two starting materials, and four products from each, two pairs reflecting the diastereoselectivity we were interested in, and two reflecting the diastereoselectivity in the protonation step, which was unlikely to be predictable. We were able to pick out the four isomers from the $^1$H-NMR signals [23], and labelled them **A**, **B**, **C** and **D**. They were formed in ratios such that **B** and **C** were the major pair from the $Z$-isomer, and **A** and **D** from the $E$-isomer. The isomers **A** and **D** were separable, free of the others, but the isomers **B** and **C** were only obtained as a mixture. To cut a long story short, we were able, by silyl-to-hydroxy conversions, and cyclic acetal syntheses, to identify them as the isomers **69-72**, respectively.

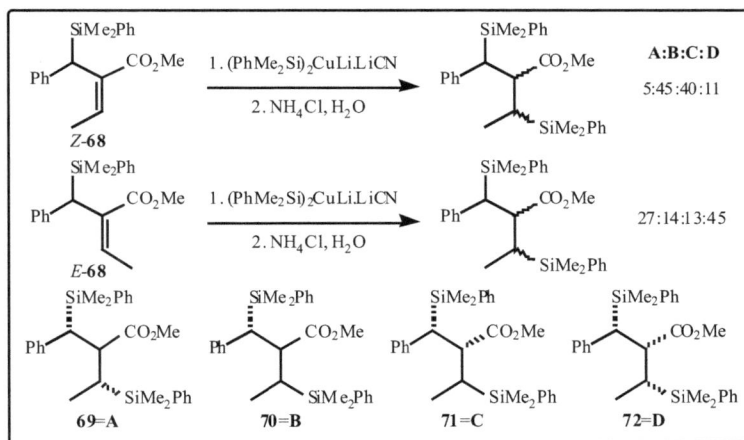

The unexpected outcome again is that the major products are those that appear to follow from attack syn to the silyl group. We suggest that there may be an electronic component resembling the 'inside oxygen' effect. Electrophilic attack when there is a neighbouring electronegative group has the O—C bond 'inside', since it would be deactivating if it were conjugated. Nucleophilic attack when there is a neighbouring electropositive group might take place more rapidly when the Si—C bond is more or less orthogonal to the double bond, since it would be deactivating if it were conjugated. To explain our results it would have to be 'outside', summarised in **73**, **74**, and **75**, which is not unreasonable, since the silyl group is surely too large to sit 'inside'.

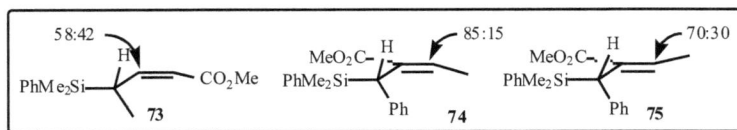

## CONCLUSIONS

Of the four systems **1-4**, only the third, electrophilic attack on a double bond with an adjacent stereogenic centre carrying a silyl group, is consistent and satisfyingly well explained. Some of the others are highly effective and reliable in total synthesis, and have all been much used, provided that there is good literature precedent. But they are not well explained, and the precedents must be close. The last system **4**, nucleophilic attack on a double bond with the stereogenic centre carrying a silyl group, has been examined with all too few reactions, and most of those cuprates—it needs more study before generalisations are safe.

## REFERENCES

[1]     Burgess, E. M.; Liotta, C. L. *J. Org. Chem.*, **1981**, *46*, 1703.
[2]     Most of them are represented in a special issue of *Chem. Rev.*, **1999**, 1067-1480.
[3]     Anh, N. T.; Eisenstein, O. *Nouv. J. Chim.*, **1977**, *1*, 61.
[4]     Frenking, G.; Köhler, K. F.; Reetz, M. T. *Tetrahedron*, **1991**, *47*, 8991 and 9005.
[5]     Allen electronegativities: Si (1.92), C (2.54), Cl (2.87).
[6]     Wong, S. S.; Paddon-Row, M. N. *Aust. J. Chem.*, **1991**, *44*, 765.
[7]     Fleming, I.; Hrovat, D.; Borden, W. T. *J. Chem. Soc., Perkin Trans. 2*, **2001**, 331.
[8]     Yamamoto, Y.; Chounan, Y.; Nishii, S.; Ibuka, T.; Kitahara, H. *J. Am. Chem. Soc.*, **1992**, *114*, 7652.
[9]     Magid, R. M.; Fruchey, O. S. *J. Am. Chem. Soc.*, **1979**, *101*, 2107.
[10]    Cha, J. K.; Christ, W. J.; Kishi, Y. *Tetrahedron*, **1984**, *40*, 2247.
[11]    Still, W. C.; Barrish, J. C. *J. Am. Chem. Soc.*, **1983**, *105*, 2487.
[12]    Vedejs, E.; McClure, C. K. *J. Am. Chem. Soc.*, **1986**, *108*, 1094.
[13]    Summarised in Fleming, I. *J. Chem. Soc., Perkin Trans. 1*, **1992**, 3363.
[14]    Buckle, M. J. C.; Fleming, I.; Gil, S. *Tetrahedron Lett.*, **1992**, *33*, 4479.
[15]    Fleming, I.; Lawrence, N. J. *J. Chem. Soc., Perkin Trans. 1*, **1992**, 3309.
[16]    Crump, R. A. N. C.; Fleming, I.; Hill, J. H. M.; Parker, D.; Reddy, N. L.; Waterson, D. *J. Chem. Soc., Perkin Trans. 1*, **1992**, 3277.
[17]    Fleming, I.; Henning, R.; Parker, D. C.; Plaut, H. E.; Sanderson, P. E. J. *J. Chem. Soc., Perkin Trans. 1*, **1995**, 317.
[18]    Ahmar, M.; Chow, H.-F.; Duyck, C.; Fleming, I.; Ghosh, S. K.; Higgins, D.; Kilburn, J. D.; Lawrence, N. J.; Lee, D.; Terrett N. K.; Winter, S. B. D. 10 papers in *J. Chem. Soc., Perkin Trans. 1*, **1998**, 2645.
[19]    Fleming, I.; Mandal, A. K.; Mandal, A. K.; in *Natural Products Chemistry at the Turn of the Century*, ed. Atta-ur-Rahman; Choudhary, A. I.; Khan, K. M. Karachi, **2002**, pp. 1-10.
[20]    Behrens, K.; Kneisel, B. O.; Noltemeyer, M.; Brückner, R. *Liebigs Ann.*, **1995**, 385.
[21]    Linderman, R. J.; Anklekar, T. V. *J. Org. Chem.*, **1992**, *57*, 5078. See also, for allylsilanes as the nucleophiles, Cossrow, J.; Rychnovsky, S. D. *Org. Lett.*, **2002**, *4*, 147.
[22]    Fleming, I.; Maiti, P.; Ramarao, C. *Org. Biomol. Chem.*, **2003**, *1*, 3989.
[23]    Betson, M.; Fleming, I.; Ouzman, J. V. A. *Org. Biomol. Chem.*, **2003**, *1*, 4017.

Atta-ur-Rahman/Choudhary/Khan (Eds.) *Frontiers in Natural Product Chemistry, Vol. 1*          65

# Natural Photoreceptors: Structure, Function and Applications

Uma S. Palkar*

*S.I.E.S College , Sion (W), Mumbai 400022, India*

**Abstract:** Natural photoreceptors evoke a biological response on absorption of light signal. A reversible change in the structure of photoreceptors occurs by energy or sensory transduction. Chemically they are conjugated trans-membrane proteins with retinal or tetrapyrrole based chromophores in most of them. Photosynthesis, photomorphogenesis, photoperiodism, vision and phototaxis are various functions of photoreceptors.

Bacteriorhodopsin (bR), from H. salinarium acts as a light driven proton pump for the synthesis of ATP. bR undergoes an interesting reversible photocycle. During the photocycle, retinylidene chromophore undergoes a reversible all-trans-to 13-cis- isomerisation, and proton translocation takes place.Chemical modifications of bR and 3D – structure of bR at 1.5-Angstrom resolution help to know the binding site of chromophore and proton translocation at molecular level. Many colour control mechanisms have been suggested for bR. A large number of bR analogues can be made as follows:

bR + $NH_2OH.HCl$ -→ Bacterial opsin (bOP) + Retinal, and bOP + retinal analogue → bR analogue, which can be used to study structure, function and likely applications. bR can act as a bistable photobiological switch with potential applications in optical memory, optical data processing.

Photoactive Yellow Protein (PYP), a cytosolic photoreceptor from E. halophila also undergoes a photocycle and can be put to similar uses. PYP uses p-hydroxy cinnamoyl thioester, a novel chromophore that isomerises with change in conformation of protein during the photocycle, resulting in a signalling state in yet unknown sensory path.

Natural photoreceptors constitute a novel and unique field of natural product chemistry.

## INTRODUCTION

A natural photoreceptor is one that evokes a biological response like germination of seeds, flowering of plants, photosynthesis, vision etc. on absorption of light signal. Chemically it is a trans-membrane conjugated protein with generally tetrapyrrole or retinal based chromophore.

On absorption of light photoreceptors get excited with a reversible change in electronic or chemical structure resulting in energy or sensory transduction. Chlorophyll, Phycobilisomes, Phytochromes, Rhodopsin, Bacteriorhodopsin, and Photoactive Yellow Protein are some of the examples of photoreceptors.

The well-known chromophore chlorophyll is complexed with proteins in light harvesting and photoreaction centre complexes to effect photosynthesis [1,2].

*Corresponding author: Fax – 91-22-24096633; E-mail: umapalkar@yahoo.com

Red marine algae and cyanobacteria have phycobilins in light harvesting complexes to absorb bluish green light. Chemically phycobilins are linear tetrapyrrole chromophores e.g. Phycoerythrobilin, phycocyanobilin. These combine with trimers\ hexamers of dipeptides to form phycoerythrocyanins, phycocyanins and allophycocyanins, as antena pigments. These are intricately arranged in phycobilisomes in hemidiscoidal structure with linker poteins.They transfer light energy to Chlorophyll-a at the photoreaction centre complex by exciton transfer [1,2].

Phytochromes too have linear tetrapyrrole chromophore viz. 3 E phytochromobilin[3a], two of which are attached covalently to two Sulphurs of cysteine of a homodimer polypeptide[M=124KDa]. Phytochromes are amazing photoreceptors of plant, which optimize the photosynthetic machinary, at the concentration of just 0.2% by weight.

There is a reverible switching between its biologically active, far red light absorbing, greenish blue $P_{FR}$ form and biologically inactive, red light absorbing, blue $P_R$ form involving s-cis to s-trans isomerisation of chromophore analogue with a change in conformation of protein.

Phytochromes control tissue differentiation in photomorphogenesis i.e. germination of seeds, flowering of plants and also act as biological clocks in photoperiodicity based on circadian rhythms e.g. leaf senescence, seasonal flowering, ripening of fruits, etc. They are believed to alter gene expression of photoregulatory genes [2,3a].

Cryptochromes are U.V. or blue light absorbing photoreceptors of plants which control stomatal opening and phototropism in plants,e.g.Arabidopsis[3b]

Retinal based photoreceptor in rod cells of our eyes is Rhodopsin(Rh), [4], with λmax 550nm in humans. It has 11-cis-retinylidene chromophore covalently linked to the apoprotein, opsin. Rhodopsin (Rh), is a hepta helical trans-membrane protein responsible for the gray vision in dim light. Rh has high sensitivity and a G protein coupled receptor [4,5].

**Sensory rhodopsins** (sR)in many microorganisms including Halobacterium salinarium(sR-1and2) also have **retinylidene moiety** as chromophore and are responsible for photo attractant or photophobic phototaxis [5].

The other two photorecepors:- Halorhodopsin (hR) in H.salinarium acts as a chloride pump and maintains osmotic equilibrium while bacteriorhodopsin (bR) in a novel way, acts as a photon driven proton pump for the synthesis of ATP, in photosynthesis. Both hR and bR have retinylidene chromophore.

H. Salinarium is a rod shaped, flagellar, motile, oldest, archaebacterium with traits of both animal and plant. In natural brines,in intense light and at low levels of oxygen it develops purple patches for photosynthesis, which contain bR [1,5].

## Structure of Bacteriorhodospin(bR) [6]

A protein of M = 26kDa, with 247 amino acid residues, consists of seven trans-membrane helices A to G circularly arranged; helices B, C, F, G forming a trans-membrane pore. Retinylidene moeity is covalently linked to ε− amino group of Lys-216 of helix G, *via* Schiff's base linkage and lies halfway in the barrel shaped pore with its cyclohexenyl ring perpendicular to the membrane and its long axis tilted by 21 degrees towards the extracellular channel. Structure of bR is now available at 1.5A° resolution and so the binding site of retinal is well characterised.

## The bR Photocycle [7]

When exposed to light bR undergoes a series of reversible changes in its structure associated with changes in $\lambda$max of absorption, forming intermediates or transitory states, 'J to O'.

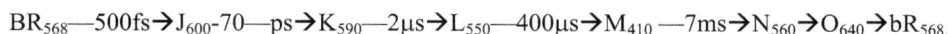

$BR_{568}$—500fs$\rightarrow J_{600}$-70—ps$\rightarrow K_{590}$—2$\mu$s$\rightarrow L_{550}$—400$\mu$s$\rightarrow M_{410}$—7ms$\rightarrow N_{560}\rightarrow O_{640}\rightarrow bR_{568}$.

The numerical subscripts indicate $\lambda$max in nm, along with transition time during the photocycle; which has been studied by variety of spectroscopic, chemical and biochemical methods. During the cycle

all-trans- Retinylidene moeity reversibly photoisomerises to 13-cis- form alongwith proton translocation across the membrane with quantum yield of 0.67and proton motive force of 800 mV is developed.

## Details of Photocycle

1. 'J'and'O' states, are probably twisted trans? Not known completely.

2. 'K' and' L' are dipolar, excited states with twisted 13-cis-C=C- .

3. During 'L'$\rightarrow$M transition, H-bond bridges between Trp-86 and Asp-85 break,with change of conformation and lowering of pKa; a proton is transferred from Schiff's base 'N' to Asp-85 COO⁻ via water molecules to extracellular side. Arg-82, Glu-194 also participate in transfer.

4. ' M' state has chromophore in 13-cis- geometry and deprotonated Schiff's base,disconnected to the extra cellular side and connected to the cytoplasmic side.

5. In 'M' $\rightarrow$ N' transition, H-bonding of Asp-96 becomes weaker. Intricate pK changes occur on breaching of hydrophobic barrier. Finally $H^+$ of Asp-96-COOH is transferred to Schiff's base nitrogen via water molecules.

6. 'N' is the relaxed state with 13-cis- geometry and protonated Schiff's base nitrogen.

Finally original state of bR is regained by retroisomerisation.

## Analogues of bR [5,8]

Two types of bR analogues have been made to study, the active site interactions and the role of various protein residues, in structure, function and potential applications of bR.

### I. Modification of Bacterial Opsin (bOP)

a) By site directed mutagenesis of bOP followed by incubation with retinal.

- Asp-96-Asn, mutant of bR,has increased life time of M state to 750 ms,with 50% increase in photosensitivity and two fold increase in diffraction efficiency in thin films.

- Interesting absorption properties have been observed for some bR variants obtained by UV induced mutagensis.

- The chemical modification studies reveal the role of , amino groups and of ionized and non-ionized carboxylic acid groups during photocycle in proton translocation.

II. A large number of **synthetic retinal analogues** have been made.First a retinal analogue *that binds* bOP is made,purified, characterised and then bound to bOP.

The following method describes the preparation of bR analogues,I and II.

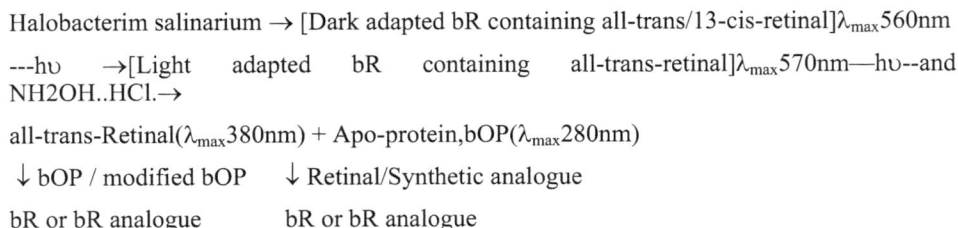

Halobacterim salinarium → [Dark adapted bR containing all-trans/13-cis-retinal]$\lambda_{max}$560nm

---hʋ →[Light adapted bR containing all-trans-retinal]$\lambda_{max}$570nm—hʋ--and NH2OH..HCl.→

all-trans-Retinal($\lambda_{max}$380nm) + Apo-protein,bOP($\lambda_{max}$280nm)

↓ bOP / modified bOP    ↓ Retinal/Synthetic analogue

bR or bR analogue         bR or bR analogue

Some of the bR analogues made in recent years are included in Table **1**.

bR analogues can be studied by various spectral techniques UV – Vis, CD, fluorescence, NMR, FTIR Raman etc and characterised by their ability of light induced proton translocation. Recent spectroscopic studies reveal [5].

1. Energy transfer couplings between retinal and Trp- residues at 86, 138, 182 and 189 present in the retinal pocket.

2. Retinal pocket of bR has specific binding sites for $Ca^{+2}$ and $Mg^{+2}$.

3. Role of divalent metal cations in colour transition of bR.

**Colour Control Mechanisms in bR [5,8]**

Nakanishi gave chemical basis for the opsin shift with his external point charge model,for the interaction between chromophore and opsin.Counter ion near Schiff's base linkage, charged amino acid residues other than counter ions, twisting of chromophore, aromatic amino acid residues, amino acids with –OH groups and structured water molecules also control colour of bR.

**Chromophore Binding Site and Mechanism of Proton Pumping in bR [2,5]**

• Asp-212, Trp, Tyr, Arg, Glu, Thr and water molecules have been found at the binding site.

• The latter stabilise the active site of protein.

• **Route of Proton Hops:-**Trp-182-Ala-215-Lys—216-Thr-46-Thr-178-Asp-96,H-bonded along with 4 structured and2 outside water molecules, on cytoplasmic side of channel andAsp-85-Asp-212-Arg-82-Tyr-57- Tyr79-Tyr185-Ser-193-Glu-204,along with 7 water molecules H-bonded on extracellular side of cannel.

• **Barrier Mechanism for Proton Movement in bR, in Dark**: There is a discontinuity in H bonded network on cytoplasmic side due to π helical turn in helix-G at Ala-215.

**Applications of Bacteriorhodopsin and its Analogues [9]**

1) Applications are based on photocycle of bR. bR can function as a photobiological switch. Optical information storage and processing exploits bR570 → K590 → bR570 and bR570 → M410 → bR570 reversible, fast phototransformations. Prof. Robert Birge of Syracuse Univ., NY has developed Bacteriorhodopsin optical memory (RAM) from Halobacterium halobium.

• as bistable red/green switch, bR $\xrightarrow{\lambda1,l1}$ K $\xrightarrow{\lambda2,l2}$ bR

**Table 1.** UV-Vis Data for Retinal, some Selected Modified Retinals, Corresponding Protonated Schiff Bases and the Corresponding bR/bR Analogues, [5, 8].

| Str.No. | Chromophore (Retinal analogue) X-Y | U.V.-Vis- Absorption $\lambda$ max in nm | | | | |
|---|---|---|---|---|---|---|
| | | Aldehyde | BuSBH[+a] | bR | OS (cm$^{-1}$)[b] | Ref. |
| I |  | 381 | 440 | 560 | 4870 | 8a |
| II |  | 373 | 455 | 480 | 1150 | 8a |
| III |  | 442 | 550 | 535 | -510 | 5 |
| IV |  | 461 | 504 | 597 | 3091 | 5 |
| V |  | 410 | 418 | 545 | 5575 | 5 |
| VI |  | 386 | 465 | 576 | 4140 | 8b |
| VII |  | 366 | 440 | 547 | 4480 | 8b |
| VII |  | 490 | 640 | 795 | 3050 | 8c |
| IX |  | - | - | - | - | 9 |

[a]BuSBH$^+$: Protonated Schiff base of chromophore with *n*-butylamin.

[b]OS: Opsin shift, i.e. $\lambda$max of n-BuSBH$^+$ (in cm$^{-1}$) minus $\lambda$max of bR (in cm$^{-1}$).

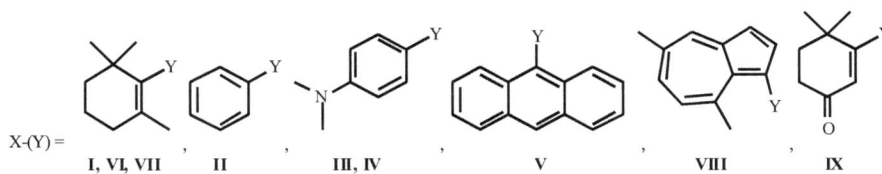

X-(Y) =   I, VI, VII ,   II ,   III, IV ,   V ,   VIII ,   IX

- (intensities $I_1$ and $I_2$ are adjusted, to exactly compensate, with no net change in population distribution)

- in the form of bR protein coat at 77K, $10^7$ to $10^8$ cycles, 10000 molecules per bit, switching time $\rightarrow$ 500fs (1000 times faster than fastest Ga/As).

- Monolayer of bR fabricated by self assembly.

II) Laser based FT holographic associative memory, Read/Write FTH memory using thin polymer films of bR has been described recently.

- FTH associative memories have significant potential applications in optical computers, optically coupled neutral networks, robotic/synthetic vision and generic pattern recognition systems.

- The Fuji Photo Film company has made a device equivalent to an eye.

- Door locks that can recognise faces of people can be developed and by changing the structure of bR, different visions can be developed.

III) Preparation of photoactive bioconjugates.

Photoactive Yellow Protein (PYP)[10,11]

PYP is a small cytosolic photoreceptor(M=14 KDa),from Halorhodospira halophila and Ectothiorhodospira halophla,a purple alkalophilic bacterium.

## Function

Phototaxis for directional motion and -ve phototaxis from blue light.

## Dark structure of PYP [12]

It has four helices A to D, a central antiparallel $\beta$ sheet and a chromophore containing loop which contains p-hydroxycinnamic thioester linked to cyst-69 residue in hydrophobic core.

Site directed mutagenesis study reveals that phenoxide group of chromophore is stabilised by H-bonding by Glu-46 and Tyr-42.While ,

Arg-52 shields the chromophore, acting as the gate and provides electrostatic complementarity.

## Photocycle of PYP[10 to14]

pG (trans-) 446-- o.21ms-->pR--1.23ms--->pB(cis-)355---405ms--->pG(trans-)446. Where the numbers indicate _-max of absorption, of ground state 'pG' and intermediates 'pR' and'pB'along with time of transition in milliseconds(ms).

During the photocycle on absorption of light, the ground state pG undergoes trans- to cis-isomerisation of ionised p-hydroxy cinnmoyl ester chromophore by flipping of thioester linkage with protein to form pre-**pR** state and then Red shifted pR state.Entire molecule undergoes conformational changes and the chromophore gets protonated to form blue shifted pB state.Conformational changes in pB state are little in the crystalline state. But in solution there is as if a protein quake and pB state exists as a family of multiple conformers that exchange on ms time scale in solution. Stuctural changes, lag behind the.conformational changes, as revealed by 'Nile Red' a polarity sensitive flourescent probe that binds pB but not pG state of PYP [Hedrickson *et al*.; **2001**]. The biological signalling state of photoreceptor 'pB' is likely to bind a partner in yet unknown sensory path. During the reconversion of pB to pG state, by retroisomerisation and protonation of chromophore,Glu-46 acts as a buffer for a complicated network of ionisation groups, controlling the rate of back reaction. 'Glu-46 –Gln' mutant, has 700 times faster rate of return to pG state. While 'Met-100-Ala' mutant, has life time of minutes, for the pB state.

## Applications

1) PYP photocycle holds promise for its applications in optical data storage and computing. 2) PYP is a model laboratory for detailed study of biological light detection and the relation of structural change to protein function.

## CONCLUSION

Natural photoreceptors constitute a novel and unique field of natural product chemistry involving biological light energy and signal transduction. It requires a new perspective and interdisciplinary approach for its study. It has facinating applications in development of biosensors, optical computers, photoactive bioconjugates and so on. There is a lot of scope for research in this field.

## ABBREVIATIONS

bR  =  Bacteriorhodopsin

bOP  =  Bacterioopsin

Rh  =  Rhodopsin

PYP  =  Photoactive yellow protein

hR  =  Halorhodopsin

sR  =  Sensory rhodopsin

## ACKNOWLEDGEMENTS

The author is extremely thankful to Dr. A.K. Singh of I.I.T. Mumbai, India, for his review article on Bacteriorhodopsin. I am indebted to Mrs. Amita Gaokar and Rahul Palkar for assistance in the preparation of manuscripts.

## REFERENCES

[1]    Nelson, D. and Michael, M., *Lehninger Principles of Biochemistry 3rd. Ed.*, Macmillan Worth, **2000**, 694-696 and 713.

[2]    Hall, D.O. and Rao, K.K., *Photosynthesis 5th Ed.,* Cambridge, University Press, **1994**, 44-46 and 145-146

[3]    (a) Bhoo, S.H. *et al.*, Nature, **2001**, *414*, 776-779. (b) Toshinorf, K. *ibid* **2001**, *414*, 656-659

[4]    Grahm Solomans, T.W. *Organic Chemistry*, 3rd Ed. Jhon Wiley and sons, **1983**, 437-443.

[5]    Singh, A.K., *Proc. Nat. Acad. Sci. India,* **2000**, Sec. A, Part-II, 70, 107-128 and references therein.

[6]    Khorana, H.G., *J. Biol. Chem.*, **1988**, *263*,7439.

[7]    Luecke, H. *et al.*, *Science,* **1999**, *286*, 255-264

[8]    Nakanishi, K., *et al., J. Am. Chem. Soc.* **a) 1980**, *102*, 7945and 7949, b) ibid, *105*, 5162, c) Asato, *et al.*, ibid **1983**, *112*, 7398.

[9]    Birge, R.R., *Annu. Rev. Phy. Chem.,* **1990**, *41*, 383.

[10]    Genick, *et al., Science,* **1997**, *275*, 1471-1475 and *Nature,* **1998**, *392*, 206.

[11]    Borgstahl, G.E.O. *et al.*, *Biochemistry,* **1995**, *34*, 6278-6287

[12]    Schilichting, and Berendezen, *Structure,* **1997**, *5*, 735-739.

[13]    Craven, C.J. *et al.*, *Biochemistry,* **2000**, *39*, 14392-14399 and references therein.

[14]    Hoff, W.D. *et al.*, *Bichemistry,* **1999**, *38*, 1009-1017 .

Atta-ur-Rahman/Choudhary/Khan (Eds.) *Frontiers in Natural Product Chemistry, Vol. 1*     73

# Molecular Cloning of Cellulase Genes from *Trichoderma harzianum*

Sibtain Ahmed[1], Nighat Aslam[1], Farooq Latif[2], M.I. Rajoka[2] and Amer Jamil[1],*

[1]*Molecular Biochemistry Lab., Dept. of Chemistry, University of Agriculture, Faisalabad, Pakistan,* [2]*National Institute of Genetic Engineering and Biotechnology, Faisalabad, Pakistan*

**Abstract**: Cellulases are attractive source for utilization of the agro-industrial waste materials. Exoglucanase (EC; 3.2.1.91), Endoglucanase (EC. 3.2.1.4) and β-glucosidase (EC. 3.2.1.21) were isolated from *Trichoderma harzianum* (E-58 strain). The fungus was grown on Vogel's medium with different carbon sources. Maximal production of the enzymes was achieved at 28 $^0$C, pH 5.5 under continuous shaking at 120 rpm for 5 days. Glucose repressed the synthesis of the enzymes whereas carboxymethylcellulose (CMC) produced the enzymes in substantial amounts. Maximum activity of cellulases (exoglucanase, endoglucanase and β-glucosidase) were found to be 2.764, 14.4 and 0.629IU mL$^{-1}$, respectively. Corresponding genes for cellulases were isolated with the help of RT-PCR. RNA was isolated from mycelia of *T. harzianum* grown on CMC and xylan. First strand of cDNA was synthesized using oligo dT (18) primer and subjected to PCR with specific primers. The amplified products were purified through agarose gel electrophoresis and ligated into SmaI site of pUC18. The plasmids containing *exg, egl* and *bgl* genes were transformed into *E. coli* for further characterization.

## INTRODUCTION

Despite the fact that the world community is no longer pre-occupied with fossil fuel shortage, there is still a considerable research and development directed towards understanding and commercializing enzymatic hydrolysis of cellulose [1]. Cellulose is the most abundant organic polymer in this planet and is an important renewable energy source along with sugars and starches [2]. Energy production from cellulosic raw material involves its hydrolysis into glucose. Highly ordered cellulose substrates are converted into soluble sugars only when exoglucanase, endoglucanase and β-glucosidase are present in solution simultaneously in right proportion. A number of fungal species are known for the production of cellulases such as *Aspergillus niger*, *Sporotrichum spp*, *Chaetomium thermophile*, *Trichoderma* species etc [3]. Gene cloning is recently being employed for studying the structure and function of a number of enzymes and proteins and their over expression. This strategy has been found very efficient as compared to other traditional methods. Present study was designed to layout strategy for enhanced production of cellulases. In this paper we have reported the isolation and cloning of cellulase genes *(exg ,egl* and *bgl)* from *T.harzianum* (E-58 strain).

## MATERIALS AND METHODS

### Growth Conditions and Enzyme Assay

*Trichoderma harzianum* (E58) was grown at 28°C with shaking at 120 rpm in Vogel's medium (0.5% *Trisodium citrate*, 0.5% $KH_2PO_4$.0.2% $NH_4NO_3$, 0.4% $(NH_4)_2SO_4$, 0.02%

*Corresponding author: amerjamil@yahoo.com

$MgSO_4$, 0.1% peptone, 0.2% yeast extract pH 5.50), containing 1% glucose or carboxymethylcellulose or xylan as a carbon source [4]. Enzymes assays for *exg*, *egl* and *bgl* were performed as described by Shamala and Sreekantiah [5].

### RT-PCR (Reverse Transcription Polymerase Chain Reaction)

Total RNA was isolated by Hot Phenol method [6]. First strand synthesis of cDNA was made with the help of cDNA synthesis kit form MBI Fermentas, Lithuania. The RT reaction was amplified by PCR using following primers.

*exg* (1) 5$^/$ATGTATCGGCGGAATTGGCCGTC 3$^/$ (2)5$^/$ CAGGCACTGAGAGTA 3$^/$

*egl* (1)5 $^/$ATGGCGCCCTCAGTTACACTG 3$^/$ (2)5$^/$ AAGGCATTGCGAGTA 3$^/$

*bgl* (1)5$^/$ ATGTTGCCCAAGGAGTTTCAG 3$^/$ (2) 5$^/$CGCCGCCGCAATCAGCTCGTC 3$^/$

PCR was done with following conditions. 10x buffer (MBI fermentas), 200 μM dNTPs each, 1U Taq polymerase were added to DNA template, 500 nM each primer and various concentrations of $MgCl_2$ (1.0–9.0 mM) were used. Thermocycler (Perkinelemer) conditions were set as: Melting 95°C for 90 sec; Annealing 50°C for 60 sec; Extension 72°C for 60 sec. PCR products were separated by electrophoresis on agarose gel and visualized by ethidium bromide staining.

### Ligation of the Genes into Plasmid

The RT-PCR amplified cellulase genes (*exg, egl , bgl*) were ligated into the pUC18 plasmid digested at *SmaI*. Insert vector ratio of 3:1 was used for ligation. The reaction was incubated in DNA ligase buffer (MBI Fermentas) for 24 hours at 18°C.

### Transformation into *E. coli*

The ligated vector was transformed into *E. coli* (10b) competent cell by Heat shock method [7] and plated on agar-ampicillin plates.

### RESULTS AND DISCUSSION

#### Growth of *T. harzianum*

Spores of *T. harzianum* were maintained on agar slants containing 0.2% CMC or 0.2% xylan. *T. harzianum* was grown in Vogel's medium for 5 days at 28°C at 120 rpm [8]. The pH of the medium was adjusted to 5.5 to obtain maximal production of cellulases from *T. harzianum*. After getting growth, the medium was filtered, residue containing growth was stored for the isolation of RNA and from the filtrate *exg*, *egl* and *bgl* assays were performed.

Present results (Table **1**) suggest that when glucose was used as a carbon source, the production of cellulases from *T. harzianum* was inhibited. Maximum activity of *exg* was achieved when 1% carboxymethylcellulose was used as a carbon source whereas *egl* and *bgl* were produced maximally with 1% xylan as a carbon source. Similarly it was found earlier that most cellulase-induced cellulases were repressed by glucose [9].

#### Gene Amplification by RT-PCR

Reverse transcription was performed on RNA isolated from *T. harzianum*. First strand cDNA synthesis was done by using oligo $(dT)_{18}$ primer from MBI Fermentas. It was directly

**Table 1.    Cellulase Activities Produced from *T. harzianum.***

|  | ENZYME ACTIVITY(1U mL$^{-1}$) | | |
|---|---|---|---|
| Substrate | Exoglucanase | Endoglucanase | β-Glucosidase |
| 1% glucose | 0.293 | 9.04 | 0.0635 |
| 1% CMC | 2.764 | 11.2 | 0.1209 |
| 1% xylan | 1.056 | 14.4 | 0.629 |

applied to PCR for amplification in which sequence specific primers for cellulase genes were used. Significant amplification was achieved from the cDNA. The corresponding bands were excised form gel and purified for ligation into pUC18. Techniques used in the present study are performed earlier [10,11]. Similarly earlier pUC18 vector was used for cloning of β-glucosidase gene [12].

## Ligation and Transformation

The amplified cellulase genes (*exg, egl* and *bgl*) were ligated into pUC18 plasmid with the help of DNA ligase. The ligated products were transformed into *E. coli* (10 b) competent cells. Earlier cellulase genes have been cloned into *E.coli* to get the better production of large quantities of pure cellulases [13].

Cellulase genes (*exg ,egl* and *bgl*) from *T.harzianum* were therefore, successfully amplified with the help of RT-PCR, cloned into pUC18 and transformed into *E. coli*.

## ACKNOWLEDGEMENTS

The authors gratefully acknowledge grants from Pakistan Science Foundation and Higher Education Commission, Government of Pakistan.

## REFERENCES

[1]     Walker, L.P. and Wilson, D.B. *Bioresource Technology*, **1991**, *36*, 3-14.
[2]     Goyal, A., Ghosh , B. and Eveleigh, O. *Bioresource Technology*, **1991**, *36*, 37-50.
[3]     Szodark, J. *Acta Biotechnol.*,**1988**, *816*, 509-515.
[4]     Ahmed, S., Qurrat-ul-Ain, Aslam, N., Naeem, S., Rahman S., and Jamil, A. *Pakistan Journal of Biological Sciences,* **2003***, 6*, 1912-1916.
[5]     Shamala, T. R., and.Seerekanth, K.R. *Enzyme. Microbiol. Technol.*, **1985**, *8*, 178-182.
[6]     Dudler, R., and Hertig, C. *Journal of Biological Chemistry*, **1992**, Vol-*267*, pp. 5882-5888.
[7]     Ausubel, F.M.; Brent, R.; Kingstone, R.E.; Moore, D.D.;. Seidman, J.A. Smith and Struhl, K. Current protocols in molecular Biology. Wiley and Sons, New York, **1988**.
[8]     Ikram-ul-Haq, Khurshid, Ali, S., Ashraf, H., Qadeer, M.A., and Rajoka, M.I. *World Journal of Microbiology and Biotechnology*, **2000**, *17*, 35-37.
[9]     Ximenes, E.A.; Felix, C.R. and Ulhoa, J. *Current Microbiology*, **1996**, *32*,199-123.
[10]    Bashir, A.,. Ashraf, S. R, Rajoka, M. I., Malik K. A. and Batt, C. A. *Proc. Int. Symp* Biotechnology for Energy Dec. 16-21, Faisalabad, **1989**.
[11]    Rajoka, M. I.; Bashir, S. R. A.; Hussain, M. T.; Ghauri, M. T.; Parvez S. and Malik, K. A. *Folia. Microbiol.*, **1998**, *43*, 129-135.
[12]    Winters, A.; Galiagher, J.; Barron, N.; Rollan, A.; and Mcltate, A. P. *Biotechnology Letters*, **1996**, *18*, 1387-1390.
[13]    Benguin, P.; Gilkes, N, R.; Kilburn, D .G.; Miller, R.C. Jr.; O'Neill, G. P. and Warren, R. A. J. U. *CRC Crit. Rev. Biotechnol*, **1987**, *6*, 129-162

Atta-ur-Rahman/Choudhary/Khan (Eds.) *Frontiers in Natural Product Chemistry, Vol. 1*      77

# Binding of Betamethasone, Prednisolone and Theophylline to Bovine Serum Albumin: Plausible Explanations for Mode of Binding and Drug-drug Interactions

Nurun N. Rahman[1,*], S. Huda[1], Khondaker M. Rahman[1] and Mohammad H. Rahman[2]

*[1]Department of Pharmaceutical Chemistry, Faculty of Pharmacy, University of Dhaka, Dhaka-1000, Bangladesh, [2]Department of Pharmaceutics and Pharmaceutical Technology, Faculty of Pharmacy, University of Dhaka, Dhaka-1000, Bangladesh*

**Abstract:** The binding of betamethasone sodium phosphate and prednisolone, two steroidal antiinflammatory drugs and theophylline sodium glycinate, a bronchodilator, to bovine serum albumin (BSA), has been studied by equilibrium dialysis (ED) method at different temperature and pH values for characterizing the binding of these drugs to BSA. Binding was exothermic, entropically driven and spontaneous, as indicated by the thermodynamic analysis. The major part of the binding energy at site II results from electrostatic and hydrophobic interactions. The free fraction of either betamethasone or prednisolone in the presence of theophylline sodium glycinate and vice versa was monitored in the presence and absence of site specific probes. The free fraction of betamethasone sodium phosphate by theophylline sodium glycinate and vice versa was increased during concurrent administration causing reduced binding of these drugs to BSA. This increment of free fraction was more prominent in the presence of site I specific probe, which suggested that in the absence of site I specific probe, betamethasone after being displaced by theophylline from its high affinity site rebound to its low affinity site. Similar type of result was observed in case of prednisolone-theophylline interaction.

## INTRODUCTION

Serum albumin, the most abundant protein in blood, plays a very important role in the binding phenomenon and serves as a depot protein and transport protein for numerous endogenous and exogenous compounds [1]. Displacement of drug is defined as reduction in the extent of binding of a drug to protein caused by competition of another drug, the displacer. This type of interaction may occur when two drugs, capable of binding to proteins, are administered concurrently. Competitive displacement is more significant, when two drugs are capable of binding to the same sites on the protein. From different investigations, it has been suggested that human serum albumin (HSA) has limited number of binding sites [2-4]. Since number of protein binding sites are limited, competition will exist between two drugs and the drug with higher affinity will displace the other causing increased free drug concentration leading to higher toxicity [5].

---

*Corresponding author: Tel: 9661900-59/4842; Fax: 880-2-8615583; E-mail: duregstr@bangla.net

The ability of one drug to inhibit the binding of another is a function of their relative concentrations, binding affinities and specificity of binding [6]. Since only a small fraction of the drug would ordinarily be available in the free form, the displacement of even a small percentage of the amount that is bound to proteins could produce considerable increase in activity. Thus when studying the drug-drug interactions, more specifically the drug-displacement, the possibility of the occurrence of site-to-site displacement should also be considered, as there will be a difference between the free concentrations of a displaced drug with or without site-to-site displacement. The purpose of our work is to see the mechanism of binding of these drugs to BSA and to observe the effect of the free concentration of either betamethasone or prednisolone by theophylline and vice versa when used concurrently.

## MATERIALS AND METHODS

Betamethasone sodium phosphate and prednisolone were kindly supplied by Organon(Bangladesh) Ltd. Theophylline sodium glycinate and ranitidine hydrochloride were obtained from Jayson Pharmaceuticals Ltd., Dhaka and Drug International Ltd., Dhaka respectively. Dialysis membrane was purchased from Medicell International Ltd., 239 Liverpool Road, London and BSA was purchased from the Sigma Chemical Co Ltd.

### Estimation of Thermodynamic Parameters

Thermodynamic parameters of betamethasone sodium phosphate and theophylline sodium glycinate were calculated by the method of Pedersen [7] using the Van't Hoff plots at three specified temperatures $10^0$, $25^0$ and $40^0$C. From the temperature dependence of association constants it is possible to calculate the values for thermodynamic parameters involved in the binding process.

### Drug-Drug Displacement Study

Displacement of either betamethasone or prednisolone by theophylline and vice versa in absence and in presence of site specific probe when bound to BSA at $25^0$C and pH 7.4 was carried out by equilibrium dialysis method [8].

### Effect of Theophylline on Betamethasone Binding to BSA and Vice Versa in the Absence and Presence of Ranitidine, a Site-I specific Probe

Five ml of previously prepared $2 \times 10^{-2}$ M betamethasone solution was added to the five out of six test tubes. Thus the final ratio between the protein and betamethasone was 1:1 ($2 \times 10^{-5}$ M: $2 \times 10^{-5}$ M) in each of the five test tubes. The sixth test tube containing only BSA solution was marked as "blank". Theophylline solution was added with increasing concentrations into four out of the five test tubes containing 1:1 mixture of the protein and betamethasone. The final ratios between theophylline and protein were 1:1, 3:1, 5:1 and 7:1. Theophylline was not added into the fifth test tube containing the protein and betamethasone mixture (1:1).

Five ml of previously prepared $2 \times 10^{-5}$ M BSA solution was taken in each of the five test tubes. Twenty microliter of $1 \times 10^{-2}$ M ranitidine solution was added in each test tube, so that the final ratio between protein and ranitidine was 1:1 ($2 \times 10^{-5}$ M: $4 \times 10^{-5}$ M) in each of the five test tubes. Thus site I of BSA was sufficiently blocked by ranitidine. Then 10 microliter of $1 \times 10^{-2}$ M betamethasone solution was added to the five test tubes. Thus the final ratio among protein, ranitidine and betamethasone was 1:2:1 ($2 \times 10^{-5}$ M: $4 \times 10^{-5}$ M: $2 \times 10^{-5}$ M) in each test tube. Theophylline solution was then added with increasing concentrations into four out of the five test tubes containing 1:2:1 mixture of the protein, ranitidine and betamethasone. The final ratios between theophylline and the protein were 1:1, 3:1, 5:1, and 7:1. Theophylline was not added in the fifth test tube. After proper mixing and shaking in a metabolic shaker at $25^0$C(room temperature) and 20 rpm, the free concentrations of betamethasone were measured by a UV spectrophotometer (SP8-400 UV/VIS spectrophotometer, Pye Unicum, England) at a wavelength of 328nm [9].

Similarly, effects of betamethasone on theophylline binding to BSA in the absence and presence of ranitidine were observed. The free concentrations of theophylline were measured by a UV spectrophotometer at a wavelength of 274 nm [10].

Effects of theophylline on prednisolone binding to BSA and vice versa in the presence and absence of ranitidine, a site I specific probe were observed. The experiment was carried out in the same way as described previously. The free concentrations of prednisolone were measured by a UV spectrophotometer at a wavelength of 243 nm [10].

## RESULTS AND DISCUSSION

The pharmacokinetic properties of exogenous as well as endogenous compounds can be influenced by binding to serum albumin in a reversible manner. In order to evaluate possible interaction between drugs, it is self-evidently essential to be able to know the binding proteins and the identity of the binding sites of the drugs on the protein molecule [11]. Betamethasone, prednisolone and theophylline bind to BSA with a high value of association constant to site II and with a low value of association constant to site I.

### Estimation of Binding Parameters

The binding parameters of betamethasone, prednisolone and theophylline bound to BSA at $25^0$C & pH 7.4 were calculated using Scatchard plots (Figures 1-3).

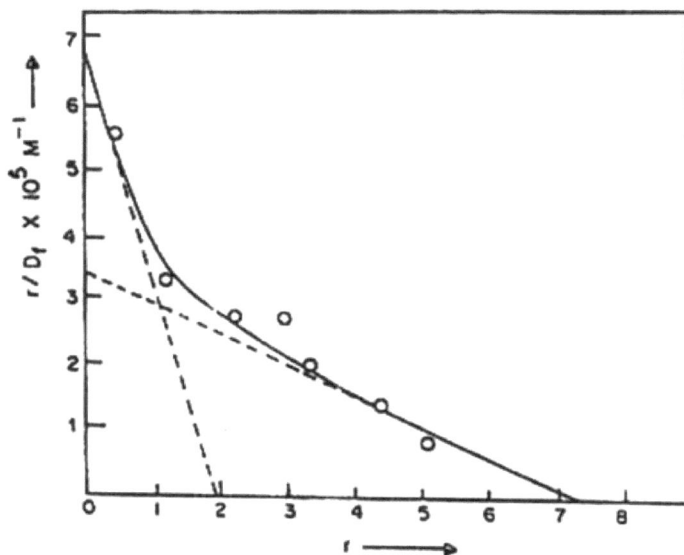

**Fig (1).** Scatchard plot of Betamethasone sodium phosphate bound to BSA at pH 7.4 and $25^0$C Following concentrations were used:

[BSA], $2\times10^{-5}$ M; [betamethasone sodium phosphate], $1\times10^{-5}$M - $23\times10^{-5}$M.

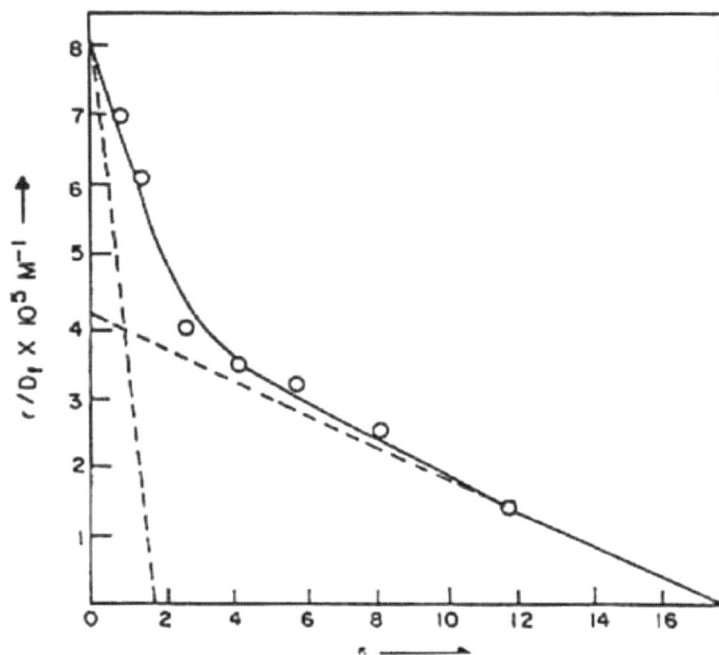

**Fig (2).** Scatchard plot of Prednisolone bound to BSA at pH 7.4 and $25^0$C. Following concentrations were used:

[BSA], $2\times10^{-5}$ M; [prednisolone], $2\times10^{-5}$M - $40\times10^{-5}$M.

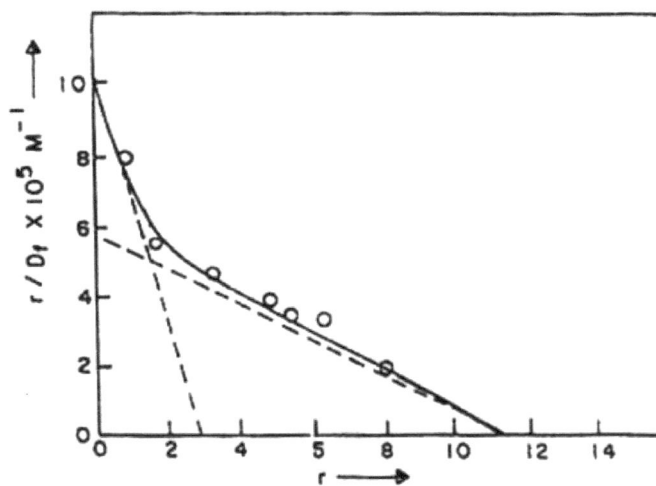

**Fig (3).** Scatchard plot of Theophylline sodium glycinate bound to BSA at pH 7.4 and $25^0$C

Following concentrations were used:

[BSA], $2\times10$-5M; [theophylline sodium glycinate], $2\times10^{-5}$ - $24 \times 10^{-5}$M.

Values are given in Table **1**.

Table. 1.   Binding Parameters of Sodium Phosphate, Prednisolone and Theophylline Sodium Glycinate Bound to BSA at pH and 25°C.

| Drugs | Association Constants | | Number of binding sites | |
|---|---|---|---|---|
| | $K_1$ (high affinity) x $10^5 M^{-1}$ | $K_2$ (low affinity) x $10^4 M^{-1}$ | $n_1$ high affinity | $n_2$ low affinity |
| Betamethasone sodium phosphate | 3.84 ±0.04 | 4.70 ± 0.05 | 1.9 ± 0.03 | 7.2 ± 0.9 |
| Prednisolone | 5.10 ± 0.07 | 2.3 ± 0.03 | 1.6 ±0.04 | 17.6 ± 3 |
| Theophylline | 3.5 ± 0.05 | 5.08 ± 0.04 | 2.8 ± 0.05 | 11.4 ± 2 |

## Binding Mode

The binding mode of betamethasone sodium phosphate and prednisolone and theophylline sodium glycinate was evaluated with respect to thermodynamic data. There are essentially four types of non-covalent interaction that can play a role in ligand binding to proteins. These are hydrogen bonds, Van Der Waals forces, hydrophobic forces and electrostatic interactions [12, 13]. The binding of betamethasone sodium phosphate and theophylline sodium glycinate with a high association constant made it seem worthwhile to investigate the entropy, enthalpy and free energy change at this site. The thermodynamic parameters as shown in Table 2 indicate that for high affinity binding of both betamethasone sodium phosphate and theophylline sodium glycinate $\Delta H$ is negative and $\Delta S$ is positive. The binding is, thereby always spontaneous as evidenced by the negative sign of the $\Delta G$ values for both drugs.

Table 2.   Theophylline Sodium Glycinate BSA Interactions at pH 7.4 and 25°C.

| Drug | $\Delta G$, cal/mole | $\Delta H$, cal/mole | $\Delta S$, cal/mole/°K |
|---|---|---|---|
| Betamethasone | (-) 7923.17+8.90 | (-) 1.34+0.40 | (+) 26.58+0.032 |
| Theophylline | (-) 8169.99+10.70 | (±) 1.42+0.15 | (±) 27.41+0.037 |

Each value represents the average value ± S.D (n=3).

It is known that for typical hydrophobic interactions, both $\Delta H$ and $\Delta S$ are positive, while negative enthalpy and entropy changes arise for Vander Waals forces and hydrogen bonding formation in low dielectric media [14]. Negative enthalpy might however play a role in electrostatic interactions, but for actual and true electrostatic interactions, $\Delta H$ is expected to be very small or almost zero [15].

Therefore, the high affinity of betamethasone sodium phosphate and theophylline sodium glycinate to BSA might involve electrostatic interactions as evidenced by very low value of $\Delta H$ (Table 2). Furthermore, it is found that $\Delta S$ is positive for binding of both betamethasone sodium phosphate and theophylline sodium to BSA and that the major contribution to $\Delta G$ arises from $\Delta S$ term rather then from $\Delta H$. Consequently, for both cases, the binding process is neurotically driven. However, the overall thermodynamic parameters for the binding of these two drugs cannot be explained on the basis of single intermolecular interaction model.

Positive value of $\Delta H$ indicates that the reaction is endothermic whereas negative value of $\Delta H$ indicates that the reaction is exothermic. In this study we find negative value of $\Delta H$, indicating that the reactions may be exothermic in both cases. The possibility of unfolding of the protein molecule during the binding process due to high positive $\Delta S$ value can be rejected because this unfolding of proteins requires bending or breaking of several bonds resulting in an endothermic reaction [16]. But reasons already exist in favor of exothermic reaction.

It is more likely that electrostatic interaction and hydrophobic interaction play a significant role in the high affinity binding of betamethasone sodium phosphate and theophylline sodium glycinate to BSA. However, Van Der Waals forces and hydrogen bonding are also expected in the binding of these two drugs of BSA due to negative value of enthalpy changes. All these indicate that the BSA binding site for betamethasone sodium phosphate and theophylline sodium glycinate probably consists of a hydrophobic patch on BSA.

In case of prednisolone we could not measure the thermodynamic data as there the van't Hoff plot was not linear.

**Drug-Drug Interaction**

Figure **4** shows the changes in free concentration of betamethasone bound to BSA in the presence of theophylline at pH 4.4 and $25^{0}$C. As evident in Fig. **1**, the free fraction of betamethasone bound to BSA was increased from 17.5% to 40% by theophylline in the absence of ranitidine, a site I specific probe. When site I of BSA was blocked by sufficient amount of ranitidine, theophylline increased the free fraction of betamethasone from 25% to 54%. This suggested that betamethasone was displaced to a greater extent by theophylline in the presence of ranitidine.

Similarly, Fig. **5** shows the changes in free concentration of theophylline bound to BSA by the addition of betamethasone in the absence and presence of ranitidine. In the absence of ranitidine, the free fraction of theophylline was increased by betamethasone from 12.5% to 54% while in presence of ranitidine, betamethasone in the same concentration range increased the free fraction of theophylline from 23.5% to 92.5%.

Similar type of change in the free fraction of prednisolone in the presence of theophylline and vice versa was obtained in the presence and absence of site specific probe as shown in Figures **6** & **7**.

Figure **6** shows the changes in free concentration of theophylline sodium glycinate bound to BSA in the presence of prednisolone at pH 7.4 and $25^{0}$C. As evident in Fig. **1**, the free fraction of theophylline sodium glycinate bound to BSA was increased from 13% to 52% by prednisolone in the absence of ranitidine, a site I specific probe, whereas, in the presence of site I specific probe, ranitidine, prednisolone increased the free fraction of theophylline sodium glycinate from 25% to 82%. This suggested that theophylline sodium glycinate was displaced to a greater extent by prednisolone in the presence of ranitidine.

Similarly, Fig. **7** shows the changes in free concentration of prednisolone bound to BSA by the addition of theophylline sodium glycinate in the absence and presence of ranitidine. In the absence of ranitidine, the free fraction of prednisolone was increased by theophylline sodium glycinate from 8% to 63% while in presence of ranitidine, theophylline sodium glycinate in the same concentration range increased the free fraction of prednisolone from 23% to 83%.

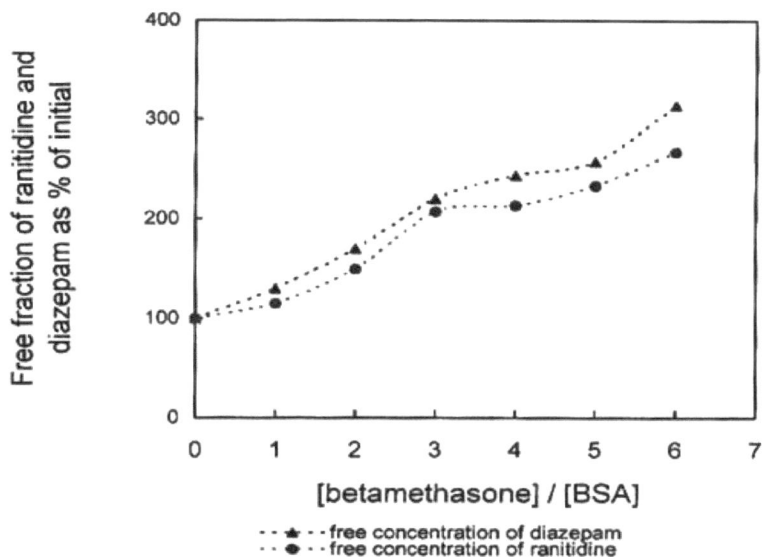

Fig (4). Free fraction (as % of initial) of ranitidine (●) or diazepam (▲) upon the addition of betamethasone sodium phosphate at $25^0$C and pH 7.4.

Concentrations used:

[BSA] = [ranitidine]= $2 \times 10^{-5}$ M;        [BSA] = [diazepam]= $2 \times 10^{-5}$ M

For both curves, [Betamethasone sodium phosphate] = 0-12 $\times$ 10 $^{-5}$ M.

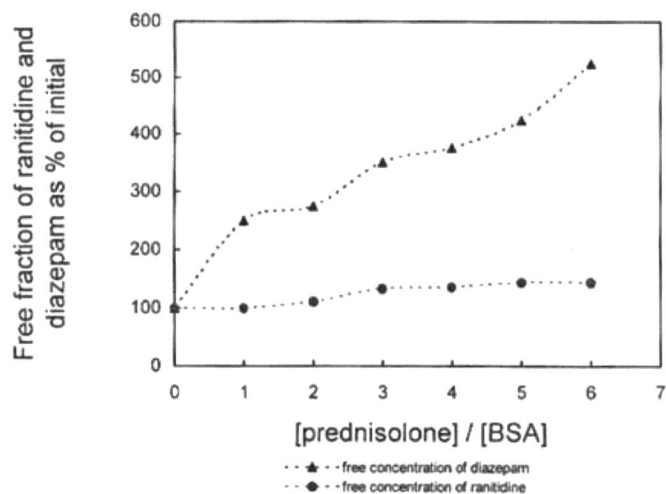

Fig. (5). Free fraction (as % of initial) of ranitidine (●) or diazepam (▲) upon the addition of prednisolone at $25^0$C and pH 7.4.

Concentrations used:

[BSA] = [ranitidine]= $2 \times 10^{-5}$ M; [BSA] = [diazepam]= $2 \times 10^{-5}$ M   For both curves, [prednisolone] = 0-12 $\times$ 10 $^{-5}$ M.

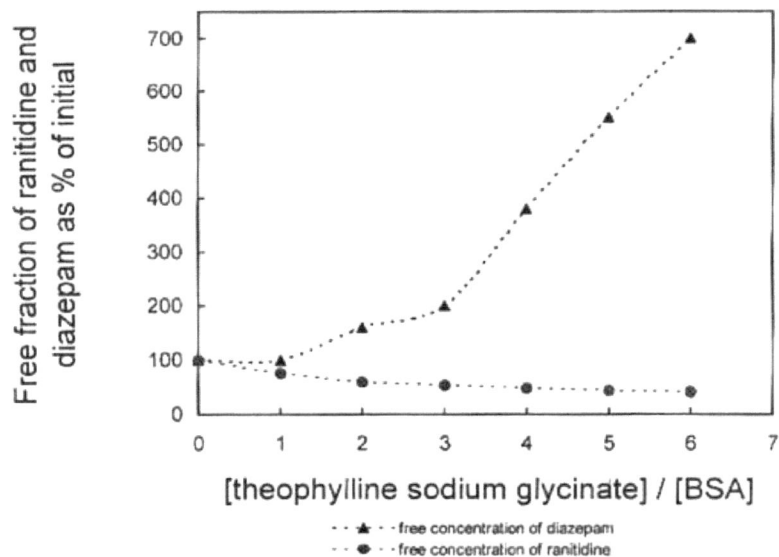

**Fig. (6).** Free fraction (as % of initial) of ranitidine (●) or diazepam (▲) upon the addition of theophylline sodium glycinate at $25^0$C and pH 7.4.

Concentrations used:

[BSA] = [ranitidine]= $2 \times 10^{-5}$ M,; [BSA] = [diazepam]= $2 \times 10^{-5}$ M

For both curves, [theophylline sodium glycinate] = $0-12 \times 10^{-5}$ M.

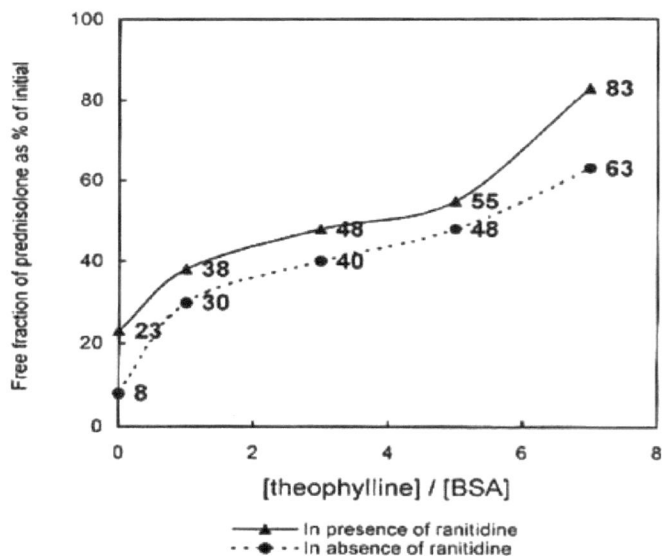

**Fig. (7).** Free fraction of prednisolone as % of initial bound to BSA (1:1) upon the addition of theophylline sodium glycinate in the presence and in the absence of ranitidine.

Concentrations used:

[BSA]=[prednisolone]=$2 \times 10^{-5}$ M; [ranitidine]=$4 \times 10^{-5}$ M; [theophylline]=$0 -14 \times 10^{-5}$ M.

On the basis of above results obtained during concurrent administration of either betamethasone sodium phosphate or prednisolone and theophylline sodium glycinate in the presence and absence of ranitidine different models of interaction have been proposed in Figures **8, 9, 10 & 11**.

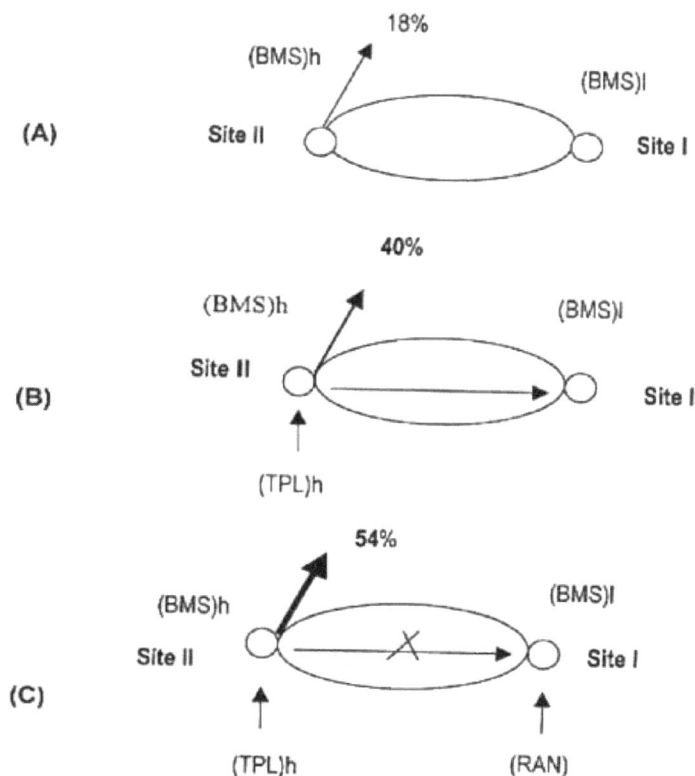

**Fig. (8).** Proposed models of the betamethasone-BSA-theophylline interactions in the presence and absence of site-I specific probe

BMS, betamethasone; TPL, theophylline; RAN, ranitidine, site I specific probe; h, high affinity; l, low affinity;

(A) = normal binding of betamethasone to BSA.

(B) = effect of theophylline on BMS bound to BSA in absence of RAN.

(C) = effect of theophylline on BMS bound to BSA in presence of RAN.

As observed from the models, during concurrent administration, theophylline displaced betamethasone & prednisolone, which then rebound to their low affinity sites due to transfer of the drugs from site II to site I. When site I was blocked by sufficient amount of ranitidine (site I probe), this transfer of drugs from site II to site I was not possible. For this reason, the free fraction of betamethasone or prednisolone by theophylline was higher in presence of site I specific probe than in the absence of this probe. This modified form of displacement pattern is tentatively referred to as site-to-site displacement. The reverse experiment i.e. effect of betamethasone or prednisolone on theophylline in presence and absence of site I specific probe showed the similar result.

RAHMAN *et al.*

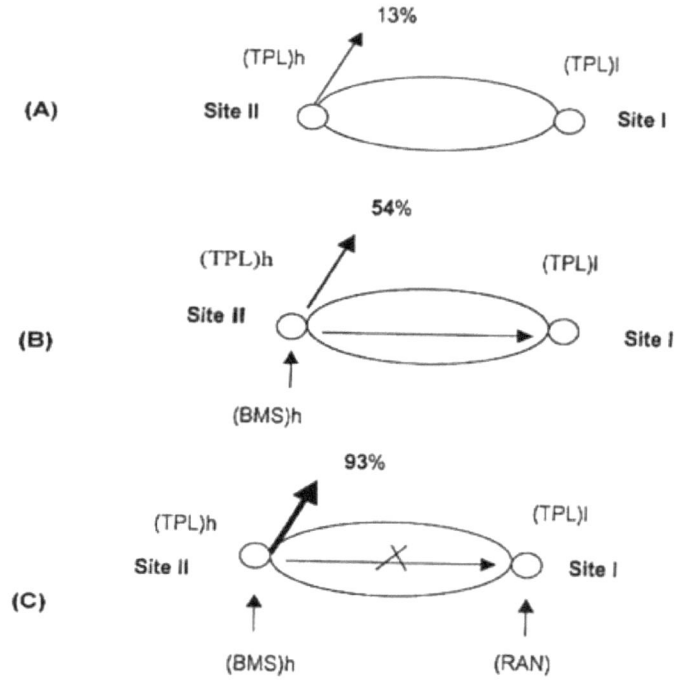

**Fig. (9).** Proposed models of the theophylline-BSA-betamethasone interactions in the presence and absence of site-I specific probe

BMS, betamethasone; TPL, theophylline; RAN, ranitidine, site I specific probe; h, high affinity; l, low affinity;

(A) = normal binding of betamethasone to BSA.

(B) = effect of theophylline on BMS bound to BSA in absence of RAN.

(C) = effect of theophylline on BMS bound to BSA in presence of RAN.

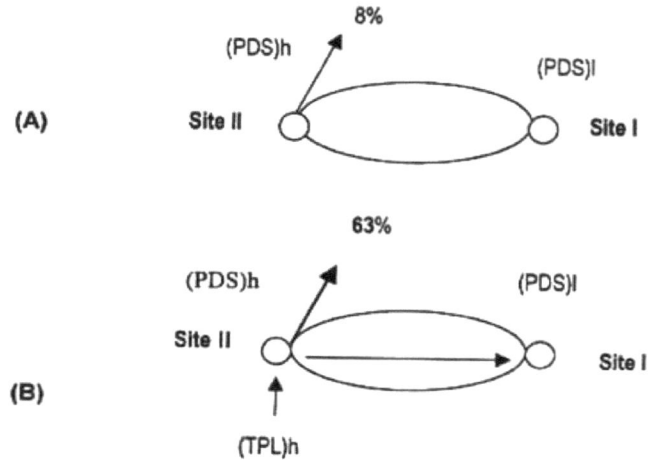

(Fig. 10. Contd....)

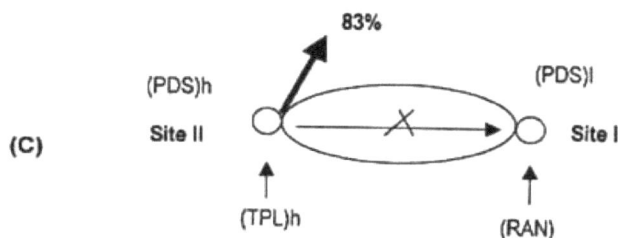

**Fig. (10).** Proposed models of the prednisolone-BSA-theophylline interactions in the presence and absence of site-I specific probe

PDS, prednisolone; TPL, theophylline; RAN, ranitidine, site I specific probe; h, high affinity; l, low affinity;

(A) = normal binding of prednisolone to BSA.

(B) = effect of theophylline on PDS bound to BSA in absence of RAN.

(C) = effect of theophylline on PDS bound to BSA in presence of RAN.

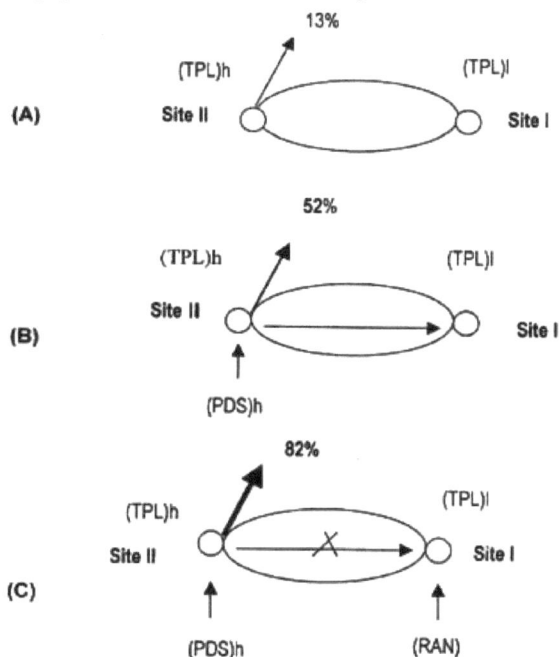

**Fig. (11).** : Proposed models of the theophylline-BSA-prednisolone interactions in the presence and absence of site-I specific probe

TPL, theophylline; PDS, prednisolone; RAN, ranitidine, site I specific probe; h, high affinity; l, low affinity;

(A)= normal binding of theophylline to BSA.

(B) = effect of prednisolone on PDS bound to BSA in absence of RAN.

(C) = effect of prednisolone on PDS bound to BSA in presence of RAN.

## Pharmacokinetic Implications

Free drug concentration is the primary determinant of pharmacokinetic/ pharmacodynamic properties of drug. The extent to which a drug binds to serum albumin is an important pharmacological variable, depending on the free drug concentration form 0 to 100% [17].

The concurrent administration of betamethasone sodium phosphate and theophylline sodium glycinate is a good idea. They can give synergistic activity due to the elevated level of these drugs during concurrent administration. They compete for a common binding site on the albumin molecule. Therefore, the free concentration of both drugs is increased to a significant level compared to the level obtained when the drugs are given individually.

The quantitative change of even few percentage in binding might exert a profound effect on the disposition of drugs. So care must be exercised in calculating the free concentration of these drugs, which show site-to-site displacement in the presence of another drug.

## REFERENCES

[1]     Kragh-Hansen, U. *Pharm. Rev.,* **1981,** *33,* 17-53.
[2]     Fehske, K.J.; Muller, W.E. And Wollert, U. *Biochem. Biophys. Acta.,* **1979,** *577,* 346-359.
[3]     Hansen, K.U. *J. Biochem.,* **1981,** *195,* 603-613.
[4]     Nahar, Z.; Rahman, M. H. And Hasnat, A. *Bangladesh J. Physiol. Pharmaco.,* **1977,** *13(1),* 18-20.
[5]     Rahman, M.H. *Characterization of binding of non-steroidal anti-inflammatory drugs on human serum albumin: Site-to-site displacement with respect to high affinity binding site.* Ph.D Thesis. Kumamoto University, Japan, **1994,** pp. 2-8.
[6]     Koch-Weser, J. And Sellers, E.M. *New Engl. J. Med.,* **1976,** *294,* 526-531.
[7]     Pedersen, A. O.; Honore, B. And Brodersen, R. *Eur. J. Biochem.,* **1990,** *190,* 497-502.
[8]     Singlas, E. *Protein binding of drugs: Definition, modalities, effects, changes,* 2$^{nd}$ ed. F. Hoffmann-La Roche & Co. Limited Company, Basle, Switzerland. **1987,** pp: 25-33.
[9]     The Merck Index. Eleventh Edition. Merck & Co. Inc. Rahway. N.J.U.S.A. **1989,** pp: 184.
[10]    The Merck Index. Eleventh Edition. Merck & Co. Inc. Rahway. N. J. U.S.A. **1989,** pp: 1461.
[11]    Kober, A. And Sjoholm, I.; *Mol. Pharmacol.,* **1980,** *18,* 421-426.
[12]    Klotz, I. M. *Ann. N.Y. Acad. Sci.,* **1973,** *226,* 18.
[13]    Timaseff, S N. *Thermodynamics of protein interactions. In: Proteins of Biological fluids (Ed. Peeters).* Pergamon Press, Oxford, **1972,** pp. 511-519.
[14]    Aki, H. And Yamamoto, M. *J. Pharm. Pharmacol.,* **1989,** *41,* 674-679.
[15]    Ross, P. D. And Subramanian, S. *Biochemistry,* **1981,** *20,* 3096-3102.
[16]    Klotz, I. M. And Urquhart, J. M. *J. Am. Chem. Soc.,* **1949,** *71,* 847-851.
[17]    Wilding, G. B.; Blumberg, S. And Vesell, E.S. *Science,* **1977,** *195,* 991-994.

Atta-ur-Rahman/Choudhary/Khan (Eds.) *Frontiers in Natural Product Chemistry, Vol. 1*

# Iron Acquisition and Iron Transport by Bacteria

Herbert Budzikiewicz*

*Institut für Organische Chemie der Universität, Greinstr. 4, 50939 Köln, Germany*

**Abstract**: Most bacteria have developed specific systems to procure sufficient amounts of iron which is not generally available in water soluble form. One possibility is the production of $Fe^{3+}$ chelating substances, so-called siderophores. Structural varieties, the transport mechanism through the cell wall, and the importance of siderophores in health, agriculture and environment will be discussed.

## INTRODUCTION

In the beginning, life on earth developed in a reductive atmosphere where iron was available abundantly in its divalent form. Salts of $Fe^{2+}$ are sufficiently water soluble for an adequate supply. But as a consequence of the photolytic cleavage of water initiated by cyanobacteria, oxygen was set free, and soon only trivalent iron abounded. Due to the low dissociation constants of its oxide hydrates in the soil the concentration of free $Fe^{3+}$ at pH-values around 7 is at best $10^{-17}$ mol/liter, while about $10^{-6}$ mol/liter would be needed to maintain the necessary supply for living cells. Microorganisms infecting animals or man are in a similar situation: here iron is bound strongly to peptidic substances such as transferrins. Bacteria developed two strategies to circumvent this problem, viz. reduction of $Fe^{3+}$ to $Fe^{2+}$ and the production of $Fe^{3+}$ chelating substances, so-called siderophores. In the following discussion examples will be taken predominantly from the bacterial genus *Pseudomonas* (*P.*, other bacterial names will not be abbreviated).

## IRON ACQUISITION BY SIDEROPHORES

Siderophores are secondary metabolites with a molecular mass below 2000 Da. Due to its high charge density, small ion radius, and low polarisability $Fe^{3+}$ is a hard Lewis acid and can bind strongly hard Lewis bases such as oxide ions. It forms octahedral $d^5$ high spin complexes providing six coordination sites. There is a number of small compounds with low complexing constants such as salicylate or citrate, but the ligands most commonly produced by bacteria are bidentate species such as catecholates, hydroxamates and as α-hydroxy-carboxylates. Three bidentate ligands are often connected by aliphatic segments keeping them in place for complexation. This results in an entropic advantage over three non-connected ligands. Typical examples will be given.

### Catecholate and Salicylate Siderophores [1]

Because of the high charge density due to the aromatic system, catecholates form strong complexes at pH values around 7, but they are acid labile since the phenolate anions get readily protonated. The typical bacterial catecholate siderophores are derived from 2,3-dihydroxybenzoic acid (DHB) attached to amino acids, amino alcohols, or aliphatic diamines.

*Corresponding author: E-mail: H.Budzikiewicz@Uni-Koeln.DE

Enterobactin (also called enterochelin) comprises three units of $N$-2,3-dihydroxybenzoyl-L-serine in a cyclic structure, Fig. (**1**). It was isolated first from culture filtrates of *Escherichia coli* [2] and from various *Salmonella* spp. [2, 3]. It forms an 1:1 complex with $Fe^{3+}$ with a complexing constant of $10^{-49}$ [4]. With decreasing pH the *m*-phenolate oxygens get protonated stepwise. At values below 3 also the *o*-oxygen functions become protonated and the complex starts to dissociate. Enterobactin is one of the rare examples where iron is set free in the bacterial cell not by reduction to $Fe^{2+}$ (see below) but by hydrolytic cleavage of the ester bonds. Though *P. aeruginosa* can not produce enterobactin by itself it can use it as a siderophore [5].

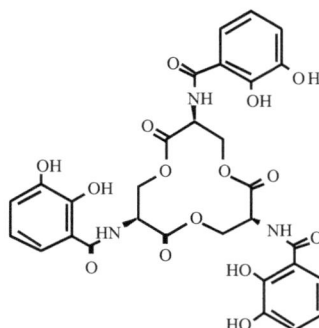

**Fig. (1).** Enterobactin.

Enterobactin binds to serum albumin. This limits the iron supply of the producing bacterium when infecting higher organisms, and thus its growth is restricted [6]. A bacterial strategy against this defense mechanism could be the formation of salmochelins produced by *Salmonella enterica* [7], glucose derivatives of $N$-2,3-dihydroxybenzoyl-L-serine.

An interesting group of catecholate siedrophores are protochelin and its constituents, Fig. (**2**), produced by *Azotobacter vinelandii*, viz. 2,3-dihydroxybenzoic acid, the monocatecholate aminochelin [8], the dicatecholate azotochelin [9, 10] and the combination product of the two, the tricatecholate protochelin [11]. Which species is actually produced depends on the amount of $Fe^{3+}$ available: At concentrations >7 μ DHB, and in a range between 7 and 3 μmol the di- and tricatecholate siderophores are used. When the iron

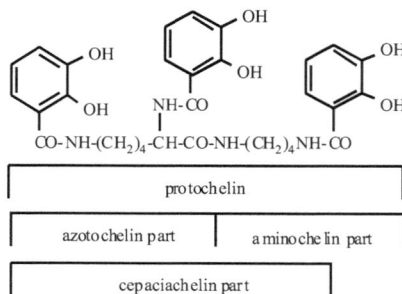

**Fig. (2).** The protochelin family.

concentration drops still lower, the high-affinity peptidic azotobactins (see below) are resorted to [11]. To the same family belongs cepaciachelin obtained from *P.* (*Burkholderia*) *cepacia* which lacks the 2,3-dihydroxybenzoyl residue from the aminochelin part of protochelin [12]. The amino acid incorporated in these catecholates is L-Lys.

When DHB is bound to a β-hydroxy amino acid such as L-threonine, oxazoline rings are formed as in the case of vibriobactin [13] produced by *Vibrio cholerae*. As apparently $Fe^{3+}$ chelation is possible by the -N=C-C=C-O⁻ partial structure, DHB can be replaced by salicylic acid as in vulnibactin [14] from *Vibrio vulnificus*, Fig. (3).

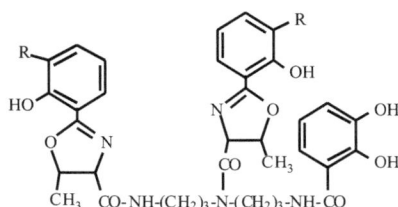

**Fig. (3).** Vibriobactin (R = OH) and vulnibactin (R = H).

Analogous condensation of *N*-salicylyl-L-cystein leads to a thiazoline system as in pyochelin, the siderophore second in importance of *P. aeruginosa*, Fig. (4). Related siderophores are produced by other bacteria. Pyochelin is actually a mixture of two easily interconverting stereoisomers epimeric at C-2". Several explanations have been invoked for this phenomenon [15].

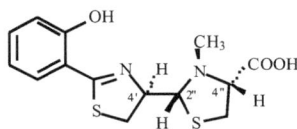

**Fig. (4).** Pyochelin I (4'R, 2" R, 4" R), pyochelin II is 2" S.

As an X-ray analysis showed pyochelin I forms a 2:2 complex with $Fe^{3+}$. Binding sites are the phenolate and the cartboxylate anions together with the adjacent nitrogen atoms. The two moieties are bridged by an acetate and a hydroxyl ion [15].

## Hydroxamate Siderophores

Cepabactin, Fig. (5) produced by *P. alcaligenes* [16] and by several *P.* (*Burkholderia*) *cepacia* strains [17] forms a red 3:1 complex with $Fe^{3+}$. More important as siderophores are the norcardamines E, consisting of alternating three molecules each of oxalic acid and of *N*-hydroxy-1,5-diaminopentane, and $D_2$ where one 1,5-diaminopentane segment is replaced by 1,4-diaminobutane, Fig. (5) from *P. stutzeri* [18].

## α-Hydroxy-carboxylate Siderophores

α-Hydroxy-carboxylate units can be embedded in various surroundings as e.g. in corrugatin [19] from *P. corrugata* which contains two β-hydroxyaspartic acid residues in an lipopeptide chain, Fig. (6).

$$[\text{-CO-CH}_2\text{-CH}_2\text{-CO-NOH-(CH}_2)_5\text{-NH-}]_3$$

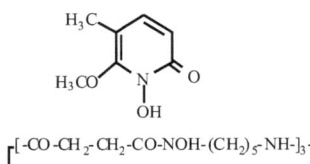

**Fig. (5).** Cepabactin (above) and norcardamine E (below).

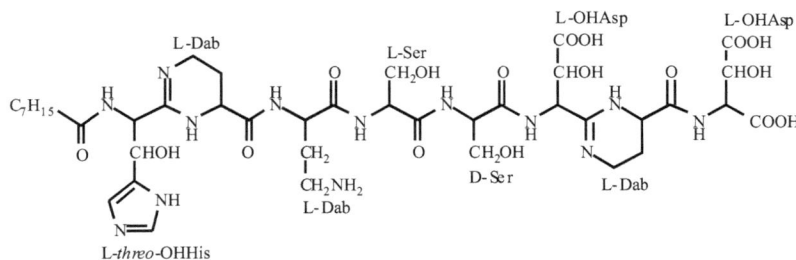

**Fig. (6).** Corrugatin.

Another group of α-hydroxy-carboxylate siderophores are those derived from citric acid. Citric acid can bind $Fe^{3+}$, but of greater importance are those derivatives where two additional ligand sites are bound to the outer carboxyl groups. Examples are schizokinen [20] from *P. (Ralstonia) solanacearum* (with two hydroxamic acid units, and achromobactin [21] from *Erwinia chrysanthemi*, the only known siderophore with three α-hydroxycarboxylate ligands, Fig. (7).

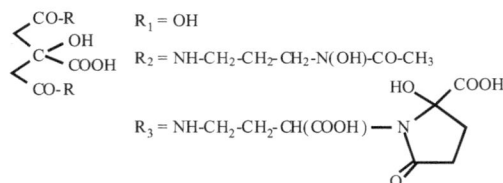

$R_1 = OH$

$R_2 = NH\text{-CH}_2\text{-CH}_2\text{-CH}_2\text{-N(OH)-CO-CH}_3$

$R_3 = NH\text{-CH}_2\text{-CH}_2\text{-CH(COOH)} \longrightarrow N$

**Fig. (7).** Citrate siderophores. With $R_1$ citric acid, with $R_2$ schizokinen, with $R_3$ achromobactin.

## Pyoverdins and Azotobactins [22]

The most elaborate siderophores are the pyoverdins and the structurally related azotobactins produced by fluorescent *Pseudomonas* spp. and by *Azotobacter vinelandii*. The pyoverdins and related siderophores consist of three distinct structural parts, *viz.* a so-called chromophore, a dicarboxylic acid or its monoamide attached amidically to the amino group of the chromophore, and a peptide chain bound to the carboxyl group of the chromophore usually by its N-terminal α-amino group (N-terminal lysine can also be connected by its ε-amino group). The biogenetic precursor of the pyoverdin chromophore is a condensation product of tyrosin and 2,4-diaminobutanoic acid, the ferribactin chromophore. Azotobactins have instead of the side chain an urea type additional ring, Fig. (8).

Usually pyoverdins with varying side chains are found to co-occur in the fermentation broth. So far glutamic acid, α-ketoglutaric acid, succinic acid (amide), and malic acid (amide) were found. They are elements of the citric acid cycle. The peptide chain of the

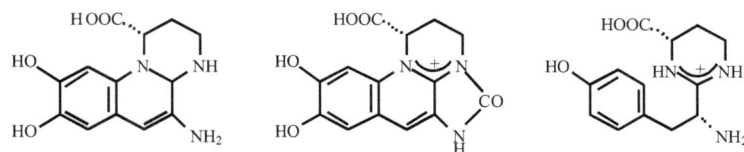

**Fig. (8).** Pyoverdin chromophore (left), azotobactin chromophore (middle), ferribactin chromophore (right).

pyoverdins and their congeners comprises 6 to 12 amino acids, both D- and L-configured. It provides two of the binding sites for $Fe^{3+}$ (the third one is the catecholate system of the chromophore). They are either β-hydroxy amino acids (mostly *threo*-β-hydroxy aspartic acid) or hydroxamic acids derived from ornithine. Either its δ-amino group is transformed into an *N*-acyl-*N*-hydroxy residue (where the acyl group can be formyl, acetyl or rarely (*R*)-β-hydroxybutanoyl) or ornithine is cyclized and hydroxylated giving 3-amino-1-hydroxy-piperidone-2 (*N*-hydroxy-*cyclo*-ornithine) which then forms the C-terminus. The last three or four C-terminal amino acids can form a cyclic substructure, Fig. (**9**).

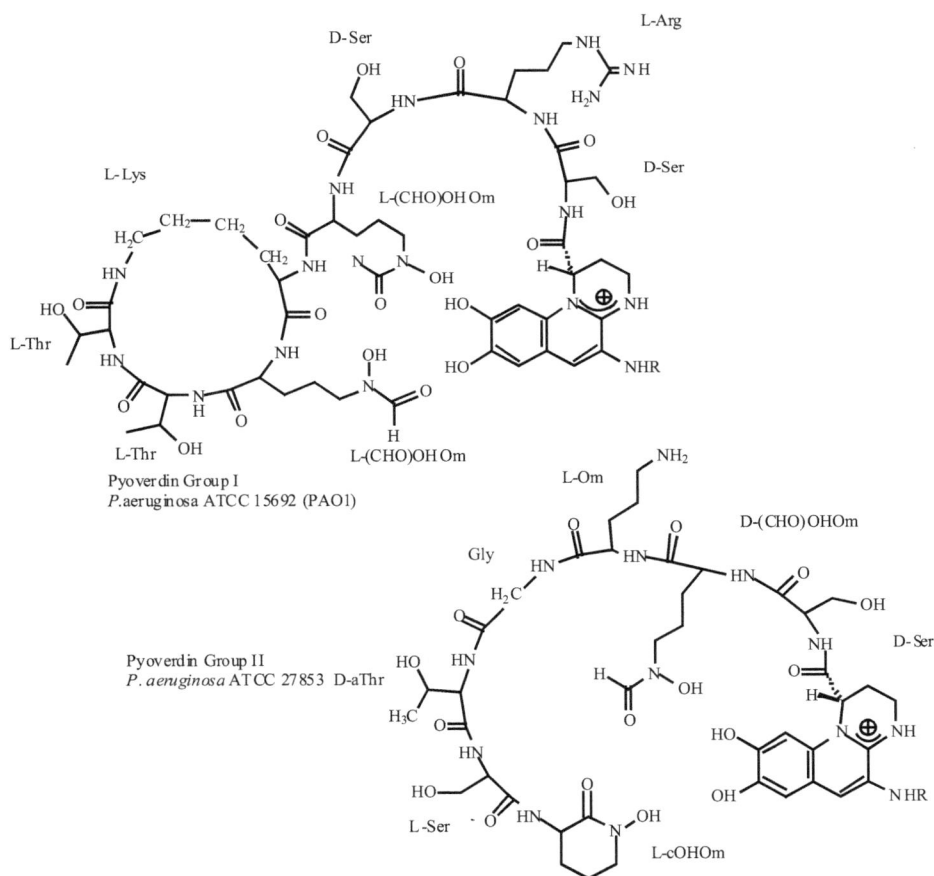

(Fig. 9. Contd....)

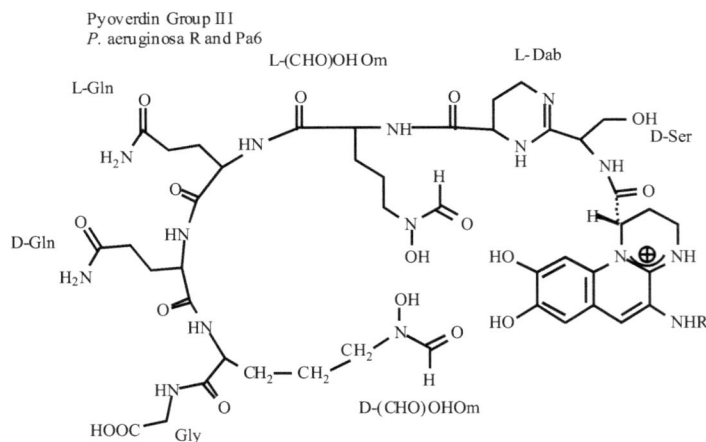

Pyoverdin Group II I
P. aeruginosa R and Pa6

**Fig. (9).** Pyoverdins of *P. aeruginosa* with different C-termini (open, *N*- hydroxy-*cyclo*-ornithine, cyclopeptide).

Determination of the amino acid sequence [23] is achieved today mainly by collision-activated decomposition of the protonated molecular ions obtained by electrospray ionization mass spectrometry, Fig. (10). The chirality of the various amino acids has to be determined after hydrolysis. If one amino acid is present both in its D- and in L-form, peptide fragments obtained by partial hydrolysis have to be analysed.

## IRON TRANSPORT INTO THE CELL [24]

The transport of the $Fe^{3+}$-siderophore complexes through the outer cell membrane takes place either (if small carrier compounds are concerned) via non-specific porins or (for larger units) via specific receptor barrel proteins. A hydrophilic portion at the cell surface recognises and binds the strain-specific siderophore complex. The receptor protein and the siderophore are produced concomitantly under iron starvation, the siderophore acting as an autoinducer controlling thus its own production. Recently evidence has been presented that pyoverdins bind strongly to the receptor protein. The first step of iron uptake is a replacement of the bound iron-free pyoverdin by the ferri-pyoverdin approaching from the medium [25, 26]. This induces a change of conformation of the receptor protein allowing the intrusion of the ferri-pyoverdin into the barrel and an active transport into the periplasmic space.

The last step for all transport systems is the release of the bound iron. The large difference in the affinity of $Fe^{3+}$ and $Fe^{2+}$ to most siderophores suggests a reductive process which is strictly anaerobic. Large amounts of free $Fe^{2+}$ in the cell have to be avoided since they can initiate the so-called Fenton process resulting in the formation of deleterious hydroxyl radicals. Such complications are possibly avoided by a transfer of $Fe^{2+}$ to ferrochelatin, *ca.* 2.2 kDa phosphorylated sugar derivatives [27].

A second way of iron acquisition by bacteria is the reduction to $Fe^{2+}$ by extracellular iron reductases as well as by low molecular weight agents such as pyridine-2,6-di(monothiocarboxylic acid) which forms $Fe^{2+}/Fe^{3+}$ redox systems, Fig. (11) [28].

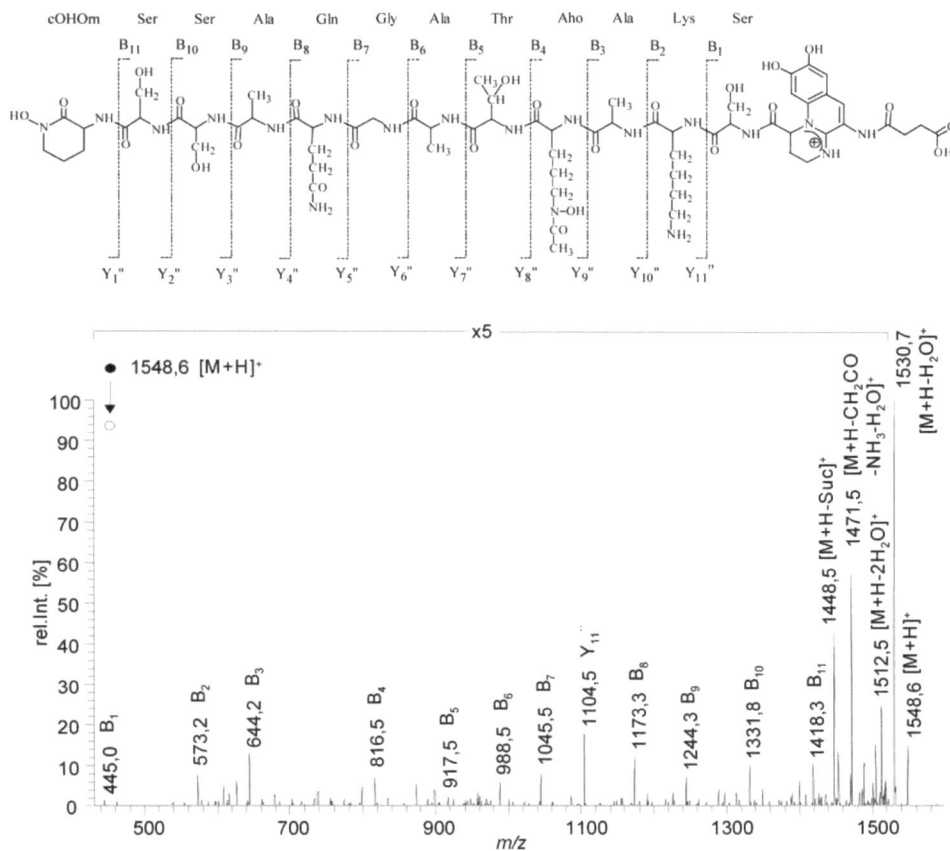

**Fig. (10).** Collision-induced fragmentation of the [M+H]$^+$ ion of the pyoverdin 1547. The sequence-characteristic B-ions obtained by cleavage of the amide bonds can be seen.

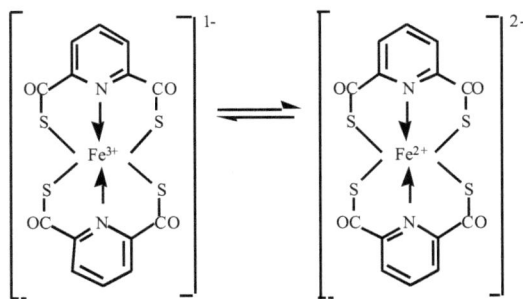

**Fig. (11).** Redox system of pyridine-2,6-di(monothiocarboxylic acid).

Little is known about the transport of Fe$^{2+}$ into the cell. For fluorescent pseudomonads it was suggested that Fe$^{2+}$ is bound by the proper pyoverdin and subsequently oxidised to Fe$^{3+}$.

The only specific $Fe^{2+}$ chelators are ferrorosamine produced by *P. roseus fluorescens* [29]and other *Pseudomonas* spp. [30] and siderochelin from a *Nocardia* sp. [31], Fig. (12).

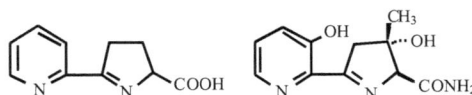

**Fig. (12).** Ferrorosamine (left) and siderochelin (right).

## PRACTICAL APPLICATIONS

### Health [32]

*P. aeruginosa* is feared as an opportunistic human pathogen responsible for frequently lethal hospital (nosocomial) infections. It is insensitive to many desinfecting agents and – more important – an increasing number of strains of *P. aeruginosa* especially from hospital isolates proves to be highly resistant against most antibiotics and also against therapeutic agents such as fluoroquinolones. An alginate film frequently surrounding the bacteria, the low permeability of their outer membrane, and an active export mechanism for low molecular weight substances are the main reasons for the resistance. β-Lactamase activity affects in addition β-lactam antibiotics which can also be specifically exported through the outer cell membrane. *P. aeruginosa* endangers especially severely injured patients suffering from large wounds or severe burns as well as persons whose immune system is weakened. An extremely critical situation exists for patients suffering from mucoviscidosis (cystic fibrosis), when *P. aeruginosa* infects the bronchial tubes.

An approach to circumvent the resistance problem of *P. aeruginosa* is to target the transport system of siderophores for drug delivery into the bacterial cell. This can be affected by binding an antibiotic molecule to a strain-specific pyoverdin ("Trojan Horse" strategy). The *prima facie* problem is that *P. aeruginosa* comprises three so-called siderovars producing different pyoverdins (see Fig. (9)) which are not accepted mutually. The second problem is that derivatisation must not interfere with the recognition of the ferri-complex at the bacterial cell surface. Hence promising site for the attachment of an antibiotic molecule is an amino acid in the peptide chain which is not involved in the recognition process. Synthesis problems are that for solubility reasons chemical reactions have to be conducted in an aqueous medium, and that the various functional groups of the pyoverdin must not be attacked during the synthesis.

For a derivatization with ampicillin the pyoverdin of *P. fluorescens* ATCC 13525 which is accepted by *P. aeruginosa* ATCC PAO1 (see Fig. (9) was used. To the ε-amino groups of their lysine residues a decandioic acid spacer was attached, to the second carboxyl group of which ampicillin was bound amidically, Fig. (13). Ferri-complexed conjugates with a hydrolysed ampicillin residue (which does not exhibit antibiotic activity) restore the bacterial growth in an iron deficient medium in the same way as the underivatized ferri-pyoverdin. This shows that the derivatisation does not interfere with the uptake of the ferri-siderophore. Upon supplementation with the ampicillin conjugate no bacterial growth was observed for about 24 hours [33].

### Agriculture [34]

Various *Pseudomonas* spp. are associated with higher plants. They can be phytopathogens while others especially when colonising the rhizosphere can suppress plant-

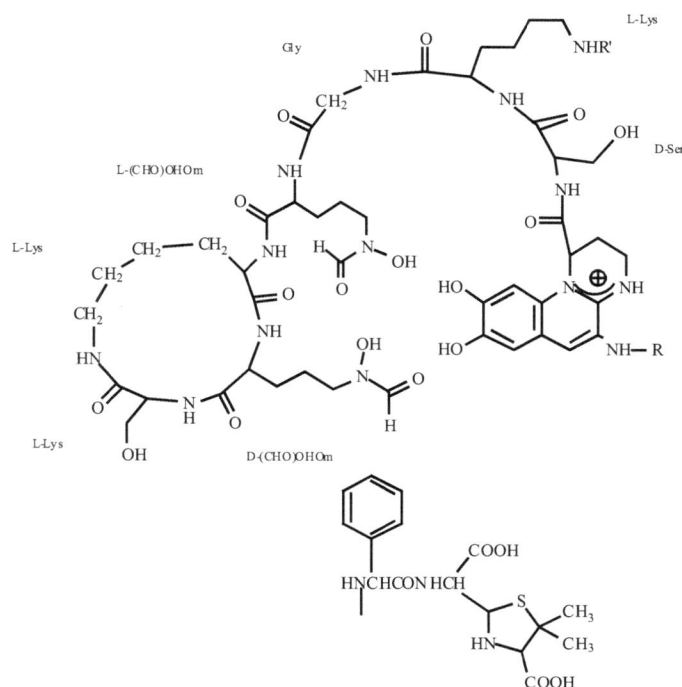

**Fig. (13).** Pyoverdin of *P. fluorescens* ATCC 13525 (R = dicarboxylic acid residue, R' = H) and ampicillin comjugate (R' = -CO-(CH$_2$)$_8$-CO + ampilcillin residue lower formula).

deleterious microorganism. The main mechanisms for the repression of phytopathogenic bacteria is the aggressive cultivation of plant roots by beneficial bacteria able to produce antibiotically active compounds and HCN, but especially their excretion of pyoverdins. Their pronounced complexation ability for Fe$^{3+}$ results in an iron starvation of the competitors.

## Degradation of Waste Materials [35]

*P. putida* can degrade many organic compounds, aromatics as well as chlorinated ones, *P. chlororaphis* polyurethane and other plastics. As a direct connection with the siderophores of this species has not been established, this aspect will not be discussed here, with one exception. It is the degradation of CCl$_4$ to CO$_2$ by *P. stutzeri*, which uses the Cu$^{2+}$ complex of pyridine-2,6-di-(monothio-carboxylic) acid (see Fig. (**11**) [36].

## ABBREVIATIONS

DHB   =   2,3-dihydroxybenzoic acid

*P.*   =   *Pseudomonas*

## REFERENCES

[1]     Budzikiewicz, H. *Mini-Rev. Org. Chem.,* **2004**, *1*, 163.
[2]     O'Brian, I.G.; Gibson, F. *Biochem. Biophys. Acta,* **1970**, *215*, 393.

[3]     Pollak, J.R.; Neilands, J.B. *Biochem. Biophys. Res. Commun.*, **1970**, *38*, 989.
[4]     Loomis, L.D.; Raymond, K.N. *InorgChem.*, **1991**, *30*, 906.
[5]     Poole, K.; Young, L.; Neshat, S. *J. Bacteriol.*, **1990**, *172*, 6991.
[6]     Konopka, K.; Neilands, J.B. *Biochemistry*, **1984**, *23*, 2122.
[7]     Hantke, K.; Nicholson, G.; Rabsch, W.; Winkelmann, G. *Proc. Natl. Acad. Sci. USA*, **2003**, *100*, 3677.
[8]     Page, W.J.; von Tigerstrom, M. *J. Gen. Microbiol.*, **1988**, *134*, 453.
[9]     Fekete, F.A.; Spence, J.T.; Emery, T. *Appl. Environ. Microbiol.*, **1983** *46*, 1297.
[10]    Corbin, J.L.; Bulen, W.A. *Biochemistry*, **1969**, *8*, 757.
[11]    Cornish, A.S.; Page, W.J. *BioMetals*, **1995**, *8*, 332.
[12]    Barelmann, I.; Meyer, J.-M.; Taraz, K.; Budzikiewicz, H. *Z. Naturforsch.*, **1996**, *51c*, 627.
[13]    Griffiths, G.L.; Sigel, S.P.; Payne S.M.; Neilands, J.B. *Biol. Chem.*, **1984**, *259*, 383.
[14]    Okujo, N.; Saito, M.; Yamamoto, S.; Yoshida, T.; Miyoshi, S.; Shinoda, S. *BioMetals*, **1994**, *7*, 109.
[15]    Budzikiewicz, H. In *Progress in the Chemistry of Organic Natural Products*; Herz, W., Falk, H., Kirby, G.W., Eds.; Springer: Wien; **2003**, Vol. *87*, pp. 178-182.
[16]    Barker, WR.; Callaghan, C.; Hill, L.; Noble, D. Acred, P.; 1096
[17]    Meyer,. J.M.; Hohnadel, D.; Hallé, F. *J. Gen. Microbiol.* **1989**, *135*, 1479
[18]    Meyer, J.M,; Stintzi, A. In *Pseudomonas;* Montie, T.C., Ed.; Plenum, New York, **1998**, 201.
[19]    Risse, D.; Beiderbeck, H.; Taraz, K.; Budzikiewicz, H.; Gustine D. *Z. Naturforsch.*, **1998**, *53c*, 295.
[20]    Budzikiewicz, H.; Münzinger, M., Taraz, K.; Meyer, J. M. *Z. Naturforsch.*, **1997**, *52c*, 496.
[21]    Münzinger, M.; Budzikiewicz, H.; Expert, D.; Enard, C.; Meyer, J. M. *Z. Naturforsch.*, **2000**, *55c*, 328
[22]    Budzikiewicz, H. In *Progress in the Chemistry of Organic Natural Products*; Herz, W., Falk, H., Kirby, G.W., Eds.; Springer: Wien; **2003**, Vol. *87*, pp. 91-174.
[23]    Fuchs, R.; Budzikiewicz, H. *Curr. Org. Chem.*, **2001**, *5*, 265.
[24]    Budzikiewicz, H. In *Progress in the Chemistry of Organic Natural Products*; Herz W, Falk H, Kirby GW, Eds.; Springer: Wien; **2003**, Vol. *87*, pp. 144-150.
[25]    Schalk, I.J.; Kyslik, P.; Prome, D.; van Dorsselaer, A.; Poole, K.; Abdallah, M.A.; Pattus, F. *Biochemistry,* **1999**, *38*. 9357.
[26]    Schalk, I.J.; Hennard, C.; Dugave, C.; Poole, K.; Abdallah, M.A.; Pattus, F. *Mol. Microbiol.,* **2001**, *39*, 351.
[27]    Matzanke, B.F. In *Transition Metals in Microbial Metabolism*; Winkelmann, G.; Carrano, C.J., Eds.; Harwood: Amsterdam; p 117.
[28]    Budzikiewicz, H. *Biodegr.,* **2003**, *14*, 65
[29]    Pouteau-Thouvenot, M.; Choussy, M.; Barbier, M.; Viscontini, M. *Helv. Chim. Acta,* **1969**, *52,* 2392.
[30]    Shiman, R.; Neilands; J:B. *Biochemistry,* **1965**, 2233.
[31]    Liu, W.C.; Fisher, S.M.; Wells jr, J.S.; Ricca, C.S.; Principe, P.A.; Trejo, W.H.; Bonner, D.P.; Gougoutos, J.Z; Toeplitz, B.K.; Sykes, R.B. *Antibiot. J.*, **1981**, *34,* 791.
[32]    Budzikiewicz, H. In *Progress in the Chemistry of Organic Natural Products*; Herz, W., Falk, H., Kirby, G.W., Eds.; Springer: Wien; **2003**, Vol. *87*, pp. 194-199.
[33]    Budzikiewicz, H. *Curr. Top. Med. Chem.,* **2001**, *1*, 73.
[34]    Budzikiewicz, H. In *Progress in the Chemistry of Organic Natural Products*; Herz, W., Falk, H., Kirby, G.W., Eds.; Springer: Wien; **2003**, Vol. *87*, pp. 200-201.
[35]    Budzikiewicz, H. In *Progress in the Chemistry of Organic Natural Products*; Herz, W., Falk, H., Kirby, G.W., Eds.; Springer: Wien; **2003**, Vol. *87*, pp. 201-202.
[36]    Lewis, T.A.; Crawford, R.L. *J. Bacteriol.,* **1995**, *177*, 2204.

Atta-ur-Rahman/Choudhary/Khan (Eds.) *Frontiers in Natural Product Chemistry, Vol. 1* 99

# Determination of Absolute Configuration of Natural Products by X-ray Diffraction: A Novel Approach of Incorporating Heavy-Atom-Containing Solvent Molecules into the Single Crystals and Refinement of Flack Parameter

Suchada Chantrapromma[1,*], Hoong-Kun Fun[2], Surat Laphookhieo[1], Saroj Cheenpracha[1] and Chatchanok Karalai[1]

[1] *Department of Chemistry, Faculty of Science, Prince of Songkla University, Hat-Yai, Songkhla 90112, Thailand,* [2] *X-ray Crystallography Unit, School of Physics, Universiti Sains Malaysia, 11800 USM, Penang, Malaysia*

**Abstract:** In this study, the method of determining the absolute configurations of 14β-hydroxy-3β-O-(L-thevetosyl)-5β-card-20(22)-enolide (I) which was isolated from the air-dried fruits of *Cerbera odollam* and 3α-feruloyl-taraxerol (II) which was isolated from the air-dried fruits of *Bruguiera cylindrica* will be presented. The novel method [1] of incorporating heavy-atom-containing solvent molecules into the single crystal structure of the compounds and refinement of the Flack parameter [2] was used to find the absolute configurations of these natural products. Compounds (I) has a cardenolide skeleton whereas compound (II) has a taraxerol skeleton. The present X-ray study shows the absolute L-form of (I) and the absolute α-form of (II). We have clearly demonstrated for the first time a novel approach which is an extremely useful and easy method to determine the absolute stereochemistry of natural products by X-ray diffraction. The importance of determining the absolute stereochemistry of natural products is emphasised in this work.

## INTRODUCTION

We present here the novel method [1] whereby besides solving the 3D structure of natural products, we also determine the absolute stereochemistry. The method consists of introducing heavy-atom containing solvent molecules into the single crystal structures of the natural products. The X-ray structure determination of these molecules would automatically determine the absolute stereochemistry by the refinement of the Flack parameter [2]. In order to establish the absolute stereochemistry of these important naturally occurring compounds, we have successfully incorporated chloroform molecules into the single crystals of (I) [1] and dichloromethane molecules into the single crystals of (II) [3] by using chloroform/ methanol and dichloromethane/methanol, respectively as solvents during crystallisation .

We have demonstrated the success of the novel method [1] by determining the absolute configurations of (I) which was isolated from the air-dried fruits of *Cerbera odollam*, Fig. (**1**) and (II) which was isolated from the air-dried fruit of *Bruguiera cylindrical*, Fig. (**2**). We intend to use this method [1] to determine the absolute configurations of other natural products. Crystal data of (I) and (II) are shown in Table **1**. The schemes and crystal

---

*Corresponding author: E-mail: suchada@ratree.psu.ac.th

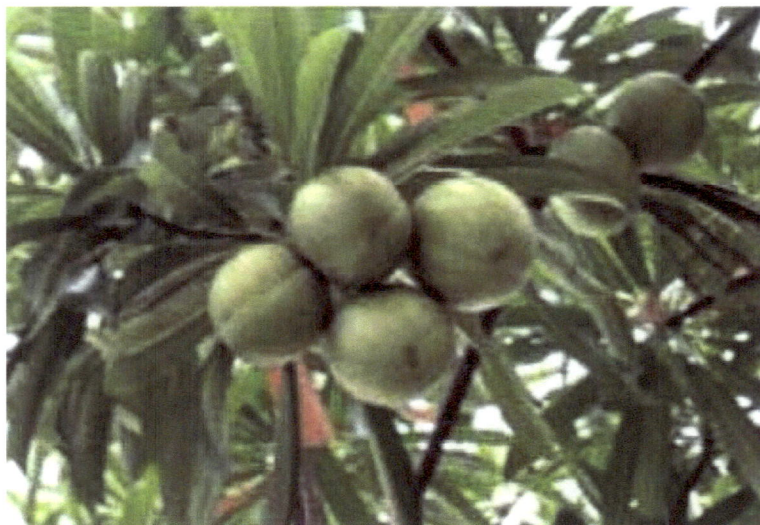

**Fig. (1).** Cerbera odollam

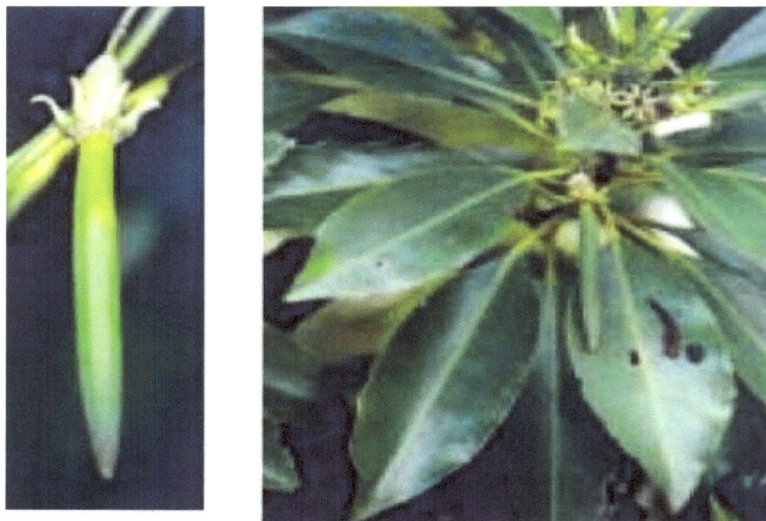

**Fig. (2).** Bruguiera cylindrica

structures are shown in Fig. (**3**) and Fig. (**4**). The absolute configurations of (I) and (II) were established on the basis of anomalous scattering effects of the heavy-atom-containing solvent molecules.

## Experimental

For compound (I), fresh seeds (940 g) of *Cerbera odollam* were extracted twice with methylene chloride (2.5 L) over periods of 5 days at room temperature. The mixture was filtered and concentrated under reduced pressure. Some white solids (0.3085 g) precipitated

**Table 1.    Crystal data of (I) and (II) at 293(2) K.**

| Compound | (I) | (II) |
|---|---|---|
| Empirical formula | $C_{30}H_{46}O_8 . 2CHCl_3$ | $C_{40}H_{58}O_4 . CH_2Cl_2$ |
| Formula weight | 773.40 | 687.79 |
| Crystal system | Orthorhombic | Monoclinic |
| Space group | $P2_12_12_1$ | $P2_1$ |
| a (Å) | 7.6426 (4) | 12.5558(1) |
| b (Å) | 9.1932 (5) | 8.5131(7) |
| c (Å) | 54.362 (3) | 18.6076(15) |
| $\alpha, \beta, \gamma$ (°) | 90.0, 90.0, 90.0 | 90.0, 104.834, 90.0 |
| V(Å$^3$) | 3819.5 (4) | 1922.7(3) |
| Z | 4 | 2 |
| $D_x$ (Mg.m$^{-3}$) | 1.345 | 1.188 |
| Cell parameters from reflection | 6197 | 4263 |
| $\theta$ (°) | 2.3-25.4 | 2.3-26.0 |
| $\mu$ (mm$^{-1}$) | 0.50 | 0.21 |
| Crystal shape and color | Block, colorless | Needle, colorless |
| Crystal size (mm) | 0.36 x 0.34 x 0.24 | 0.48 x 0.18 x 0.14 |
| Data collection : | Siemens SMART CCD diffractometer ; $\omega$ scans | Mo K$\alpha$ radiation |
| measured reflections | 18659 | 10423 |
| independent reflections | 6626 | 7198 |
| reflections with I > 2$\sigma$(I) | 4427 | 5897 |
| $R_{int}$ | 0.044 | 0.020 |
| h = | -9 → 9 | -15 → 15 |
| k = | -10 → 8 | -9 → 10 |
| l = | -62 → 64 | -14 → 22 |
| Refinement on F$^2$, R[F$^2$ > 2$\sigma$ (F$^2$)] | 0.077 | 0.062 |
| wR(F$^2$) | 0.227 | 0.152 |
| reflections | 6626 | 7198 |
| parameters H-atom parameters constrained | 422 | 445 |

(Table 1. Contd....)

| Compound | (I) | (II) |
|---|---|---|
| $(\Delta/\sigma)_{max}$ | < 0.001 | 0.002 |
| $\rho\Delta_{max}$ (eÅ$^{-3}$) | 0.33 | 0.34 |
| $\rho\Delta_{min}$ (eÅ$^{-3}$) | -0.40 | -0.48 |
| Absolute structure: Friedel pairs | 2780 | 3171 |
| Flack parameter | 0.14(14) | 0.12(13) |

and were purified by preparative TLC (eluent: 2% methanol in ether), yielding (I) ($R_F$ = 0.19, 30% acetone-hexane). Colourless single crystals of (I) suitable for X-ray diffraction were obtained by slow evaporation of a solution of (I) in chloroform-methanol (3:0.05 v/v) over a period of 3-4 days (m.p. 475-479 K).

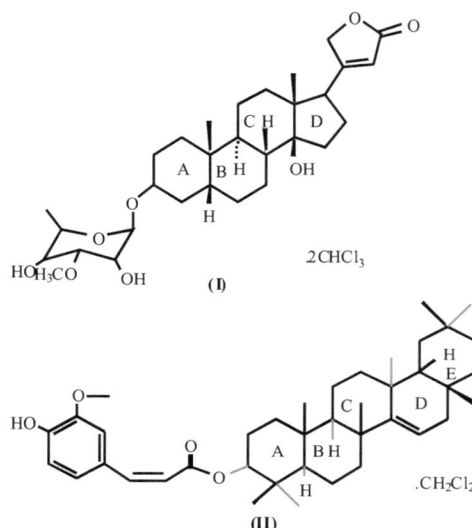

**Fig. (3).** Chemical schemes of (I) and (II).

For compound (II), air-dried fruits of *Bruguiera cylindrica* (6 kg) were milled and extracted with hexane (20 L x 2). The filtered solution was then evaporated to dryness under reduced pressure to afford 35 g of crude hexane extract. This extract was subjected to quick column chromatography (QCC) over silica gel and eluted with a gradient of hexane/acetone to afford 15 fractions (A1-A15, each fraction collecting 300 ml). Fraction A9 (2.80 g) was recrystallized from acetone/hexane (3:7 v/v, 50 ml) to give a white powder of (II). The white powder were recrystallised from dichloromethane/methanol (9:1v/v) to give colourless single crystals of (II) after a few days (m.p. 458-459 K).

## Results and Discussion

Preliminary testing of (I) showed the strong activities against human breast-cancer cells, human small-cell lung cancer and human oral epidermoid carcinoma. Compound (I) has a

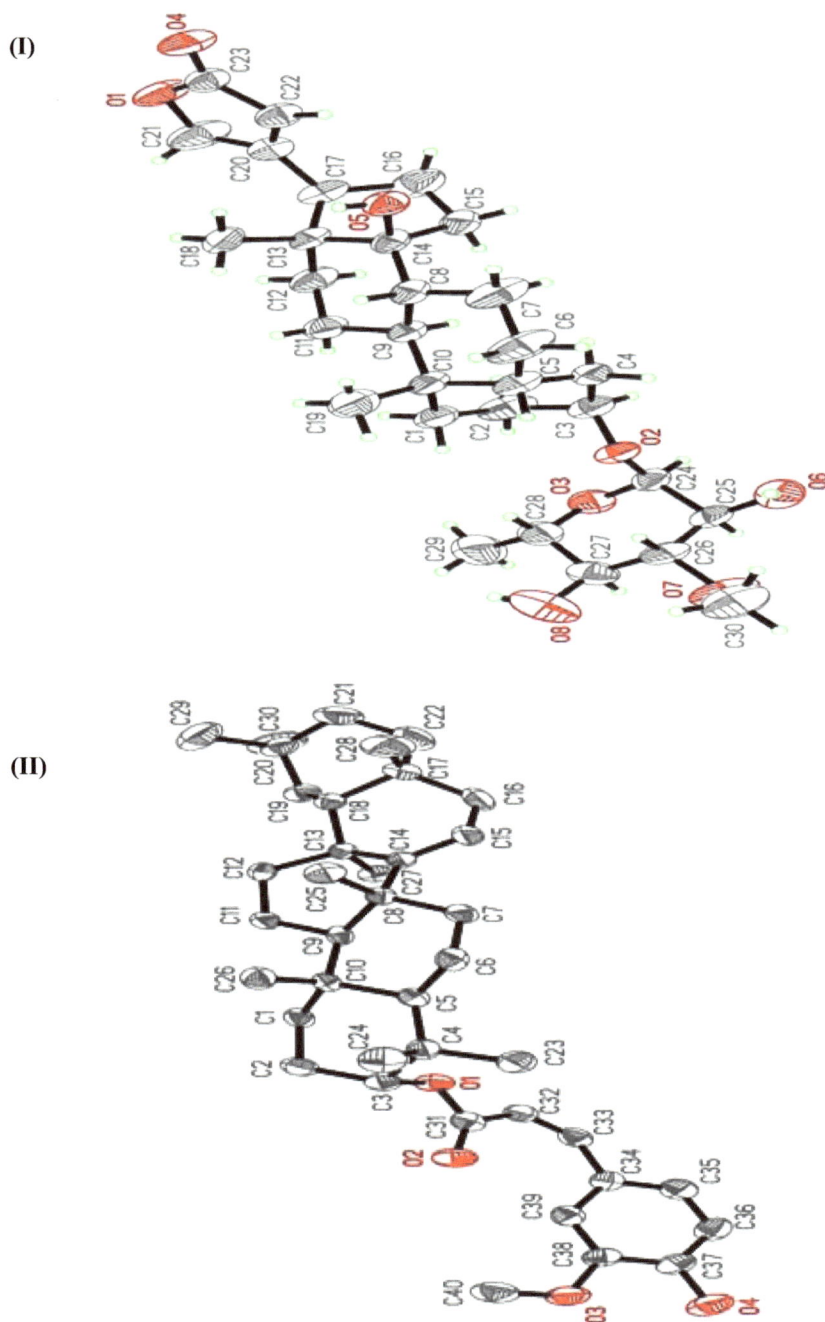

**Fig. (4).** The Ortep diagrams of (I) and (II) showing 50% probability displacement ellipsoids and atomic numbering . For clarity, the chloroform solvent molecules for (I) and the H atoms and dichloromethane molecule for (II) have been omitted.

cardenolide skeleton. The asymmetric unit of (I) contains one cardenolide molecule and two chloroform molecules, Fig. (**4**). The geometries of the steroid nucleus, lactone ring and glycoside are in agreement with those reported earlier for the unsolvated structure [4]. The steroid nucleus has a cis/trans/cis configuration for the A-B/B-C/C-D rings and the cyclohexane A, B and C rings have standard chair conformations; the cyclopentane ring D has an envelope conformation. The lactone ring (O1/C20-C23) attached at atom C17 is essentially planar, mainly due to conjugation of the C=C and C=O bonds. Selected bond lengths and angles of (I) are shown in Table **2**. The molecular structure is stabilised by C-H...O interactions. The solvent molecules are linked to the cardenolide through C-H...O hydrogen bonds. Screw-related molecules are linked together by O-H...O hydrogen bonds, Fig. (**5**).

**Table 2.    Selected Geometric Parameters (Å ,$^{\circ}$ ) of (I).**

| O1-C23 | 1.329 (7) | O1-C21 | 1.439 (7) | O2-C24 | 1.398 (6) | O2-C3 | 1.426 (6) |
|---|---|---|---|---|---|---|---|
| O3-C24 | 1.403 (7) | O3-C28 | 1.433 (7) | O4-C23 | 1.213 (6) | O5-C14 | 1.430 (5) |
| O6-C25 | 1.405 (8) | O7-C30 | 1.394 (8) | O7-C26 | 1.423 (7) | O8-C27 | 1.399 (8) |
| C20-C22 | 1.313 (7) | C20-C21 | 1.453 (9) | C22-C23 | 1.444 (7) | | |

| C24-O2-C3-C4 | -156.0(4) | C24-O2-C3-C2 | 82.0 (6) | C16-C17-C20-C22 | -42.9 (9) |
|---|---|---|---|---|---|
| C13-C17-C20-C22 | 78.3 (8) | C16-C17-C20-C21 | 133.9 (7) | C13-C17-C20-C21 | -104.9 (7) |
| C3-O2-C24-O3 | -84.3 (6) | C3-O2-C24-C25 | 154.2 (5) | | |

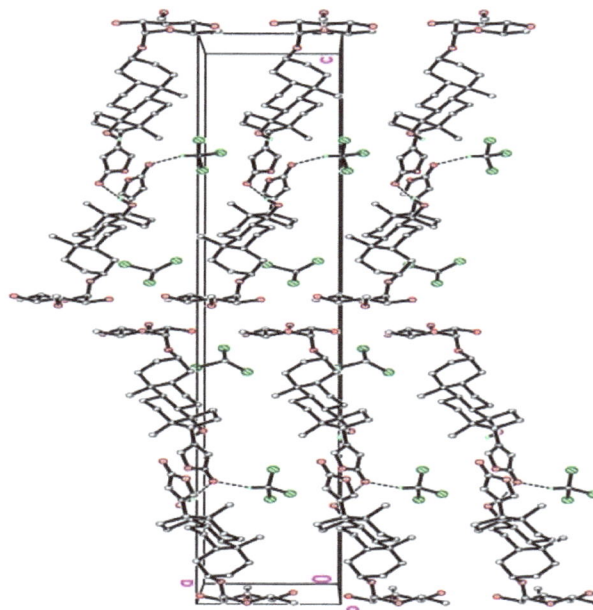

**Fig. (5).** Packing diagram for (I), showing the molecular ribbons. H atoms have been omitted, except for those involved in hydrogen-bond interactions (dash lines).

Compound (II) was isolated for the first time from *Bruguiera cylindrica*, and also for the first time from natural product resources. It is found to exhibit cytotoxicity against human small lung-cancer cell lines. (II) has a taraxerol skeleton and its structure contains five fused six-membered rings, with two rings (A and B) in chair, two rings (C and D) in twist-boat and one ring (E) in a slightly twisted boat conformation. The D and E rings are cis-fused, Fig. (4). The feruloyl substituent group is axially attached to the skeleton. O-H...O hydrogen bonds and C-H...O interactions are observed in the structure. Selected bond lengths and angles of (II) are shown in Table 3. The methoxy and carbonyl O atoms are involved in O-H...O hydrogen bonding and C-H...O weak interactions, respectively. The molecules are interlinked through O4-H4...O2$^i$ (i = 1-x, y-1/2, 1-z) hydrogen bonds into chains parallel to the *b* axis, Fig. (6).

**Table 3.    Selected Geometric Parameters (Å ,° ) of (II).**

| O1-C31 | 1.349 (4) | O1-C3 | 1.457 (4) | O2-C31 | 1.211 (4) | O3-C38 | 1.369 (4) |
|---|---|---|---|---|---|---|---|
| O3-C40 | 1.410 (4) | O4-C37 | 1.357 (4) | C14-C15 | 1.328 (4) | C32-C33 | 1.324 (5) |

| C31-O1-C3-C2 | -121.4 (3) | O1-C31-C32-C33 | 164.0 (3) | C31-C32-C33-C34 | 3.2 (7) |
|---|---|---|---|---|---|
| C32-C33-C34-C39 | 21.8 (6) | C40-O3-C38-C39 | -10.8 (5) | C40-O3-C38-C37 | 171.3(3) |

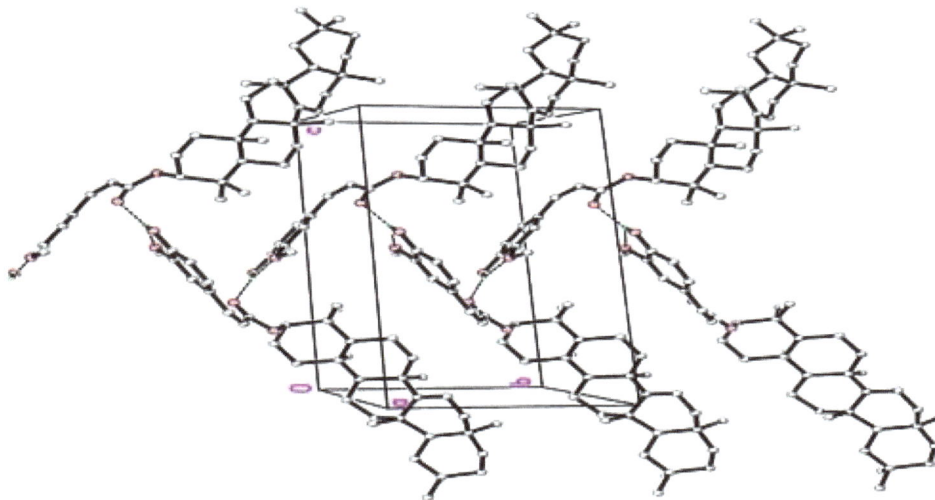

**Fig. (6).** Packing diagram for (II), showing the molecular ribbons. H atoms have been omitted,  except for those involved in hydrogen-bond interactions (dash lines).

The knowledge of the absolute stereochemistry of natural products is essential when their 3D structures are used for theoretical modelling of drug design. Drugs work by binding to the hosts (e.g enzymes) *via* hydrogen-bonding through the "lock and key" concept. If the absolute stereochemistry of the drugs are not known, the "mirror-image keys" may be used and the resulting prediction of the drugs' effectiveness would be erroneous and misleading. The novel method[1] illustrated in this work is an extremely easy and convenient way of determining the absolute stereochemistry of natural products.

## CONCLUSION

The novel method[1] of determining the absolute stereochemistry of natural products have been successfully demonstrated with two examples. In general the knowledge of the absolute stereochemistry of natural products is very important especially when their 3D structures are used for theoretical modelling as in the example of drug designs. Without the experimental knowledge of the real absolute stereochemistry, the modelling may have been conducted using their enantiomorphs and the results of these predictions would be at best unreliable or at worst entirely wrong.

## ACKNOWLEDGEMENTS

SC would like to thank Prince of Songkla University for financial support. The authors also thank the Malaysian Government and Universiti Sains Malaysia for research grant R&D No.305/PFIZIK/610961.

## REFERENCES

[1]     Fun, H.-K.; Chantrapromma, S.; Cheenpracha, S.; Karalai, C.; Anjum, S.; Chantrapromma, K.; Azhar, A. R. *Acta Cryst*. E59, **2003**, 1694–1696.
[2]     Flack, H. D.; Bernardinelli, G. *Acta Cryst*. A55, **1999**, 908-915.
[3]     Chantrapromma, S.; Fun, H.-K.; Ibrahim, A. R.; Laphookhieo, S.; Karalai, C. *Acta Cryst*. E59, **2003**, 1864–1866.
[4]     Chantrapromma, S.; Usman, A.; Fun, H.-K.; Laphookhieo, S.; Karalai, C.; Rat-a-pa, Y.; Chantrapromma, K. *Acta Cryst*. C59, **2003**, 68-70.

Atta-ur-Rahman/Choudhary/Khan (Eds.) *Frontiers in Natural Product Chemistry, Vol. 1*

# Researches on the Technology and Bioactive Properties of Phenolic Lipids

## J.H.P. Tyman*

*Centre for Environmental Research, Brunel University, Uxbridge, Middlesex, UB8 3PH, UK*

**Abstract:** *Anacardium occidentale* (cashew) containing the principal component phenols, anacardic acid, cardol, 2-methylcardol and cardanol is a unique source of materials useful both for industrial technology, in semi-synthesis and for biological/pharmaceutical applications. Thus, by industrial decarboxylation, anacardic acid in the natural cashew gives predominantly cardanol in the product; technical cashew nutshell liquid (CNSL) together with cardol/2-methylcardol and the cashew kernel is the valuable desired main edible commercial product. Anacardic acid itself together with cardol is best recovered by cold cutting of raw cashew shells followed by solvent extraction to afford natural CNSL. Either from technical or natural CNSL, the individual component phenols, cardanol, anacardic acid, cardol, 2-methylcardol, respectively can be separated by several different techniques notably by phase separation. Each separated component phenol contains saturated, 8(Z)-monoene, 8(Z),11(Z)-diene and 8(Z).11(Z),14-triene constituents. Subsidiary chromatographic separation can give the individual constituents. Technical CNSL without separation is widely used in the production of friction dusts for the automobile industry and in certain polymeric/surface coating applications. Cardanol separated from technical CNSL has uses in semi-synthesis, e.g. in the formation of polyethoxylate surfactants, chelatants for metals and for boron. Natural CNSL and anacardic acid separated from it, has potential industrial applications in semi-synthesis and in biological studies. Cardol separated, either from technical or natural CNSL also has potential interest in semi-synthesis, and its homologues, more recently as a potential biological marker.

## INTRODUCTION

*Anacardium occidentale* (cashew) grows in sub-equatorial regions of the world notably India, Brazil, E. Africa, Indonesia and production, once thought to be by 2000, $10^6$ tonnes, is probably much less, namely 0.5 x $10^6$ tonnes [1-4], while technical CNSL production is probably about 5x $10^4$ tonnes. Edible kernel production is the chief commercial interest and probably reaches more than $10^5$ tonnes worldwide. The kernel is approximately 50%, natural CNSL is 25% and the remaining weight comprises shell material and testa. The formulae of the component phenols in natural CNSL, are shown in Fig. (**1**) which depicts anacardic acid (**1**), cardol (**2**), 2-methylcardol (**3**) and cardanol (**4**) present to approximately 70%, 20%, 5%, 3%, respectively together with polymeric material. Each phenol exists as a saturated, an 8(Z)-monoene, an 8(Z),11(Z)-diene and an 8(Z), 11(Z),14-triene.

From the chemotaxonomic aspect, anacardic acids (6-alkylsalicylic acids), cardols (5-alkylresorcinols) and cardanols (3-alkylphenols) exist in many species. Thus, anacardic acids are found in *Pistacia vera* ($C_{13}$, $C_{15}$), *Spondias mombin* ($C_{17}$), Merulius spp. ($C_{15}$, $C_{17}$),

*Corresponding author: Fax: 020-8878 6314; E-mail: jhptyman@hotmail.com

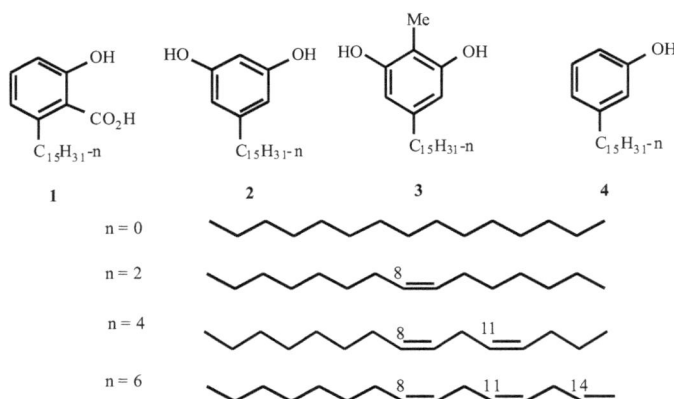

**Fig.(1).** Formulae of Component Phenols of *Anacardium occidentale*

*Kneama elegans* ($C_{11}$-$C_{17}$), *Ginkgo biloba* ($C_{15}$), *Chrysanthemum elegans* $C_6$ (methyl ether), *Philodendron scandens* ($C_{17}$), *Pelargonium xhortorum* ($C_{15}$, $C_{17}$), *Schoepfia californica* ($C_{15}$, $C_{17}$) [5].

Resorcinols occur widely botanically, in *Mangifera indica* ($C_{15}$, $C_{17}$), Grevillea spp. ($C_{11}$-$C_{15}$), *Cereale secale* ($C_{15}$-$C_{25}$), Triticale, Tritium (similar chain lengths), *Ginkgo biloba* ($C_{15}$), Ononis spp. (substituted side chains; bacterially in Mycobacterium spp. ($C_{15}$, $C_{17}$), Pseudomonas spp. ($C_{19}$, $C_{19}$), Streptomyces spp. ($C_{15}$); and in insect sources, *Anagasta kuenella*, $C_{18}$) [6,7].

Cardanols are of limited occurrence, *Anacardium occidentale*, *Ginkgo biloba*, ($C_{15}$), and in mycobacterial, and glycolipids.

## BIOSYNTHESIS

The biosynthesis of the phenolic lipids in *Anacardium occidentale* has not been fully established with respect to enzymic systems involved although the polyketide pathway to the aromatic ring is clear [8]. It appears most probable that a similar process operates as found for the anacardic acids in *Pelargonium xhortorum* [9]. In this, a $C_{16}$ fatty acid adds two malonyl CoA units and a reductive step followed by dehydration, folding, aldol reaction and dehydration affords a $C_{15}$ anacardic acid and cardanol. The addition of 3-malonyl CoA units, and similar sequences gives an orsellinic acid and thence cardol by decarboxylation as depicted in Fig. (2).

## PROCESSES FOR TECHNICAL AND NATURAL CASHEW NUTSHELL LIQUID (CNSL)

The cashew nut is the external seed of the cashew apple. A cross section of the nut itself is depicted attached to the cashew apple (Appendix i, Figs. (3a,b). Natural CNSL is contained between an inner shell (endocarp) and the outer shell (epicarp) and the kernel is protected both by a testa and the inner shell. In the current widely used industrial roasting process [1,4] at 180-190°C, for obtaining technical CNSL, cardanol, the main component, is formed by the decarboxylation of the anacardic acid in the natural CNSL of the raw nut. The outer shell is burst and the highly prized edible kernel is simultaneously roasted. In a vessel

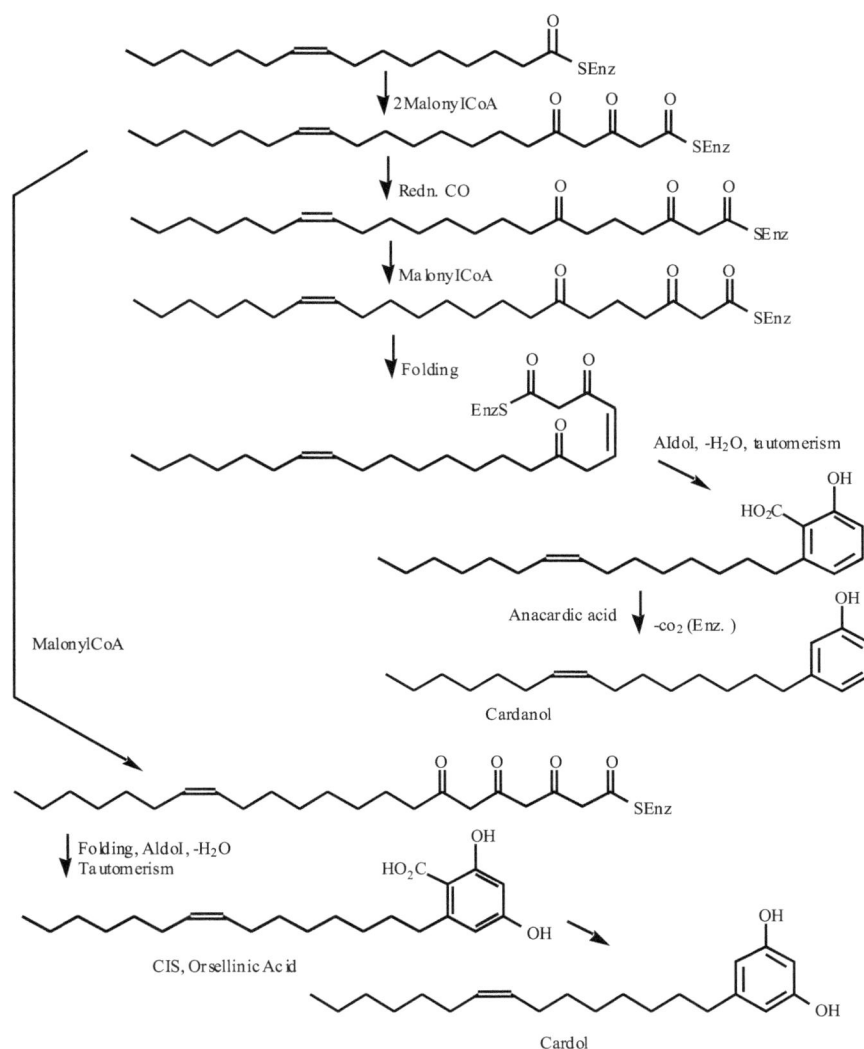

**Fig. (2).** Possible Biosynthesis of Component Phenols in *Anacardium occidentale*.

(Appendix, i Fig. (**4**) in which raw cashew nuts are drawn submerged through hot CNSL. In subsequent manual or automatic techniques, the kernel is retrieved by careful fracture of the inner shell. Natural CNSl with 70% anacardic acid gives technical CNSL containing cardanol (60-70%), cardol and 2-methylcardol, relatively unchanged (20-25%), and polymer (5-10%). The proportion of polymeric material is dependent on the skill of the operator and temperature control. (Appendix, ii Fig. (**5**) depicts the aerial oxidative and thermal effect of temperature at 180°C and at 245°C on the saturated (15:0), monoene (15:1), diene (15:2) and triene (15:3) constituents, determined by HPLC analysis [10] and (Appendix ii, Fig. (**6**) the influence of a nitrogen atmosphere. Although the release of carbon dioxide affords an inert blanket, a sharp rise in temperature above 190°C in the industrial process is adverse. Additionally, since the yield (ca 10%) falls short of the theoretical 25%, (based on the natural CNSL% in the raw shell), attempts have been made to improve the efficiency by first the extraction of natural CNSL followed by decarboxylation. For the extraction of natural cashew nutshell liquid, different techniques are employed. Thus, solvent extraction with carbon tetrachloride of raw half shells obtained by mechanically cutting with commercial equipment [11] gave a theoretical recovery of natural CNSL (25%) and catalysed decarboxylation at 130°C then yielded technical CNSL, free of polymeric impurities [12]. Nevertheless, although this represents a considerable improvement, the mechanical cutting method has remained of very limited commercial implementation. Alternative extraction procedures with supercritical carbon dioxide [13,14] and with carbon dioxide-isopropanol mixtures [15], have been successful. The porosity of the shell permits pressurised supercritical extraction with carbon dioxide in the equipment shown [16] in (Appendix, i Fig.(7), whereby yields of 94% have been claimed.

## SEPARATION PROCESSES FOR CARDANOL CONSTITUENTS

For semi-synthetic applications, it is desirable to employ cardanol containing the four constituents illustrated earlier, but free from cardol, 2-methylcardol and the polymeric material, which appears partly to consist of a dimer.

The (15:0), (15:1), (15:2), and (15:3) constituents separate collectively in distillation and adsorption chromatographic methods.

### Physical Methods

#### Vacuum Distillation

This has been widely used, very often with very poor results, due to excessive polymerisation [10]. Unless operated under a vacuum of 1mm.Hg with wide bore equipment to maintain a low pressure throughout the system, considerable loss of di- and tri-unsaturated constituents occurs. By continuous admission of distilland and minimisation of the temperature gradient between the heat source and distilland, recoveries of cardanol (67-69%) from technical CNSL with purity 90-95% were obtained the remainder being cardol, which itself was recoverable to only 10% [17].

#### Molecular Distillation

Short path distillation in a 10 stage Ridgeway-Watt still at $10^{-5}$ mm. Hg, gave a recovery of phenolic material in 81-87% yield, of a nearly colourless product of 99% purity with greatly reduced polymer formation [17]. Nonetheless, the scale of operation restricted the utility of this method.

#### Adsorption Chromatography

This has been conducted in large columns with TLC grade silica gel H and adsorbent/solute, 5:1, with gradient elution (light petroleum 60-80°C/diethyl ether). A complete separation of cardanol (69% yield) and cardol (11%) was obtained with four-fold reuse of the column. The scale was limited to 36g/batch with relatively high volumes of recoverable solvent [18].

#### Phase Separation

Distribution of technical CNSL between light petroleum and an alkane diol (ethane-1,2-, propane-1,2-, butane-1,4- or pentane-1,5-diols) effected a complete separation of cardanol and cardol. Thus, technical CNSL in an equal wt. of butane-1,4-diol continuously extracted with light petroleum gave a 84.2% recovery of cardanol and by aqueous dilution of the diol phase, followed by extraction, cardol, 15.8%. The method is applicable on a larger scale than the preceding methods and solvent recovery is feasible. 2-Methylcardol accompanies cardol [19].

## Chemical Methods

### Base Addition

Cardol is more acidic than cardanol and by treatment with a strong base forms a more thermally stable salt than cardanol. Thus, with Technical CNSL and diethylene triamine, the following reactions occur:

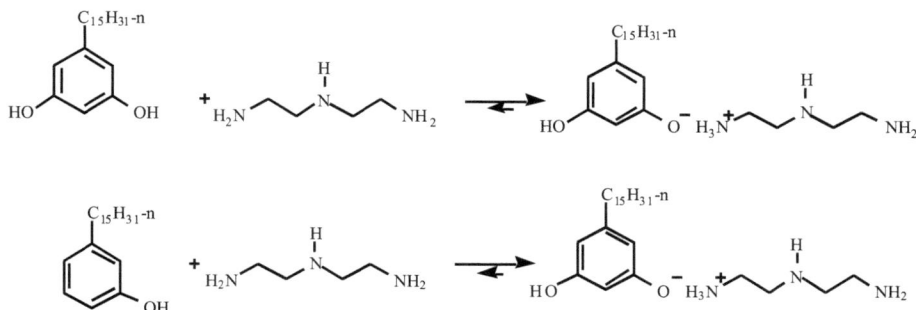

Thus technical CNSL, (0.5mol), containing cardanol (86.9%), cardol (10,3%), and 2-methylcardol (2.3%), treated with diethylene triamine (0.5mol) at ambient temperature for 24h, upon vacuum distillation afforded cardanol (62.3%) containing cardanol (97.7%) and cardol (2.0%). Other strong organic bases may be used e.g. n-butylamine [20].

### Mannich Reaction

In this method cardol more readily forms a polymer than cardanol. In the first stage, technical CNSL (1.0mol) with 40% aqueous formaldehyde (1.2mol) and diethylene triamine (0,125mol) in methanol (1250ml) are reacted at ambient temperature during 30min. A resulting polymer forms a separate lower layer which can be removed and the upper layer after concentration and vacuum distillation affords cardanol in 60% yield containing less than 2% cardol [21]. The reactions are:

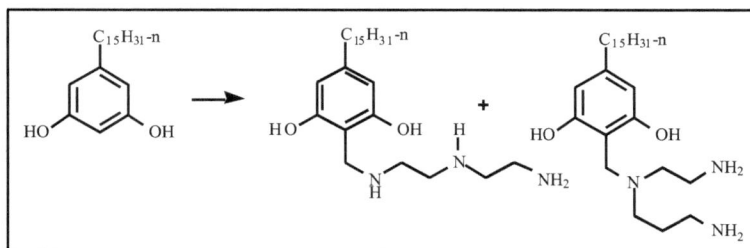

### Preferential Reaction with Ammonium Hydroxide

Technical CNSL in methanol containing ammonium hydroxide, (8:5) by extraction with hexane afforded cardanol and extraction of the methanolic ammonium hydroxide solution with ethyl acetate gave cardol [22]. The method derives from an earlier TLC separation [23].

## SEPARATION OF THE CONSTITUENTS OF PHENOLIC LIPIDS

These methods are applicable to all the phenolic lipids as well as to cardanol. In the previous methods briefly described no separation of the constituents takes place but for certain applications in technical, pharmaceutical or biological studies, the saturated (15:0), monoene (15:1), diene (15:2), or triene (15:3) constituents are required.

### Argentation Chromatography

The constituents of cardanol, cardol, 2-methylcardol and anacardic acid have been separated by argentation thin layer chromatography on silica gel G containing 5-10% silver nitrate; with the solvent chloroform-ethyl acetate (90:10v/v) for cardanol; (80:20) for cardol and 2-methylcardol; (90:10, containing 1% formic acid) for anacardic acid, to maintain the solute in the non-polar hydrogen-bonded form. These separations can be effected analytically and preparatively [24].

### Gas/Liquid Chromatography

Although analytical separations on polyethylene glycol adipate were highly effective for cardanol, both cardol and anacardic acid required conversion to methyl ethers or trimethylsilyl derivatives [25]. Preparative separations have been superseded by HPLC methods.

### High Performance Liquid Chromatography

The constituents of cardanol and of cardol have been separated readily by HPLC on a preparative scale [26], and those of anacardic acid in a similar way [27]. A recycling technique for larger scale runs has been described [28].

## SYNTHESIS OF CARDANOL UNSATURATED CONSTITUENTS

To aid structure/activity studies and in certain cases to obtain readily larger quantities of (15:1), (15:2), or (15:3) constituents, synthesis is obligatory. For the 8(Z)-monoene and 8(Z),11(Z)-diene acetylenic methodology has proved most useful [29] and selective, while for the triene a Wittig method proved of value [30] (Appendix, iii Scheme 1).

## TECHNOLOGICAL APPLICATIONS OF TECHNICAL CNSL AND OF CARDANOL

The component phenols of *Anacardium occidentale* (cashew), anacardic acid and cardol in the natural product, and cardanol with cardol in technical CNSL are both replenishable rather than fossil fuel derived. Cardanol has been employed as a replacement raw material for 4-t-nonyl and 4-t-octylphenol, obtained petrochemically. Thus, both technical CNSL and cardanol itself have wide industrial technological and semi-synthetic uses [4, 31,32] as distinct from biological applications, which have proved possible with cardol and anacardic acid.

### Friction Dusts

The chief uses of technical CNSL from industrial processing have been firstly with resins from formaldehyde for compounding in friction dusts and clutches for the automobile and transport industry and secondly in surface coatings. Major advances in recent years have been in solution rather than solid state polymerisation to avoid communication, and in the replacement of asbestos by the use of thermally stable polymers, such as polyimides (Kevlar and Aramid). Composites for brake linings contain a variety of inorganic materials in addition to phenol-formaldehyde and CNSL-formaldehyde resins.

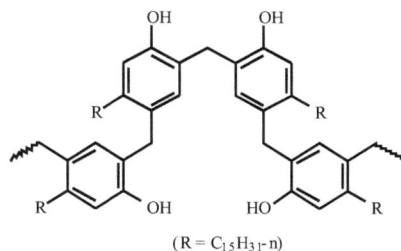

$(R = C_{15}H_{31-n})$

**Fig. (8a).** Formaldehyde/CNSL reaction.

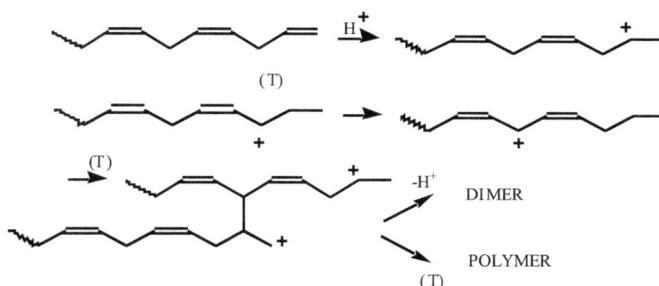

**Fig. (8b).** Side-chain polymerisation.

The latter result from aldehyde condensation at o- and p- positions as depicted in Fig. (8a), while with acidic reagents, side-chain polymerisation occurs through a carbonium ion mechanism as shown in Fig. (8b) [1,4]. A variety of composites are fabricated for friction dust products and a recent formulation [33] incorporates a wide range of materials.

### Surface Coatings

In surface coatings a lower degree of polymerisation is used than in friction dusts. The side chain remains to effect plasticity [34], and conjugation of the unsaturation, to permit Diels-Alder addition [35], leads to formation of water-soluble materials. To list a few of many applications, co-polymerisation of technical CNSL with styrene and use with alkyd resins are established procedures. More recent developments have been in the development of 'cardbisphenol'(A) [36] for polymerisation with diisocyanates, with the oxirane (B) [37], the acrylate (C) [38] for polymerisation reactions, and in phosphorylation to obtain thermally stable polymers [39]. In products requiring less colour, cardanol has been employed rather than technical CNSL.

### Cardanol Polyethoxylates in Non-ionic Surfactants

Cardanol separated from cardol is a potential replacement for p-t-nonyl and t-octylphenols, both derived from petrochemical sources. The inherent advantage of cardanol is its replenishability and potential biodegradability. Thus, cardanol and cardol polyethoxylates (A) and (B) respectively have been prepared by the base-catalysed reaction with ethylene oxide and compared with p-t-nonylphenol polyethoxylate (C).

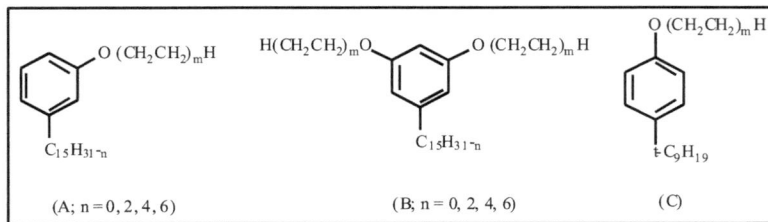

(A; n = 0, 2, 4, 6)                    (B; n = 0, 2, 4, 6)                    (C)

The structures were confirmed by independent synthesis (Appendix, iv Scheme 2 ) and spectral study. In each case, polyethoxylation led to a profile of components in which, m = 1-48. In each profile the component giving the greatest reduction in surface tension was judged to be the most surfactant and was selected for biodegradation studies. Thus, (Appendix, v Fig. (9) shows the variation of surface tension with the number of ethylene oxide groups and the maxima for (A), (B) and (C) [40]. Effective biodegradation of surfactants is an important environmental aspect. Soil bacterial degradation was examined over a month by measurement of the total organic carbon (TOC) in comparison with the reference compound, glucose. As depicted in (Appendix, v Figs. (10a and (10b), cardanol polyethoxylate is substantially degraded, cardol polyethoxylate to a lesser extent and p-t-nonylphenol polyethoxylate only very slightly [41].

**Use of Cardanol Derivatives from Ozonolysis and Reduction**

For some purposes, derivatives of cardanol having a shorter side chain have proved useful, as for example in polymer chemistry and for solvent extraction of metals.

Ozonolysis of cardanol containing unsaturated constituents each with unsaturation at the 8-position, afforded after reduction 8-(3-hydroxyphenyl)octanal, by way of the Criegee mechanism, as depicted in (Appendix, vi Fig. (11) readily separable from associated short chain aldehydes [42]. Conversion to 8-(3-hydroxyphenyl)octanol, 8-(3-hydroxyphenyl) octanoic acid or to 8-(3-hydroxyphenyl)octane, independently synthesised, gave derivatives of value in polymer chemistry.

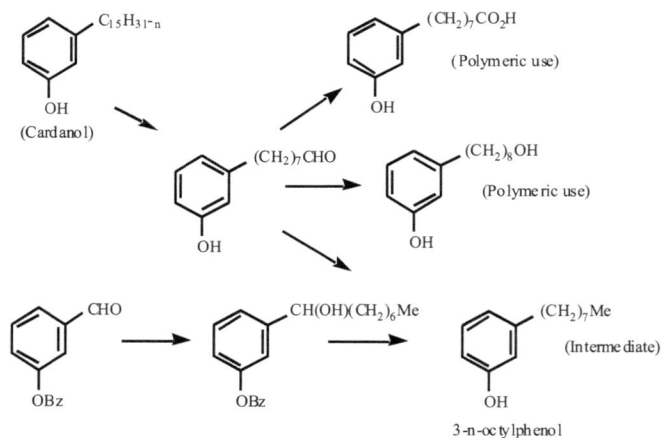

**Fig. (11).** Reaction of Ozonolysis product from Cardanol.

8-(3-Hydroxyphenyl)octane is an intermediate towards 2-formyl-5-n-octylphenol aldoxime, for comparison with the $C_{15}$ analogue from cardanol as solvent extractants for copper(II). The m-$C_{15}$ compound (n = 0,2,4,6) (S) was studied alongside the commercial p-compounds, Acorga reagent (A), Shell ketoxime (B) and the Henkel, phenyl compound (C). The results [43], for the extraction and stripping from kerosene solution for these four compounds are shown in (Appendix, vii Table 1). The m-$C_{15}$ and the m-$C_8$ analogue compared with the Acorga reagent, although of the $C_8$ structural isomers only the o- gave good phase separations at both stages.

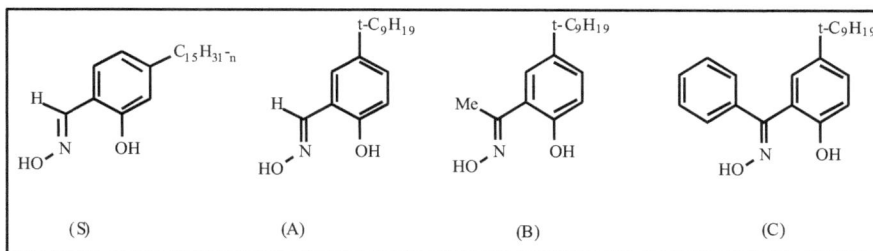

## BIOLOGICAL AND ENVIRONMENTAL APPLICATIONS OF ANACARDIC ACIDS

This review of the three main component phenols of *Anacardium occidentale* turns to the main component in natural CNSL, anacardic acid, which unlike cardanol has found uses mainly in biological/biochemical work, although some technological applications are nevertheless evident.

Unlike technical CNSL, the natural product is not commercially available despite the existence of a number of separating processes.

## SEPARATION OF ANACARDIC ACID FROM NATURAL CNSL

Precipitation of metal salts: The method involves the use of a soluble lead salt to precipitate lead anacardate, filtration to separate cardol and regeneration of anacardic acid by acidification at low temperature [44]. Other metal salts may be used and the use of lead nitrate enables the precipitant to be recycled.

### Chromatography on Alumina

In this method, anacardic acid is the last fraction eluted by acidic eluents [45].

### Cryoscopic Method

Natural CNSL cooled to -65°C in pentane containing a trace of water over 6 h affords anacardic acid [46].

### Phase Separation Method

By phase separation between light petroleum and a diol, anacardic acid enters the hydrocarbon phase due to its intramolecular hydrogen-bonding and cardol, the diol phase giving an excellent separation, which can be conducted continuously [19].

The unsaturated constituents of anacardic acid are separable by the methods for cardanol, although in structure/activity studies synthesis has proved a valuable alternative.

## CHEMICAL APPLICATIONS OF NATURAL CNSL AND OF ANACARDIC ACID

As with cardanol, natural CNSL has been used directly, as well the isolated natural acid, by the above methods [5]. Fig (12) illustrates a number of uses.

Methylation afforded (A), which upon ozonolysis and reduction gave the octanol (B), intramolecular high dilution cyclisation of which yielded the macrocycle (C, $R^1 = H$), an analogue of lasiodiploidin (C, $R^1 = OMe$) [47], a plant growth compound. Polymerisation of the sodium salt of natural CNSL with formaldehyde, in aqueous solution, gave the polymer (D) for the fabrication of particleboard, with avoidance of chlorinated and other organic solvents [48]. Reduction with lithium aluminium hydride of anacardic acid (or of natural CNSL) gave anacardic alcohol of value for the complexation of boric acid [49]. An isomer of the aldoxime formed from cardanol (43), was obtained by the oxidation of anacardic alcohol with pyridinium chlorochromate and oximation to give (F) [50].

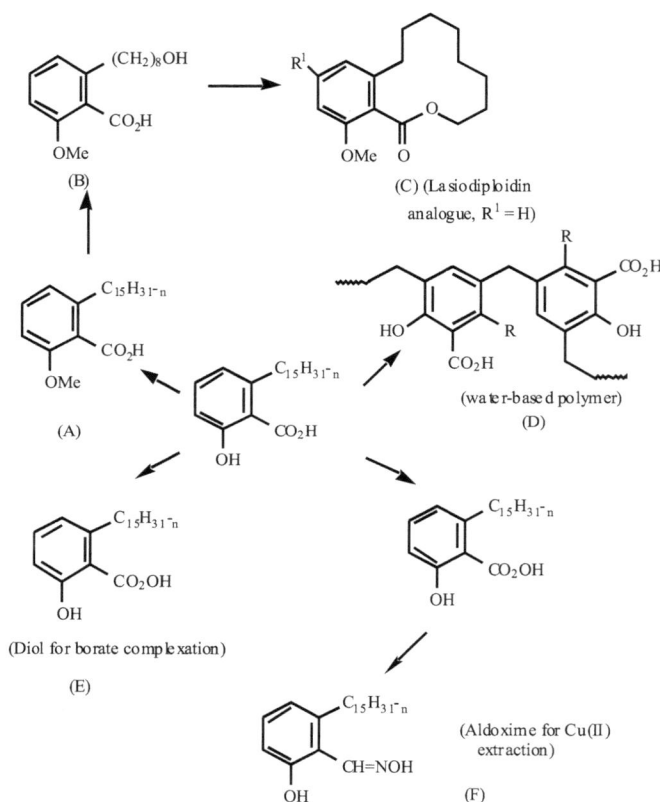

Fig. (12). Some Chemical Applications of Anacardic acid.

## BIOLOGICAL APPLICATIONS OF ANACARDIC ACIDS FROM DIFFERENT SOURCES

Enzyme inhibitory action has been a prominent activity studied with anacardic acids isolated from a variety of sources. Thus, (15:3)-anacardic acid from *Anacardium occidentale* was found to be an effective molluscicide [51] and mixed anacardic acid together with totarol combated methicillin-resistant *staphylococcus aureus* (MRSA) [52]. (15:1), (17:1) and (17:2)-anacardic acids from *Ginkgo biloba* were discovered to be inhibitors of glycerol 3-phosphate dehydrogenase (GPDH) and therefore of potential interest as controllers of obesity [53]. The 8:11:14-triene of the $C_{17}$ anacardic acid from *Spondias mombin* proved to be an inhibitor of penicillinase, the enzyme, which destroys the four-membered ring in penicillin [54]. In cancer studies the $10^1$-monene of the $C_{17}$ anacardic acid in *Schoepfia californica* was found to be an inhibitor of DNA polymerase, which repairs the damage to cancer cells subjected to cancer curing agents [55]. A carbon-based adsorbent material from pistacia shells and rubber tyres has been used in an environmental application to remove mercury and mercury (II) from power house flues [56].

## SYNTHESIS OF ANACARDIC ACIDS

For structure/activity studies availability of the four constituents of anacardic acid is required and synthesis has proved useful to meet this end. (Appendix viii, ix, x, xi, Schemes 3-6) depict the following routes.

The saturated (15:0) member obtained by the reaction of fluoroanisoles [57] and Michael addition [58], respectively. The (15:2) member was synthesised by alkylation of the carbanion from a derivative of 6-methylsalicylic acid [59].

(15:1)-Anacardic acid in 8(Z) form [60] and as the 8(E) isomer [61] has readily been obtained.

(15:3)-Anacardic acid has been synthesised [59], by an alkylation route as illustrated. In many applications the biological properties have proved dependent on the level of unsaturation and the geometrical configuration. The (15:2) dienes in the four isomeric forms have been synthesised [59], by an alkylation route, dependent on the syntheses of the four stereoisomeric tetradecadienols.

## GENETIC SIGNIFICANCE OF ANACARDIC ACIDS

Perhaps the most significant aspect of the chemistry of anacardic acids has been the discovery of the role of the (15:1 and (17:1)-anacardic acids, which occur in *Pelargonium x hortorum*. They are exuded by tall glandular trichromes of the plant and are responsible for its resistance to aphid and spider mite. The expression of a delta$^9$(14:0)-acyl carrier protein fatty acid desaturase gene is necessary for the production of these $C_{15}$ and $C_{17}$-ϖ5 anacardic acids in the geranium [62,63]. The incorporation of this gene into other species opens the possibility for similar resistance in other species

## BIOLOGICAL APPLICATIONS OF CARDOLS

With this last group of phenolic lipids, as with anacardic acids, the main utilisation of cardols, which from the chemical taxonomic view occur widely in many botanical species [6], has occurred in biological studies. The bifunctional nature of cardols alone might also be of interest in polymeric systems and their presence with cardanol in polymer applications of technical CNSL would also involve their reaction in such systems. In recent years research interest has centred on the resorcinolic lipids, which occur in cereal seeds and crops. Thus wheat bran, (triticum), contains 0.4% of $C_{19}$ and $C_{21}$ 5-alkylresorcinols [64] while whole kernels contained a low % of $C_{15}$-$C_{25}$ saturated and monoene constituents [65] together with 2-ketoalkylresorcinols. Rye (*Cereale secale*) contains approximately 1% of $C_{15}$-$C_{25}$ saturated, momene and diene constituents [66]. In barley (*Hordeum distichon*) 12 compounds, $C_{25}$-$C_{31}$ have been isolated [67] and in rice (*Oryza sativa*) from root exudates, a range of shorter chain compounds $C_{13}$-$C_{19}$ compounds [68] have been isolated.

## SYNTHESIS OF CARDOLS

The structures of this range of compounds have been confirmed by the synthesis of saturated, monoene, diene and triene constituents [6,66,69] as illustrated in (Appendix, xii, xiii Schemes **7,8**).

## ROLE OF CARDOLS IN CEREALS CEREAL SEEDS AND IN HUMAN NUTRITION

Although originally thought to be growth inhibitors, it is now recognised that resorcinolic lipids have primarily an antifungal role as secondary metabolites (phytoanticipins) [70], in cereal seeds and plants, while in mature plants, cereal whole grains are beneficial in human nutrition and health. The consumption of whole grain cereals has been linked to a decreased risk of diabetes, obesity, heart disease and some cancers [71]. Wheat and rye are the main sources of alkylresorcinols in the human diet and are absorbed at levels between 33-79%. Nevertheless, to obtain stronger evidence for a link between reduced risk of disease and consumption of whole grain cereal, a biomarker [72,73] would be valuable. Similarly to cholesterol, resorcinolic lipids may prove to be such potential biological markers of health and to this end analysis of these compounds in food products and in body fluids may establish this role.

## ACKNOWLEDGEMENTS

The author thanks K. H. Tam, P. Payne, 3M Research, Tropical Products Institute, Esso Ltd., Borax Ltd., Macphersons Ltd., BP Ltd., Wolfson Industrial Fellowship, John Vine (Peabody Sturtevant), Society of Chemical Industry and SERC.

## REFERENCES

[1]     Tyman, J.H.P. *Non-isoprenoid Long Chain Phenols, Chem. Soc. Rev.*, **1979**, *8*, 499-538.
[2]     Ohler, J. G. Cashew, Communication 71, Department of Agricultural Rsaearch, Royal Tropical Institute, Amsterdam, **1979**, pp. 21.
[3]     Nomisima, The Cashew Economy, Edizioni l'Inchiostroblu, Bologna, Italy,**1994**.
[4]     Tyman, J.H.P., Synthetic and Natural Phenols,Elsevier, Amsterdam, **1979**, ch.13, 465-546.
[5]     Tyman, J.H.P. Chemistry and Biochemistry of Anacardic acids, Recent Research in Lipids, Transworld Research Network, **2001**, *5*, 125-145.
[6]     Kozubek, A.; Tyman,J.H.P. Resorcinolic Lipida, the Natural Non-isoprenoid Phenolic amhiphiles, Chem. Rev., **1999**,*99*, 1-26.
[7]     Kozubek, A.; Tyman, J.H.P. Bioactive Phenolic Lipids, in *Studies in Natural Products Chemistry*, Atta-ur-Rahman, Ed. Elsevier Science, Amsterdam, vol.30, **2004** (in press).
[8]     Schlenk.H.; Gellerman, J.L.; Anderson, W.H. *Lipids*, **1974**, *9*, 722-725.
[9]     Hesk, D.; Craig, R.;Mumma, R.O.Biosynthesis of Anacardic acids in *Pelargonium xhortorum, J. Chem. Ecol.*, **1992**, *18*, 1349.
[10]    Tychopoulos, V.; Tyman, J.H.P. HPLC Studies of thr Thermal and Oxidative Deterioration of Phenolic Lipids, *J. Soc. Food Agric.*, **1990**, *52*, 71-83.
[11]    Hugentobler, H.; Cashew Nut processing Plants, Technical brochure, Buhler-Miag, Uzwil, Switzerland, **1984**.
[12]    Tyman, J.H.P.; Muir, M.;Johnson, R.A.; Rokhgar, R. The Extraction of Natural cashew nutshell liquid from *Anacardium occidentale, J. Am. Oil Chem Soc.*, **1989**, *66*, 553-557.
[13]    Tyman, J. H. P.;Visani, N. The Chemistry of Anacardic Acids, in *Topics in Lipid Research*, Eds. Klein, R. A.; Schmitz, B. *Royal Soc,. Chem.*, **1987**, 115.
[14]    Shobha, S.V.; Ravindranath, B. *J. Food Agric. Chem.*, **1991**, *39*, 2214.
[15]    Arie, K.; Ajiri, M.;Suzuki, S.; Nishimura, M. JPn. 0500979.

[16] Smith, R.L.; Mataluan, R.M.; Setianto, W.B.; Inomata, H.;Arai, K., Separation of cashew nut shell liquid with supercritical cabon dioxide *Bioresource Technology*, **2003**, *88,* 1-7.

[17] Davis, G.L.;Sood,S.K.; Tychopoulos, V.; Tyman. Practical Separations of the Component Phenols in Technical Cashew Nutshell Liquid: Distillation procedures for Cardanol, *J. Chem. Tech.and Biotech.*, **1982**, *323*, 681-690.

[18] Sood, S.K.; Tyman, J.H.P.; Durrani, A.A.; Johnson, R.A.. Practical Liquid Chromatographic Separations of the Phenols in Technical CNSL, *Lipids*, **1986**, *21*, 241-246.

[19] Tyman, J.H.P.; Payne, P.; Bruce, I.E. The Phase Separation of Phenolic Lipid from *Anacardium occidentale, Natural Products Letters*, **1992**, *1*, 117-120.

[20] Patel, M.; Tyman,J.H.P.; Manzara, A. The Purification of Cashew Nutshell Liquid, GB 2066820B, **1981**.

[21] Tyman, J.H.P. Chemical Purification Method, GB2152925A, **1983**.

[22] Kumar, P.P.; Vithayathil, P.J.; Rao, P.V.Subba.; Rao, A..Srinavasa. Process for Isolation of cardanol from technical CNSL, *J. Agric. Food Chem.*, **2002**, *50,* 4705-4708.

[23] Tyman,J.H.P. Quantitative analysis of Natural and Technical CNSL: by TLC, Densitometry and UV Spectrophotometry, *J, Chromatogr.*, **1978**, *166*, 159-172.

[24] Tyman, J.H.P. Quantitative Analysis of the unsaturated Constituents of Phenolic Lipids by TLC/Mass Spectrometry, *J. Chromatogr.*, **1977**, *136*. 289-300.

[25] Tyman, J.H.P. Quantitative Detemination of thr Olefinic Composition of the Component Phenols in *Anacardium occidentale, J.Chromatogr.*, **1975**, *111,* 277- 284 .

[26] Tyman, J.H.P.; Bruce,I.E.; Long, A.; Payne, P. The Preparative HPLC Separation of the Unsaturated Constituents of Phenolic Lipids, *J. Liquid Chromatogr.*, **1990**, *13*, 2103-2110.

[27] Lloyd, H. A.; Denny, C.; Krishna, B. The HPLC separation of Anacardic acid, *J. Liquid Chromatogr.*, **1980**, *3*, 1497.

[28] Naksu, T.; Kubo, I. A recycling technique for larger scale operation, 16th IUPAC Sym.Chem. Nat. Products, Kyoto, Jpn. **1988**, PA87.

[29] Caplin, J; Tyman, J.H. P. The Synthesis of Cardanol Monoene and Diene. *J. Chem. Res.*, **1982**, (S), *34-35*; (M), 0321-0351.

[30] Tyman, J.H.P. The synthesis of Cardanol triene (unpublished work).

[31] Tyman, J.H.P. The Role of Biological Materials in Synthesis, in Studies in Natural Products Chemistry, ed. Atta-ur-Rahman, Elsevier Science, Amsterdam, **1993**, *17*, 601-654.

[32] Tyman, J.H.P. Partial and Semi-synthesis with Biological Raw Materials, in Phytochemical Diversity:asource of New Industrial Products, eds. Wrigley,S.;Hayes, M.;Chrystal, E. **1997**, 195-309, Royal Society of Chemistry, Canbridge.

[33] Horiguchi, K. JP 91 237183.

[34] Gedam, P.H. ; Sampathkumaran, P.S. *Prog. In Org. Coatings*, **1986**, *14*, 115.

[35] Mahusudhan, V.; Ramalingham, T.; Murthy, B.G.K. *Eur. Coatings J.*, **1989**, *6*, 502.

[36] Kokane, S. V. *Paintindia*, **1991**, *41*, 43.

[37] O'Connor, D. *Polym. Mater. Sci, Eng.*, **1990**, *63*, 700.

[38] Sitaraman, B.S.; Chatterjee, P.C. *J. Appl. Polym. Sci.*, **1992**, *37*, 33.

[39] Pillai, C.S.K.; Prasad. V.S.; Sudha, J.D.; Bera, S.C.; Menon, A.R.R. *J. Appl. Polym. Sci.*, **1990**, *41*, 2487.

[40] Tyman, J.H.P. ; Bruce, I.E.. Synthesis and Characterisatioi of Polyethoxylate Surfactants derived from Phenolic Lipids, *J. Surf. and Detergents*, **2003***, 6*, 291- 297.

[41] Tyman, J.H.P.; Bruce, I.E. Surfactants in Lipid Chemistry, ed. Tyman, J.H.P., *Royal Soc. Chem.*, Cambridge, UK, **1992**. J. Surf and Detergents, (7,2004, in press).

[42] Graham, M.B.; Tyman, J.H.P. Ozonisation of the Component Phenols of *Anacardium occidentale* (Cashew), *J. Am. Oil Chem. Soc.*, **2002**, *79,* 725-732.

[43] Tyman, J.H.P. USP 4697038; Tyman, J.H.P.; Iddenten, S.A. (unpublished data).

[44] Stadeler, *Ann. Chim. u Pharm.*, **1847**, *63*, 147.

[45] Tyman, J.H.P, *J.Chem. Soc., Perkin trans 1* , **1973**, 1639-1647; in *Studies in Natural Products Chemistry*, ed. Atta-ur-Rahman, Elsevier, Amsterdam, **1991**, *9*, 313.

[46] Asahi Chemical Industry Co. Ltd., JP 10 259150 (Sept.19, 1998).

[47] dos Santos, M.L.; Magalhaes, G.C. *Quim Nova*, **1993**, *16,* 534

[48] Durrani, A.A.; Hawkes, A.J.; Tymen, J.H.P. PCT 0015761.

[49] Tyman, J.H.P.; Mehet, S.H. *Chem. and Physics of Lipids*, **2003**, *127*, 1771-1791

[50] Lam, S.K.; Tyman, J.H.P. *J.Chem. Soc., Perkin trans I*, **1982**, 1942-1952.

[51] Lloyd, H.A.; Denny, C.; Krishna, B. *Planta Med.*, **1982**, *44*, 175.

[52] Muroi, H.; Kubo, I. *Biosci. Biotechnol. and Biochem.*, **1994**, *58*, 1925

[53] Tsuge, N.; Mikozami, M.; Imai, S.; Shimazu, A.; Seto, H. *J.Antibiot.*, **1992**, *45*, 886.

[54] Coates, N.J.; Gilpin, M.L.; Hird, N.W.; Lewis, D.E. ; Milner, P.H. Abstract 568, 8th IUPAC Symp. *Chem. Nat. Prod.*, Strasbourg,, **1992**.

[55] Chen, J.; Zhang, Y.-H.; Wang, L.-K.; Suchek, S.J.; Snow, A.M.; Hecht, S.M. *Chem. Commun.*, **1998**, 2769.

[56]    Rostam-abadi, M. *Chem. and Ind. (London)*, **2000**, 521.
[57]    Durrani, A.A.; Tyman, J.H.P. *J.Chem. Soc. Perkin trans 1* , **1979**, 2079-2087
[58]    Tyman, J.H.P. ; Visani. N. *J. Chem. Res.*, (S), **1997**, 14-15; (M), 0241-0251.
[59]    Tyman, J.H.P.; Visani, N. *Chem. and Physics of Lipids*, **1997**, *85*, 157-174.
[60]    Tyman, J.H.P. *J. Org. Chem.*, **1976**, *41*, 894 and suppl.
[61]    Green, I.R.; Tocoli, F.E. *Synth. Commun.*, **2002**, 947-957.
[62]    Craig, R.; Medford, J.L.; Mumma, R.O.; Cox-Foster, D.L.; Schultz, D. USP 5856157 (Jan. 5 **1999**).
[63]    Schultz, D.J.; Cahoon, E.; Shanklin, J.; Craig, R.; Cox-Foster, D.; Mumma, R.O.; Medford, R.O. *Proc.Natl. Acad. Sci.*, **1996**, *93*, 8771.
[64]    Wenkert, E.; Loeser, E.-M.; Mahapatra, S.N.; Schenker, F.; Wilson, E.M. *J. Org. Chem.*, **1964**, *29*, 435.
[65]    Ross, A.B.; Shepherd, M.B.; Schupphaus, M.; Sinclair, V.; Alfaro, B.; Kamal- Eldin, A,; Aman, P. *J. Agric. Food Chem.*, **2003**, *51*, 4111-4118.
[66]    Tyman, J.H.P.; Kozubek, A. *Chem. and Physics of Lipids*, **1995**,*79,* 29-36.
[67]    Briggs, D.E. *Phytochemistry*, **1974**, *13*, 987-996.
[68]    Bouillant, M.I.; Jacoud, C.; Zanela, I.; Favre-Bonvin, J.; Baily, R. *Phytochemistry*, **1994**, *35*, 769-771.
[69]    Baylis, C.J.; Odle, S.W.D.; Tyman, J.H.P. *J. Chem. Soc., Perkin Trans I*, **1981,** 132-141.
[70]    Suzuki, S.;Yamaguchi, I. *Nippon Noyaku Gakkaishi*, **1998**, *23*, 316-321.
[71]    Slavin, J.L.; Jacobs, D.; Marquart, Wiener, K. *J. Am. Dietetics Assocn.*, **2001**, *101*, 780-785.
[72]    Branca, F.; Hanley, A.B.; Pool-Zobel, B.; Verhagen, H. *Brit. J. of Nutrition*, **2001**, *85*, 885-892.
[73]    Ross, A.B.; Kamal-Eldin, A, *Nutrition Reviews*, **2004**, *62*, 81-95.

# Development of Pharmaceuticals from Indonesian Natural Resources, Genetically Engineered Microbes and Diversification of Palm Oil Products

Ignatius Suharto[1,*] and Leonardus B.S. Kardono[2]

*[1]Faculty of Industrial Technology, Catholic University of Parahyangan (Unpar), Jl Ciumbuleuit 94-96, Bandung 40141, Indonesia, [2]Research Center for Chemistry, Indonesian Institute of Sciences (LIPI), Kawasan PUSPIPTEK, Serpong 15314, Indonesia*

**Abstract:** The **objective** of this paper is to give an overview on natural resources in terms of renewable resources as well as non-renewable resources for the development of new pharmaceuticals, chemical and food products, the roles of microbial cells in solid substrate fermentation and submerged fermentation. **The benefit** of this paper is to present current information on the role of traditional and modern biotechnology.

**The methods** used, namely traditional and modern biotechnology and chemical synthesis are developed and implemented to produce pharmaceutical and chemical products. **Results** can be shown that microorganisms have been engineered to commercially produce such substances as the hormone insulin, the virus fighting compound interferon, and a new vaccine against foot-and-mouth disease. Traditional fermentation technology has been done to produce low cost protein food using natural product as a substrate and the development of palm oil derived products for food, oleo chemicals, bio-plastic, bio-diesel and lubricants, respectively.

**Key Words:** Natural resources, traditional and modern biotechnology, chemical synthesis, palm edible oils derived products.

## INTRODUCTION

Indonesia has a number of natural resources in terms of renewable resources and non-renewable resources, it can be said that those two resources can be used as raw material for the production of chemical and biotechnological products. Therefore, chemical synthesis and development of synthetic methodologies and biotechnological approaches have made number of contributions to the industrial sector growth in Indonesia as well as in other developing countries.

**Renewable Resources** such as ginger, *curcuma xanthohorrohiza, curcuma domestica, kaempferia galanga, alpina galanga, animirta occulenes, eucalyptus, cinchona pubescens,* can be used to produce traditional medicines and rice, corn, cassava, sweet potato, peanut, sugar cane, palm oils, coconut, banana, coffee, cacao bean, oils seed such as rice bran, soybean oils, coconut oil, rice bran oils for foods and also, water hyacinth, mushroom, rubber, and other agricultural wastes and agricultural-by products can be used as a substrate in the fermentation process for foods, animal feed, and chemicals product. Those substrate

---

*Corresponding author: Tel/ Fax: 62. 22. 2032700; E-mail: suharto@bdg.centrin.net.id

can acts as carbohydrates that not only contribute carbon atom, but serve as source of energy for microbial growth. Nitrogen sources, fats, antifoaming agent, mineral and trace elements, precursor and special materials can be supplied by adding those elements to the fermentation medium.

**Non–renewable Resources** such as coal, natural gas, Liquified Petroleum Gases (LPG), industrial gases, carbon black, lampblack, activated carbon, natural graphite, lime, gypsum, salt, aluminum, magnesium, phosphate rock, potassium, sulfur, Iodine, iron and steel, can be used for raw material in chemical processing using chemical synthesis approaches. Therefore, clean technology and eco-technology as well as biotechnological approaches can be used as a platform for the strategic application of biotechnology and chemical synthesis to produce industrial chemicals products.

## DEVELOPMENT OF PHARMACEUTICALS FROM INDONESIAN NATURAL PRODUCTS

Chemical synthesis and purification processes on pharmaceutical product has been manufactured, but genetic engineering makes it possible to manufacture a host, a new molecules to produce new pharmaceutical product. The production of penicillin rose slowly at first, but after the second world war huge quantities were coming out of giant vat. It has been estimated that the development of new drug costs about US $ 300 million and takes somewhere between 7 and 10 years from initiation of pre-clinical development to first marketing. It is a very complex process and high-risk business requiring a great effort of coordination and communication between a wide range of different disciplines. Despite such a number of difficulties, pharmaceutical industries have been striven to introduce novel entities into the world market with the anticipation of making a profit [1]. There are four main approaches for medicinal chemists in developing new pharmaceuticals according to sources for new drug leads. These are from natural products, from drug in use, from synthetic chemicals, and from modern rational approach to drug design. Natural products provide the oldest and the most reliable source of new pharmaceuticals. Natural selection during evolution, and competition between the species, has produced powerful biologically active natural products that can serve as chemical leads. Penicillin, ginkolides and taxol are good examples of pharmaceuticals from natural products. Some examples of clinically used natural products originated from plants are showed in Table 1. They are not only excellent drugs but also important chemical leads for the drug of enhanced activity and improved safety [1,2].

## STEPS ON DEVELOPMENT OF PHARMACEUTICALS FROM NATURAL PRODUCTS

The development of new pharmaceuticals from natural products might follow the following patterns: screening of natural products for biological activity, isolation and purification of the active component, determination of chemical structure, settlement of structure-activity relationships (SARs), synthesis of analogs, structure modification, collection of information on the protein with which the drug interact, design-synthesis of novel drug structures and process improvement through genetically engineered microbes. Screening of natural products from plant and microbial sources was triggered by the discovery of penicillin, and it continues today as the never-ending quest to find new lead compounds. Search on bioactive compounds from endophytic microbes was accelerated by the possibility of anticancer taxol production through fermentation of *Taxomyces andreanae* an endophytic fungi isolated from the inner bark of *Taxus brevifolia*, plant producing taxol [1,3].

**Table 1. Clinically Used Natural Products Originated from Plants [1].**

| ACTION | PLANTS | ACTIVE COMPONENT |
|---|---|---|
| Anti cancer agents | *Catharanthus roseus* | Vindesine |
| | | Vinblastine |
| | | Vincristine |
| | *Podophyllum peltatum* | Teniposide |
| | | Etoposide |
| | *Taxus brevifolia* | Taxol |
| | *Ochrosia elliptica* | Ellipticine |
| | *Camptotheca acuminata* | Camptothecin |
| | *Cephalotaxus harringtonia* | Homoharringtonine |
| | *Colchicum atumnale* | Colchicines |
| Cardiovascular agents | *Digitalis purpurea* | Digitoxin |
| Antagonists of platelet-activating factor (PAF) | *Ginko biloba* | Ginkogolides |
| | *Piper futokadsura* | Kadsurenone |
| | *Bursera microphylla* | Burseran |
| | *Magnolia salicinale* | Magnosalicine |
| Bronchospasmic | *Ephedra sinensis* | Ephedrine |
| Anti-inflammatory | *Ananas comosus* | Bromelain |
| Anticholinestrase | *Physostigma vanesosum* | Physostigmine |
| Antimalaria | *Cinchona pubescens* | Quinine |
| | | Oquine |
| | | Quinidine |
| | *Brucea japonica* | Bruceins |
| | | Brusatol |
| | *Simarouba amara* | Glaucarubinone |
| | *Artemisia annua* | Artemisinin |
| | | Artemether |
| Analgesics | *Papaver somniverum* | Codeine |
| | | Reserpine |
| Andrenergic neuron blocking agents | *Rauvolfia serpentina* | Reserpine |

(Table 1. Contd....)

| ACTION | PLANTS | ACTIVE COMPONENT |
|---|---|---|
| Central nervous system stimulants | *Camelia sinensis* | Caffeine |
|  |  | Theophylline |
| Cholinergic agonist | *Pilocarpus joborandi* | Pilocarpin |
| Hypertension | *Veratrum viride* | Cryptenamine |

The ease with which the active component can be isolated and purified depends largely on the structure, stability and quantity of the compound. Structure determination should have been major hurdle to overcome in the past. The introduction of new analytical methods such as NMR, IR, mass spectrometry made the determination of structures of compounds remarkably easy. X-ray crystallography must have provided an invisible tool for structure determination. Once the structure of biologically active compound is known, medicinal chemists synthesize a selected number of slightly modified compounds to study the structure activity relationships, where they determine which parts of molecule are important in exhibiting activity. Then they synthesize analogs that still contain those essential parts giving activity to the compound. these works are to maximize activity, to minimize side effects, and to provide easy and efficient administration to the patient. The strategies of synthesizing analogs include variation of constituents, extension of the structure, chain extension/contraction, ring expansion/contraction, ring variation, replacement of stereo-centers, structure simplification, and structure rigidification. When the organic chemists are not able to modify the structures using the existing knowledge of organic synthesis, the work then will be take over by microbes or other living organisms through microbial transformation or genetically engineered microbial processes. From the activity data of these analogs, medicinal chemists obtain important information on protein with which the drug interacts. The information comprises the basis of rational design of drugs having novel chemical structures [1,4].

Modern concepts, such as computer-aided drug design, combinatorial chemistry, high-throughput screening and molecular biology has provided medicinal chemists powerful tools for the development of new pharmaceuticals. However, no other source than the naturally occurring biologically active substance provides us more concrete and promising starting points toward novel drugs of high potency and efficacy. Specially in Indonesia, rich in biodiversity and folk medicines, development of natural products in an area where they can have international competitiveness.

## SOME PHARMACEUTICALS DEVELOPED FROM MICROBE

Among pharmaceuticals being developed from genetically engineered microbes, antibiotics are the most frequent. Antibiotics differ widely in their chemical structure. Antibiotics can be classified into a relatively few major groups based on their chemical structure. Usually they are classified as the β-Lactam, Macrolides, Aminoglycosides, Tetracyclines, Polypeptide, Polyenes, and Other Antibiotics. The β-lactam category includes the penicillins, monobactams, cephalosporins, and carbapenems. All contain a characteristic four-membered ring, the β-lactam ring, which is composed of three carbon atoms and one nitrogen atom [5].

There are many different penicillins, but all have a core structure called *6-aminopenicillanic acid*. The differences among the various penicillins are due to differences in the side chains (portions of the molecule other than the core). Penicillins that are produced by microorganisms are called *natural penicillins*. These antibiotics are produced by certain species of molds in the genus *Penicillium*. The two most important ones are *penicillin G* and *penicillin V*. Semisynthetic Penicillins are from the core compound 6-aminopenicillanic acid, which can be produced in quantity by molds through fermentation culturing technique. Chemists have been able to add various chemical side chains to this core compound, thus creating new kinds of penicillins that are not found in nature. These penicillins are called semisynthetic penicillins, and some have advantages over natural penicillins. For instance, one of the first semisynthetic penicillin to be produced for clinical use was *phenethicillin,* which is more readily absorbed from the intestine into the body than is natural penicillin V. *Pseudomonas aeruginosa*, a frequent cause of wound and burn infections, is resistant to natural penicillins but can be inhibited by several semisynthetic penicillins [5].

Inactivation of Penicillins: Natural penicillins can be destroyed by enzymes called *penicillinases*. These enzymes destroy the β-lactam ring in the core structure of penicillins, and for this reason they are also called β-*lactamases*. Penicillinases are produced by many different bacteria including staphylococci and infections caused by these bacteria are resistant to treatment with natural penicillins. However, some semisynthetic penicillins have the advantage of being resistant to attack by penicillinases. One example is *methicillin*, which is often used to treat "penicillin-resistant" staphylococcal infections [5].

Some groups of Inhibitors of Penicillinases are also having a β-lactam ring. *Clavulanic acid* is a naturally occurring β-lactam compound produced by *Streptomyces clavuligerus*. It has relatively low antibacterial activity, but it is a potent inhibitor of penicillinases, as is *sulbactam*, a semisynthetic compound that has similar characteristic. Currently, there are commercially available products which contain clavulanic acid or sulbactam in combination with the antibiotics ampicillin, amoxicillin, or ticarcillin. These products allow the antibiotics in them to be effective against microorganisms that ordinarily would be resistant because of their ability to make penicillinases. Another class of β-lactam antibiotics called monobactams, was originally discovered to be produced by a Gram-negative bacterium, *Chromobacterium violaceum*. One of the monobactams, *aztreonam*, is now made synthetically and is active against a wide variety of aerobic Gram-negative bacteria. Aztreonam has the added advantage of not being inactivated by penicillinases or by other enzymes such as cephalosporinases [5].

Cephalosporins differ from penicillins in the structure of their core compound, 7-aminocephalosporanic acid. They are produced by species of marine fungi belonging to the genus Cephalosporium (now reclassified as Acremonium). Since the mid-1960s, when this group of antibiotics came into use, pharmaceutical companies have developed many new cephalosporins, each with new and more desirable characteristics for chemotherapy. Cephalosporins are grouped as "first-generation", "second-generation" and "third-generation" products. Second-generation cephalosporins (e. g., cefamandole, cefoxitin, and cefuroxime) and third-generation cephalosporins (e. g., cefotaxime, cefoperazone, ceftriaxone) have greater antimicrobial activity, including a broader spectrum of activity, and are much more resistant to enzymatic inactivation than are the first-generation products [5].

Carbapenems, or thienamycins, are produced by *Streptomyces cattleya*. *Imipenem*, a semisynthetic carbapenem, is produced by chemical modification of thienamycin. Imipenem has a very wide spectrum of antibacterial activity and inhibits most aerobic and anaerobic Gram-positive and Gram-negative bacteria, including those which produce β-lactamases. The macrolide category includes the well-known antibiotic *erythromycin,* which consists of a large lactone ring linked with aminoacid. Erythromycin is produced by a strain of

*Streptomyces erythreus*, which was originally isolated from soil collected in the Phillipines. The erythromycins are not destroyed by penicilinase, it is frequently used as an alternative to penicilin therapy [5].

Some of the Aminoglycosides antibiotics are Streptomycin, Neomycin. Chemically, aminoglycosides consist of amino sugars and a ring structure called aminocyclitol. Streptomycin is produced by the soil bacterium *Streptomyces griseus*. Neomycin is the most toxic aminoglycoside group. Neomycin is a component of some topical preparations. The tetracyclines include chlortetracycline, oxytetracycline, tetracycline, doxycycline, and minocycline. They all have in common a chemical structure called naphthalene ring; these antibiotics are produced by *streptomyces*; differences in the chemical groups attached to the naphalene ring. Bacitracin and the Polymyxins are included among the polypeptide antibiotics. They and the other members of this group are characterized chemically by their consisting of a chain of amino acids. Both bacitracin and the polymyxins produced bacteria in the genus of *Bacillus*. The Polyene compound is the one that contains three or more double covalent bonds which join carbon atoms. The group includes Nystatin and Amphotericin B, produced by the bacterium *Streptomyces noursei* and *Streptomyces nodosus*, respectively [5].

## GENETICALLY ENGINEERED MICROBE FOR NATURAL PRODUCTS DRUG DEVELOPMENT

Since the discovery of recombinant DNA technology in 1973, scientists have developed techniques making it possible to move genes from one cell type to another (for example, from plants and mammals to bacteria). The future of genetic engineering is considered almost unlimited in its commercial applications. It already has solved some major research problems. For instance, rather than rely on extraction of limited quantities of a valuable compound from normal plant and animal tissue, a gene that codes for production of the compound can be taken from a plant or animal cell and placed into a bacterial cell. The bacterial cell may then synthesize unlimited quantities of the gene product. As a specific example, if you place copies of the human gene coding for the hormone insulin into a cell of the bacterium *Escherichia coli*, the bacterium and its progeny can make the gene product, human insulin. The insulin is then extracted from the bacterial cultures. This industrial process produces the human form of insulin-of particular importance because a certain proportion of human diabetics must use human insulin, rather than the commonly available bovine insulin, because their immune systems react against the "foreign" bovine insulin [5].

Animal and plant cells usually cannot be cultured for the production of medicinally useful compounds such as insulin. For instance, the tissue cells that make insulin in normal humans lose their ability to produce this hormone when they are isolated and grown in the laboratory. Moreover, the cultivation of tissue cells in the laboratory is expensive and requires highly enriched complex media. The use of microorganisms to produce medicinally important compounds avoids many of the problems associated with obtaining them from higher organisms. Bacteria carrying the human insulin gene can be grown indefinitely and thus will produce human insulin indefinitely [5].

In 1974, scientists predicted that it would take from 5 to 10 years to place the human gene for insulin into a bacterium. However, it was done successfully within 1 year, and similar success with the gene for interferon was attained within 2 years. Today, the microbial production of human insulin, as well as human and bovine growth hormones, vaccines against hepatitis and foot-and-mouth disease, and certain amino acids, has moved from research-and-development laboratories through pilot plants to industrial production. In 1982, the Eli Lilly Company announced that it had approval from the Governments of Great

Britain and the United States for the sale of human insulin produced by genetic engineering (the genetically engineered microorganism that produced the human insulin was developed by Genentech, Inc., a San Fransisco based biotechnology firm). Thus molecular biology moved from the discovery of a promising research method to the marketing of an important health care product in less than a decade. It is important to recognize, however, that not all bioengineered products move this quickly from research to application. Requirements by various governmental agencies must first be met, and this can take considerable time and can cost millions of dollars [5].

## SOME RESEARCH ACTIVITIES ON DEVELOPING PHARMACEUTICALS FROM GENETICALLY ENGINEERED MICROBES

Systematic exploration of biological catalysts from unexplored realms of microbes to improve the performance of biocatalysts and new biochemical processes. This activity includes Collection and selection of enzymes producing microorganisms from natural habitats, including thermophilic organisms; Determination of optimum condition for enzyme production through Solid State Fermentation technique; Down stream processing of enzyme as products; Studies on cell and enzyme immobilization techniques; Scale up and cost evaluation for the enzyme production and its Application of the carbohydrate and protein converting enzymes for industrial processes. Significant results has been achieved in production of alpha amylase from *Aspergillus oryzae*, glucoamilase from *Rhizopus oryzae*, xylanase, dextranase, laccase from white rot fungi and Production of protease developed from tempe inoculum and papaya latex (*Carica papaya*), peroxidase from horseradish and long white radish [6]. Gen manipulation on amylase production on *Bacillus licheniformis* has been conducted. The first step of cloning is DNA chromosome isolation in single cell of *B. licheniformis*. The gen of α amylase isolated from DNA *B. licheniformis* chromosome was amplified and cloned using cloning vector of p-GemT and host cell of *E. coli* DH5α. Insertion confirmation of α-amylase gen was conducted by determination of its nucleotide sequence. Over expression was performed by recombination of α-amylase gen into expression vector PT77, expressed in *E. coli* BL21 cells.

A study of development of taxol derivates from *Taxus sumatrana* and its endophitic microbes was carried out. Evaluation of taxol contents on endophytic fungi isolated by Dr. Triadi Basuki, from inner bark of *Taxus sumatrana* has been completed. Taxol constituents in the methanol-, chloroform-, ethyl acetate- and water-soluble extracts have been evaluated using Competitive Inhibition Enzyme Immunoassay (CIEIA) and Liquid Chromatography Mass Spectrometry (LC-MS). Moreover, isolation of Baccatin III as starting materials for taxol production was performed. The Baccatin III then will be converted to the anticancer taxol. This year a program on conservation of *Taxus sumatrana* will be conducted. About 100 seedlings of *Taxus sumatrana* from Cibodas Botanical garden, will be cultivated in Arjuna Arboretum, East Java [7,8]. A number of Indonesian soil microbes have been screened for their potential antibiotic activities. A bacterium *Phanerochaeta* sp. was fermented and selected for searching the antibiotic. Two Phenazin antibiotics were isolated, and its derivatives were synthesized for more potent and saver drug candidates [9].

## THE IMPORTANCE OF DEVELOPMENT OF DIVERSIFICATION OF PALM OILSPRODUCTS IN INDONESIA

Commercial palm oil plantation in Indonesia was started with 2000 seedling palm tree in Aceh, North Sumatra in 1911. Palm oil plantation is developing in Indonesia and it was up to 2. 9 million hectares in 1999, and the crude palm oil (CPO) production about 5. 9 million tons. Palm oil commodity becomes the first priority of plantation in Indonesia due to its economic contribution to the country and regional development. To improve utilization of palm oil, many efforts need to be done to solve the current problems and to increase value-added of palm oil derive products. Palm oil tree industry in general has potential to increase government income with various palm oil products, palm oil kernel, shell, fiber and empty fruit bunch. World demand on palm oil is predicted to increase from currently 20. 2 million ton per year to 40 million ton per year in 2020. Whereas in year 2010, it is predicted that Indonesia will be the largest producer of palm oil [10].

Palm oil is competitive enough when compared to other vegetable oils because of its high productivity per ha, reliable enough to climate changes, not proven to increase the cholesterol level, moreover it contains b-carotene as pro-vitamin A. Furthermore, usage of bio-diesel in Europe and America also push Indonesia to improve palm oil down stream processing of palm oil technology. In the future, it is predicted that palm oil demand for food and non-food product will keep on increasing.

National palm oil production that is consumed locally is about 54% of total production. Palm oil is mostly used for raw material of cooking oil, margarine and other oleofood products, whereas the rest is used for oleochemistry raw material. Advantages of palm oil when compare to other vegetable oil are low production cost, well-balanced between saturated and non-saturated fatty acid, containing minor components that have health value, such as, beta-carotene, tocopherol, tocotrienol. Besides, comparing petrochemical products, oleochemical products are biodegradabel and renewable. Oleochemical products that have potential are basic oleochemical such as fatty acid, methyl ester, fatty alcohol, fatty amine and glicerol. Fatty acid is a basic product which is widely used [11].

Palm oil and palm oil cernel can be processed for various down stream products for food as well as non food/oleochemicals.

## PALM OIL FOOD INDUSTRY

Generally, for food product, CPO are fractionated to become solid fraction (stearin) and liquid fraction (olein) that can be used for cooking oil. Cooking oil is food product that mostly used CPO production in Indonesia. With population more than 200 million people and oil consumption per capita of 15 kg/capita per year, we need more than 3 million tons of cooking oil per year [11].

The problem is arisen when the cooking oils were exported to cold climate countries because the cooking oils become cloudy. This is due to low iodine number of the cooking oil. To overcome this problem, cook oil with higher iodine number through multi fractionation process. Palm oil contains beta-carotene as the source of pro-vitamin A. Food product from palm oil known as red cooking oil is an oil with high carotene content about 500 ppm. This kind of oil has higher nutrition compared to golden color oil. Because caroten content is easily degraded by high temperature, usually red cooking oil is used for cooking mix that is boiled and not used for frying.

Palm oil modification product could also be conducted by adding omega-3 fatty acid. This product is called PALMEGA (palm oil rich omega-3 fatty acid). The n-3 fatty acid is from fish oil incorporated to palm oil gliceride through enzymatic process. Omeg-3 fatty acid (*eicosapentaenoic acid*) and DHA (*docosahexaenoic acid)* are clinically proven and can prevent cardiovascular disease (*atherosclerosis and coronary disease*), and has antitumor activity and anti-inflammation. This product hopefully can overcome the horrible oil fish smell product constraint as omega-3 fatty acid raw material source for food.

Palm shortening as one of food product from palm oil can be used as replacement of shortening that usually form animal fat. Shortening used as a food product from palm oil can be used as a substitute for shortening materials made of animal fat. Shortening mainly is used for food products based on flour, such as dried and wet cookies. Application of animal food for shortening is decreasing due to its negative effect, such as cholesterol consumption and religious reason (halal and haram food) [12].

## PALM OLEOCHEMICAL INDUSTRY

In Indonesia, oleochemical raw materials that will have increasing supply are both for crude palm oil (CPO) and palm kernel oil (PKO). Other oleochemicals are available such as tallow, and coconut oil. The development of CPO and PKO is showed on Table 2.

**Table 2.  Consumption of Several Oils for Oleochemical Raw Materials [10].**

| Sources | Consumption (thousand Tons) | | | | | | |
|---|---|---|---|---|---|---|---|
| | 1950 | 1960 | 1970 | 1980 | 1990 | 1995 | 2000 |
| Soybean oil | 2. 100 | 4. 000 | 6. 100 | 12. 200 | 16. 100 | 18. 200 | 21. 000 |
| Coconut oil | 1. 900 | 2. 100 | 2. 200 | 3. 300 | 3. 100 | 3. 800 | 4. 200 |
| CPO | 900 | 1. 100 | 1. 700 | 5. 000 | 10. 800 | 11. 113 | 13. 245 |
| PKO | 400 | 400 | 400 | 700 | 1. 400 | 1. 424 | 1. 542 |
| Tallow | 2. 200 | 3. 600 | 4. 400 | 6. 000 | 6. 600 | 7. 100 | 7. 000 |
| Others | 16. 100 | 20. 900 | 25. 300 | 25. 300 | 41. 200 | 35. 200 | 50. 000 |
| Total | 23. 600 | 32. 100 | 40. 100 | 56. 800 | 79. 200 | 76. 837 | 96. 987 |

Oleochemical products in general are divided into basic oleochemicals and downstream processed products. Basic oleochemicals are fatty acid, fatty ester, fatty alcohol, fatty amine, and gliserol. Downstream process products are oleo palm derivatives such as, detergent, cleaning agent, surfactant, cosmetics, plasticizer for plastics, feed, etc.

Fatty acid is an oleochemical product required for many applications. It is a starting material for production of palm oil derivatives, such as fatty ester, fatty alcohol and fatty amines. Fatty acids can be made by splitting of CPO or PKO at high temperature and high pressure. Then palm oil fatty acid is distilled or fractionated to get pure fatty acid. Other products such as glicerols are applied as other processes. Fatty esters are downstream products applied mainly as surfactants. Further more, fatty esters can be applied as fuel materials, such as for bio-diesel as well as for plasticizer. Several surfactants are prepared by Research Center for Chemistry, Indonesian Institute of Sciences, such as gliserol monooleic (GMO), gliserol monostearic (GMS), sorbitol monostearic, sorbitol monooleic, isopropyl lauric, isopropyl palmitic, [12]. The second oleochemical products are fatty alcohol. Large portion of fatty alcohol are converted into their derivatives, such as fatty alcohol sulphate (FAS), fatty alcohol ethoxylic (FAE) and fatty alcohol ethoxy sulfate (FAES). Fatty alcohols are applied for production of nonionic and anionic surfactants. Surfactant products such as sodium lauril sulphate are applied for foaming agent for tooth paste, shampoo or other cosmetics. Fatty amines are palm oil derivatives for production of cationic surfactants. The main products are quarternary ammonium such as distearyl dimethyl ammonium, which are applied for textile softener, hair conditioners and baby shampoo. Although the production of quartenary ammonium is starting to be developed in Indonesia, however, so far none of the commercial products are developed from CPO or PKO [13].

## BIODEGRADABLE PLASTICIZER (BIOPLASTIC)

Plasticizer is a high boiling point organic compound or low melting point of solid compound having a softening function. When it is added to hard or rigid resin, such as rubber, poly vinyl chloride (PVC) plastic, polyvinyl intermolecular strength accumulation in long chain bond will be decreasing so that it becomes elastic and flexible soften, and the elongation increases. Most of the plasticizers are derived from petroleum, such as dioctyl phthalat (DOP), dioctyl phthalat (DOP) or diethylhexyl phthalat (DEHP). However, the application of DOP as PVC for food and medical products become questionable in recent days.

Efforts to develop plasticizer from palm oil has been started since early of 1990, however, palm oil plasticizers are more expensive compare to those of petroleum (DOP). Several plasticizers developed from palm oils are palm oil esters, diesters or epoxides [12 ].

## BIODIESEL LUBRICANT FROM PALM OILS

Biodiesel as an alternative fuel is a renewable energy source. Many researches have been conducted on palm oil for biodiesels. One of the advantages of biodiesel is no that sulfuric compound content and oxygen content is used up to 11%, so that the biodiesel becomes more environment friendly. Biodiesel from palm oil can be produced by using trans-esterification method from crude palm oil with methanol using acidic or basic catalysts. Nowadays, most lubricants are derived from petroleum, therefore the sources are not renewable. Lubricants from vegetable oils have been known for long time. These lubricants can be derived from vegetable oils, such as canola, rapeseed, palm oils and other vegetable oils. Lubricant from palm oil can be synthesized from esterification of fatty acid with various alcohols. Formulating those esters with various additives make then lubricants for various applications [14].

## TRADITIONAL FERMENTED FOODS

Solid substrate and submerged fermentation of renewable resources for food is a well-known process in developing countries and in Indonesia in order to produce foods such as soy sauce, tempe, fish sauce, shrimp paste, fermented shrimp, soybean paste(tauco), soybean cake, fermented rice, fermented durian, rice wine, vinegar, fermented cassava (tape).

The technological problems of solid substrate and submerged fermentation could be derived from substrate, water content, temperature, relative humidity, oxygen concentration, pH values, and inoculum. Traditional fermented food has been done by small and medium scale food industries so that there is no assurance of contamination in a substrate as a source of carbon for energy.

The problem of contamination occurs not only during the fermentation process but also during the handling and preparation of raw materials as well as in the field production area. The problem in traditional fermented food is to use a standardized inoculum using mixed cultures in order to get a stabilized population. A strict sanitation implementation in small and medium scale food industries is a must in order to prevent contamination must be done.

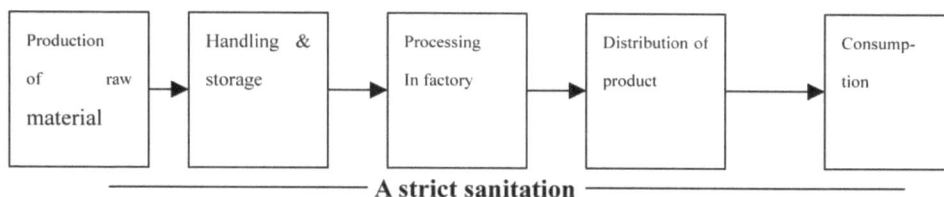

Fig. (1). A strict sanitation for preventing contamination in small and medium scale food industries.

## FUTURE PROSPECT IN INDONESIA

Indonesia is a rich country of biodiversity. However, in the global era, the richness of biodiversity is not the determination of prosperity of the people. The knowledge about how to develop biodiversity is more important. Development of pharmaceuticals from natural products is important and a hot area for Indonesian researchers. Techniques in new pharmaceuticals through genetically engineered microbes have a very good prospect for their development in Indonesia. Palm oil derived products in Indonesia are important for Indonesian industry development. The palm oil can be developed for food, oleochemicals, biodegradable plasticizers, biodiesel and lubricant industries. Palm oil may have potency for the development of Indonesian pharmaceuticals specially for intermediate products, pharmaceuticals and cosmetics supporting agents, such as surfactants, humidifiers, lubricants, and others.

## REFERENCES

[1]     Kim, Y. *How to Develop New Pharmaceuticals from Natural Products*, Proceeding National Seminar on Indonesian Medicinal Plants XVII, Bandung 28-30 March 2000, Research Center for Chemistry, **2001**, 600 pp.

[2]     Colegate, S. M. and Molyneux, R. J. *Bioactive Natural Products: Detection, Isolation and Strutural Determination*, CRC Press, Boca Racon, **1993**, 528 pp.

[3]     Borris, R. P. and Gould, S. J. *Pure Appl.. Chem.* **1998**, *70*, 1-9.

[4]     Kardono, L. B. S. *Research and Development on Bioactive Potential for Pharmaceuticals from Tropical Rain Forest Plants*, Indonesian Traditional Medicines, Endemic and Endophytic Microbes, Paper Presented at National Symposium on NaturalProducts Chemistry XIII, Bandung, 18-19 February, **2002** (**2003**).

[5]     Pelczar, M. J., Chan, E. C. S. and Krieg, N. R. *Microbiology: Concepts and Applications,* Mac Graw-Hill, Inc., New York, **1993**, 897 pp.

[6]     Pujiraharti, S., L. Z. Udin dan T. A. Budiwati. **2002**. Mutasi kapang Rhizopus Oryzae L16 dengan radiasi sinar UV untuk produksi Glukoamilase, Buletin IPT, **2002**, II, 20-25.

[7]     Basuki, T., Kardono, L. B. S., Wahyuni, W. T., Dewi, R. T. and Tachibana. S. **2002**. *Taxol Producing Endophytic Fungi of Taxus sumatrana (Miquel) Laubenfels from Cibodas Botanical Gardent*, West Java, Proc. National Seminar on Chemistry and Development, Ed. Pujiyono, *et al.,* National Chemistry Network, Yogyakarta, March 15-16, (**2002**).

[8]     Puspa Dewi, T. Basuki, R. Triana Dewi, L. B. S. Kardono and S. Tachibana. *LC-MS evaluation of taxol content from T. sumatrana extractives*, Proceeding of The Fourth International Wood Science Symposium, 2-5 September, Serpong, Indonesia (**2002**).

[9]     Hanafi, M., Kardono, L.B.S., Linar Z. Uddin, Tjandrawati and Roy Heru Trisnamurti. *Novel phenolic lactam antibiotics and their analogs from Indonesian soil microbes*, Indonesian Patent Office Application, April (**2002**).

[10]    Directorate General of Horticulture, Ministry of Agriculture, *Indonesian Statistics on Indonesian Palm Oil Plantation*, Ministry of Agriculture, Jakarta. **2000**, 52 p.

[11]    ICBS. *Study on Indonesian Palm Oil Plantation and Marketing*, Indonesian Center Bureau of Statistics, Jakarta (**1997**).

[12]    Salmiah, A. and Beng, K. Y. Oleochemicals and other non-food applications of palm oil and palm oil products. Most, **1997**, *6*(1), 24-44.

[13]    Kaufman, A. J. and Rubusch, R. J. **1990**. *Oleochemicals:* A world overview. Proceeding of World
        Conference on Oleochemicals. AOCS, Champaign, Illinois: 10-25.
[14]    Vries, R. J. *Oleochemicals Potential in the Pacific Rim.* Proceeding of World Conference on
        Oleochemicals. AOCS, Champaign, Illinois: 45-50 (**1990**).

Atta-ur-Rahman/Choudhary/Khan (Eds.) *Frontiers in Natural Product Chemistry, Vol. 1*    133

# Microbial Transformation of Natural Products- A Tool for the Synthesis of Novel Analogues of Bioactive Substances

Atta-ur-Rahman*, M. Iqbal Choudhary and S. Ghulam Musharraf

*H.E.J. Research Institute of Chemistry, International Center for Chemical Sciences, University of Karachi, Karachi-75270, Pakistan*

**Abstract:** Microbial transformation is an effective tool for the structural modification of bioactive natural and synthetic compounds. Its application in asymmetric synthesis is increasing due to its versatility and ease. The present article reviews our contributions in the field of microbial transformation of different classes of bioactive natural products. The microbial transformation of monoterpenoids [(1R, 2S, 5R)-(−)-menthol and (−)-α-pinene], sesquiterpenoids [(+)-sclareolide, 7α-hydroxyfrullanolide, nootkatone, α-santonin, (−)-ambrox and isolongifolen-4-one], sapogenins (sarsasapogenin), alkaloids (vindoline) and steroids (E-guggulsterone, withaferin-A, (+)-adrenosterone, androst-1,4-dien-3,17-dione, dehydroepiandrosterone, norethisterone, 17α-ethynylestradiol, prednisone, testosterone and danazol) are described here along with biological activities of transformed products.

## INTRODUCTION

Microbes have been used for the preparation of foods and beverages from the dawn of civilization. However the use of microorganisms for the conversion of steroids and other classes of natural products is comparatively recent [1]. Microbial transformation methodology is a blend of various fields and has yielded fruitful results, which can be applicable on laboratory as well as industrial scales.

Currently different classes of natural products including steroids, terpenoids, alkaloids, coumarins and flavonoids, have been subjected to fungal or bacterial transformation leading to the synthesis of structurally novel analogues with enhanced bioactivity profiles.

Microbial transformation reactions are catalyzed by enzymes and are highly regio- as well as sterospecific. These transformations require mild conditions of temperature and pH and show a great degree of reproducibility. This field has attracted the attention of synthetic chemists as a tool for asymmetric synthesis. Microbes and immobilized enzymes are now commonly used as synthetic reagents in chemoenzymatic syntheses [2].

Microbial transformation can be conducted by using fungal or bacterial broths in shaking or resting condition. Bacterial transformation involves changes in the structures of organic compounds through degradation pathways, while fungal enzymes interact with substrates either in a "xenobiotic" or "biosynthetic" fashion. These transformations include the insertion of oxygen into C-H and C-C bonds; addition of oxygen to alkene (C=C); transfer of acyl, or sugar units from one substrate to another; hydrolysis or formation of amide, epoxide, esters and nitriles; hydrogenation, hydration and elimination of small units; epimerization, racemization and isomerization reactions; and formation of C-C, C-O, C-S

*Corresponding author: Tel: 924 3211; Fax: 924 3190; E-mail: hej@cyber.net.pk

and C-N bonds. Michael and Bayer-Villiger reactions are also commonly observed [3]. In brief the microbial transformation of various classes of organic compounds have been successfully employed as a powerful synthetic tool for introducing chemical functionalies into often inaccessible site of molecule, thus producing new analogous of natural and synthetic compounds which may be difficult to synthesize otherwise.

We have investigated the microbial transformation of various classes of bioactive natural products, mainly terpenes, alkaloids, sapogenins and steroids by using various fungal strains such as *Cephalosporium aphidicola*, *Botrytis cinerea*, *Aspergillus niger*, *Aspergilus quadrilineatus*, *Rhizopus stolonifer*, *Curvularia lunata*, *Gibberella fujikuruoi*, *Cunninghamella elegans*, *Fusarium lini*, *Fusarium monolinum*, *Pleurotus oestreatus* and *Mucor pulumbeus*. This work has resulted in the formation of structurally interesting transformed products, summarized in Table-1.

**Table 1.    Microbial Transformation of Different Classes of Bioactive Natural and Synthetic Compounds.**

| | Class of Compound | Substrate | Transformed Products | Ref. |
|---|---|---|---|---|
| 1 | **Terpene** a) Monoterpene | (−)-Menthol (1) | 10-Acetoxymenthol (2), 7-hydroxymenthol (3), 4α-Hydroxymenthol (4), 3α-hydroxymenthol (5), 9-Hydroxymentol (6),10-hydroxymenthol (7) | [6] |
| | | (−)-α-Pinene (8) | Verbenone (9), 3β-hydroxy-(-)-α-pinene (10), 9β-Hydroxy-(-)-α-pinene (11), 4β-Hydroxy-(-)-α-pinene-6-one (12) | [7] |
| | a) Sesqueterpene | (+)-Sclareolide (13) | 3-Oxosclareolide (14), 1β-hydroxysclareolide (15) 2α-Hydroxysclareolide (16) 3β-hydroxysclareolide (17), 1β,3β-Dihydroxysclareolide (18) 1α,3β-Dihydroxysclareolide (19), 2α,3β-Dihydroxysclareolide (20) 3β-Hydroxyepisclareolide (21) | [10, 11] |
| | | 7α-Hydroxyfrullanolide (22) | 11,13-Dihydro-7α-hydroxyfrullanolide (23) 13-Acetyl-7α-hydroxyfrullanolide (24) | [13] |
| | | Nootkatone (25) | 9α-Hydroxynootkatone (26), 9α-hydroxynootkatone (27) | [14] |
| | | A-Santonin (28) | 1,2-Dihydrosantonin (29) | [15] |
| | | (−)-Ambrox (30) | 1α-Hydroxyambrox (31), 1α,11α-dihydroxyambrox (32), 1α,6α-Dihydroxyambrox (33),1α,6α,11α-Trihydroxyambrox (34), 3-oxoambrox (35), 3β-Hydroxyambrox (36), 3β,6β-dihydroxyambrox (38), Tetranor-12, 8-diol-labdane (39) | [11] |
| | | Isolongifolen-4-one (40) | (7R)-12-Hydroxyisolongifolen-4-one (41) (7S)-12-Hydroxyisolongifolen-4-one (42), (11S)-9-Hydroxyisolongifolen-4-one (43), (9S)-9-Hydroxyisolongifolen-4-one (44), (10R)-9-Hydroxyisolongifolen-4-one (45) | [17] |

(Table 1 Contd....)

| | Class of Compound | Substrate | Transformed Products | Ref. |
|---|---|---|---|---|
| 2 | **Sapogenin** | Sarsasapogenin (**46**) | 3β-Acetoxysarsasapogenin (**47**), 7α-Hydroxysarsasapogenin (**48**). | [18] |
| 3 | **Alkaloid** | Vindoline (**49**) | 17-Deacetylatedvindoline (**50**) | [15] |
| 4 | **Steroids** | *E*-Guggulsterone (**51**) | 11α-Hydroxy-*E*-guggulsterone (**52**), 7β-Hydroxy-*E*-guggulsterone (**53**), 11α-Hydroxy-*Z*-guggulsterone (**54**), 7β-Hydroxy-*Z*-guggulsterone (**55**), 7β-Hydroxypregn-4-ene-3,16-dione (**56**), 11α, 15β-Dihydroxy-*E*-guggulsterone (**57**), 11α, 15β-Dihydroxy-*Z*-guggulsterone (**58**), 15β, 7β-Dihydroxypregn-4-ene-3,16-dione (**59**) | [20] |
| | | Withaferin-A (**60**) | 2,3-Dihydrowithaferin-A (**61**) | [21] |
| | | (+)-Adrenosterone (**62**) | Androsta-1,4-dien-3,11,17-trione (**63**), 17β-Hydroxyandrost-4-en-3,11-dione (**64**), 17β-Hydroxyandrosta-1,4-dien-3,11-dione (**65**) | [22] |
| | | Androsta-1,4-dien-3,17-dione (**66**) | Androst-4-en-3,17-dione (**67**), 17β-Hydroxyandrosta-1,4-dien-3-one (**68**), 11α-Hydroxyandrosta-l,4-dien-3,17-dione (**69**), 11α-Hydroxyandrost-4-en-3,17-dione (**70**), 17β,11α-Dihydroxyandrost-4-en-3-one (**71**), 17β,11α-Dihydroxyandrosta-l,4-dien-3-one (**72**) | [23] |
| | | Dehydroepiandrosterone (**73**) | 3β,17β-Dihydroxyandrost-5-ene (**74**), 3β,17β-dihydr-oxyandrost-4-ene (**75**), 17β-hydroxyandrost-4-ene-3-one (**76**), 3β,11β-Dihydroxyandrost-4-ene-17-one (**77**), 3β,7α-Dihydroandrost-5-ene-17-one (**78**), 3β,7α,17β-trihydroxyandrost-5-ene (**79**), 11β-hydroxyandrost-4,6-diene-3,17-dione (**80**), 3β-Hydroandrost-5-ene-17-one (**81**), 3β,7α-dihydroandrost-5-ene-17-one (**82**) | [24, 25] |
| | | Norethisterone (**83**) | 17α-Ethynylestradiol (**84**) | [26] |
| | | 17α-Ethynylestradiol (**84**) | 19-*Nor*-17α-pregna-1,3,5 (**10**)-trien-20-yne-3,4,17β-triol (**85**), 19-*Nor*-17α-pregna-1,3,5(**10**)-trien-20-yne-3,7α,17β-triol (**86**), 19-*Nor*-17α-pregna-1,3,5(**10**)-trien-20-yne-3,11α,17β-triol (**87**), 19-*Nor*-174α-pregna-1,3,5 (**10**)-trien-20-yne-3,6β,17β-triol (**88**), 19-*Nor*-17α-pregn--1,3,5(**10**)-trien-20-yne-3,17β-diol-6β-methoxy (**89**) | [26] |
| | | Prednisone (**90**) | 17α,21-Dihydroxy-5α-pregn-1-ene-3,11,20-trione (**91**), 17α,20S,21-Trihydroxy-5α-pregn-1-ene-3,11-dione (**92**), 1,4-Pregnadiene-17α,20S,21-triol-3,11-dione (**93**) | [27] |

(Table 1 Contd....)

| | Class of Compound | Substrate | Transformed Products | Ref. |
|---|---|---|---|---|
| | | Testosterone (94) | 17-Dehydrotestoesterone (95), 15β-Hydroxytestosterone (96) | [28] |
| | | Cortisol (97) | 11β-Hydroxyandrost-4-en-3,17-dione (98), 11β, 17α, 20 (S), 21-Tetrahydroxy-pregn-4-en-3-one (99), 11β, 17α, 21-trihydroxy-5α-pregnan-3, 20-dione (100), 3β, 11β, 17α, 21-tetrahydroxy-pregnan-20-one (101) | [29] |
| | | Danazol (102) | 17β-Dydroxy-2-hydroxymethyl-17α-pregn-4-en-20-yne-3-one (103), 17β-Hydroxy-2-hydroxymethyl-17α-pregna-4-dien-20-yne-3-one (104) | [30] |

## 2. MICROBIAL TRANSFORMATION OF TERPENOIDS

Terpenoids are widely distributed in plants and fungi with various skeletal arrangements and exhibit a wide range of biological activities. Terpenes are good substrate models for fungal enzymatic system and mostly terpenes are transformed in a "xenobiotic" fashion [4].

### 2.1. Monoterpenoids

Monoterpenes normally possess a C-10 skeleton and they can be subdivided into three basic types: acyclic, monocyclic and bicyclic. A problem associated with monoterpenes is difficulty in handling due to their high volatility. Microbial transformation is the best way to reduce their volatility through introducing polar functionalites in their structures.

A monoterpenoid, menthol (1) is the main constituent of peppermint oil, and it exhibits anaesthetic, disinfectant and photoprotective effects [5]. Microbial conversion of (1R, 2S, 5R)-(−)-menthol (1) by *Cephalosporium aphidicola* (IMI 68981) yielded six polar metabolites characterized as (−)-10-acetoxymenthol (2), (−)-7-hydroxymenthol (3), (−)-4α-hydroxymenthol (4), (−)-3α-hydroxymenthol (5), (−)-9-hydroxymentol (6) and (−)-10-hydroxymenthol (7) (Scheme 1) [6].

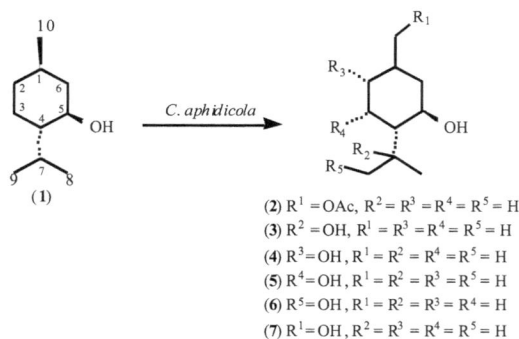

(2) R$^1$ = OAc, R$^2$ = R$^3$ = R$^4$ = R$^5$ = H
(3) R$^2$ = OH, R$^1$ = R$^3$ = R$^4$ = R$^5$ = H
(4) R$^3$ = OH, R$^1$ = R$^2$ = R$^4$ = R$^5$ = H
(5) R$^4$ = OH, R$^1$ = R$^2$ = R$^3$ = R$^5$ = H
(6) R$^5$ = OH, R$^1$ = R$^2$ = R$^3$ = R$^4$ = H
(7) R$^1$ = OH, R$^2$ = R$^3$ = R$^4$ = R$^5$ = H

**Scheme 1.**

(−)-α-Pinene (8), a bicyclic monoterpene, is a major flavor and fragrance constituent of many essential oils and aromatic plants. (−)-α-Pinene was biotransformed by the plant pathogenic fungus, *Botrytis cinerea* to afford four metabolites [7], characterized as verbenone (**9**), 3β-hydroxy-(−)-β-pinene (10%) (**10**), 9-hydroxy-(−)-α-pinene (12%) (**11**), 4β-hydroxy-(−)-β-pinene-6-one (16%) (**12**) (Scheme **2**).

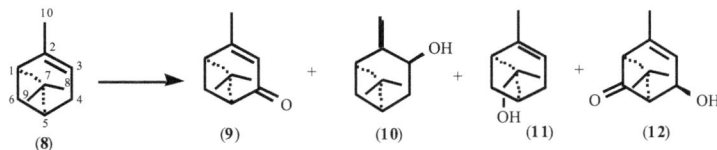

**Scheme 2.**

## 2.2. Sesquiterpenoids

Sesquiterpenes have a C-15 framework and they can be classified into four groups according to the number of rings present in the structure. Sesquiterpene lactones and alcohols are easy to handle and are excellent candidates for the microbial transformations.

(+)-Sclareolide (**13**), a sesquiterpene lactone, a constituent of *Arnica angustifolia*, *Sideritis nutans* and *Kyllinga erecta* [8], has exhibited phytotoxicity and cytotoxicity against human cancer cell lines [9]. Incubation of compound **13** with various fungal strains showed enantioselective hydroxylations at C-1, C-2, C-3 and epimerization at C-8 (Scheme **3**), affording polar oxidized metabolites, namely: 3-oxosclareolide (**14**), 1β-hydroxysclareolide (**15**), 2α-hydroxysclareolide (**16**), 3β-hydroxysclareolide (**17**), 1β,3β-dihydroxysclareolide (**18**), 1α,3β-dihydroxysclareolide (**19**), 2α,3β-dihydroxysclareolide (**20**), and 3β-hydroxyepisclareolide (**21**) [10, 11]. The inversion of stereochemistry encountered in is compound **21**, a rare phenomenon in biotransformation. Metabolite **19** showed cytotoxicity against various human cancer cell lines [10]. Metabolites **14**, **17** and **18** showed significant phytotoxicity at higher doses against *Lemna minor* L. [11].

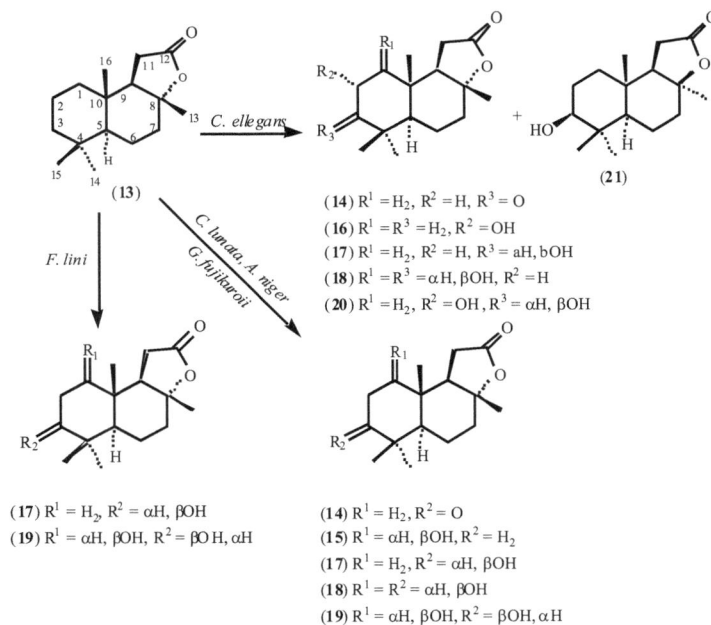

**Scheme 3.**

7α-Hydroxyfrullanolide (22) is a major constituent ($2.5 \times 10^{-2}$%) of *Sphaeranthus indicus* L. (Compositae) which exhibited pronounced cytotoxicity and antitumor activity against a number of human cell lines [12]. Microbial transformation of 7α-hydroxyfrullanolide (22) with *Aspergillus niger* yielded 11,13-dihydro-7α-hydroxyfrullanolide (23) (4.3%), while *Aspergilus quadrilineatus* transformed the substrate into 13-acetyl-7α-hydroxyfrullanolide (24) (5.8 %) and to compound 23 (3.1 %) [13] (Scheme 4).

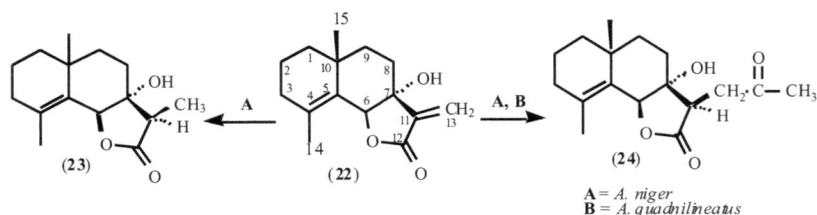

**Scheme 4.**

Nootkatone (25) is a mildly pungent, cytotoxic ketone isolated from *Citrus paradise* and *Chamaecyparis nootkatensis*. The fermentation of 25 with *C. aphidicola* afforded two hydroxylated products, 9α-hydroxynootkatone (26) and 9α-hydroxynootkatone (27) [14] (Scheme 5).

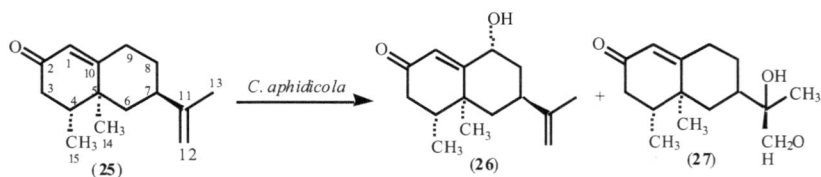

**Scheme 5.**

α-Santonin (28), a sesquiterpene lactone, is a constituent of various *Artemisia* spp. (Compositae). It has been used in the treatment of nervous complaints and as an anthelmintic. Incubation of 28 with *Aspergillus niger* has yielded 1,2-dihydrosantonin (29) (Scheme 6) [15].

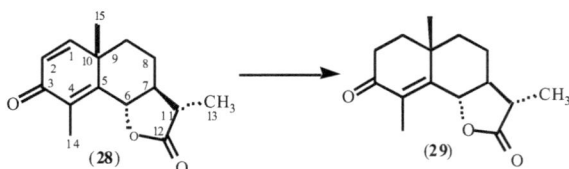

**Scheme 6.**

(–)-Ambrox (30), a perfumery sesquiterpene, has a strong amber-like odor. It is a major constituent of ambergris (a metabolite of the sperm whale). In animal perfumes, (–)-ambrox (30) is graded to be as good as "Civet" and "Musk" [16]. We have carried out a microbial transformation of (–)-ambrox (30) to obtain several interesting metabolites with new fragrances. Fermentation of (–)-ambrox (30), with *Fusarium lini* (Scheme 7) afforded mono-, di- and tri-hydroxylated metabolites such as 1α-hydroxyambrox (31), 1α,11α-dihydroxyambrox (32), 1α,6α-dihydroxyambrox (33) and 1α,6α,11α-trihydroxyambrox (34). Enantioselective α-hydroxylation occurred at C-1, C-6 and C-11 [11].

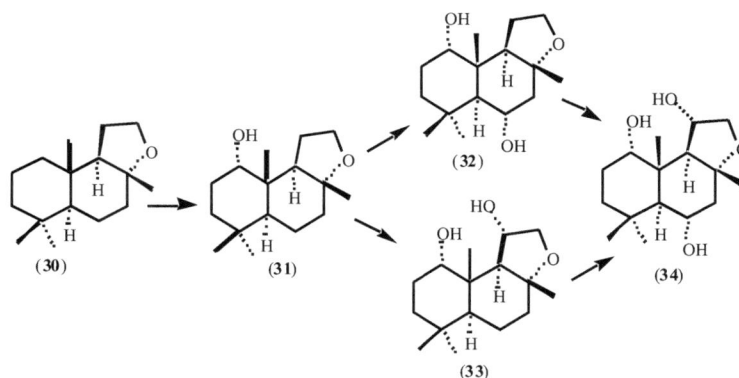

**Scheme 7.**

On incubation of compound **30** with *Rhizopus stolonifer*, 3-oxoambrox (**35**), 3β-hydroxyambrox (**36**), 3β,6β-dihydroxyambrox (**38**) and its ether cleaved product, tetranor-12, 8-diol-labdane (**39**) were obtained. Ether cleavage by biotransformation is a relatively rare reaction. Fermentation of compound **30** with *Curvularia lunata* yielded metabolites **35** and **36**, while biotransformation of **30** with *Cunninghamella elegans* afforded compounds **35**, **36** and **37** (Scheme **8**) [11].

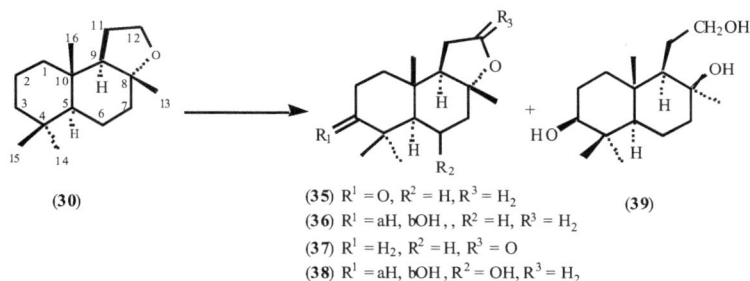

(30)

(35) $R^1 = O$, $R^2 = H$, $R^3 = H_2$
(36) $R^1 = aH$, $bOH$, , $R^2 = H$, $R^3 = H_2$
(37) $R^1 = H_2$, $R^2 = H$, $R^3 = O$
(38) $R^1 = aH$, $bOH$, $R^2 = OH$, $R^3 = H_2$

(39)

**Scheme 8.**

Isolongifolen-4-one (**40**), a tricyclic sesquiterpene, was found to be active against the enzyme tyrosinase with an $IC_{50} = 51$ μM [17]. Biological derivatization of compound **40** was carried out in order to obtain new derivatives with increased potency against tyrosinase and to understand the structure-activity relationships. The transformation of compound **40** with *Aspergillus niger* (ATCC 10549) afforded three new metabolites, (7R)-12-hydroxyisolongifolen-4-one (**41**), (7S)-12-hydroxyisolongifolen-4-one (**42**) and (11S)-9-hydroxyisolongifolen-4-one (**43**) were obtained after 12 days of fermentation. Incubation of compound **41** for 8 days with *Fusarium lini* (NRRL 68751) afforded (9S)-9-hydroxyisolongifolen-4-one (**44**) and (10R)-9-hydroxyisolongifolen-4-one (**45**). Metabolites **41** and **42** were also obtained on incubation with *Rhizopus stolonifer* (ATCC 10404) after 12 days of fermentation, while incubation with *Cephalosporium aphidicola* (IMI 68689) afforded compound **43** after 8 days of fermentation. Metabolite **43** showed potent tyrosinase inhibitory activity, while its benzyl ether derivative was found to be more potent than the standard used for tyrosinase inhibition (Scheme **9**) [17].

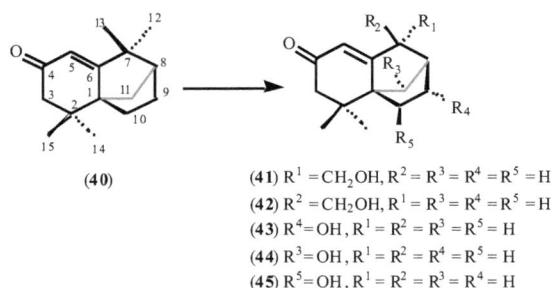

(40)

(41) $R^1 = CH_2OH$, $R^2 = R^3 = R^4 = R^5 = H$
(42) $R^2 = CH_2OH$, $R^1 = R^3 = R^4 = R^5 = H$
(43) $R^4 = OH$, $R^1 = R^2 = R^3 = R^5 = H$
(44) $R^3 = OH$, $R^1 = R^2 = R^4 = R^5 = H$
(45) $R^5 = OH$, $R^1 = R^2 = R^3 = R^4 = H$

Scheme 9.

## 3. MICROBIAL TRANSFORMATION OF SAPOGENIN

Sapogenins are the aglycon part of saponins and are characterized by the presences of a spiroketal side chain. Sarsasapogenin (46), a spirostan-type steroidal sapogenin, has been isolated from *Yucca sckudigeria*. Microbial transformation of sarsasapogenin (46) with *Fusarium lini* yielded 3β-acetoxysarsasapogenin (47) and 7α-hydroxysarsasapogenin (48). Metabolites have shown spasmolytic activity in the rat duodenum [18] (Scheme 10).

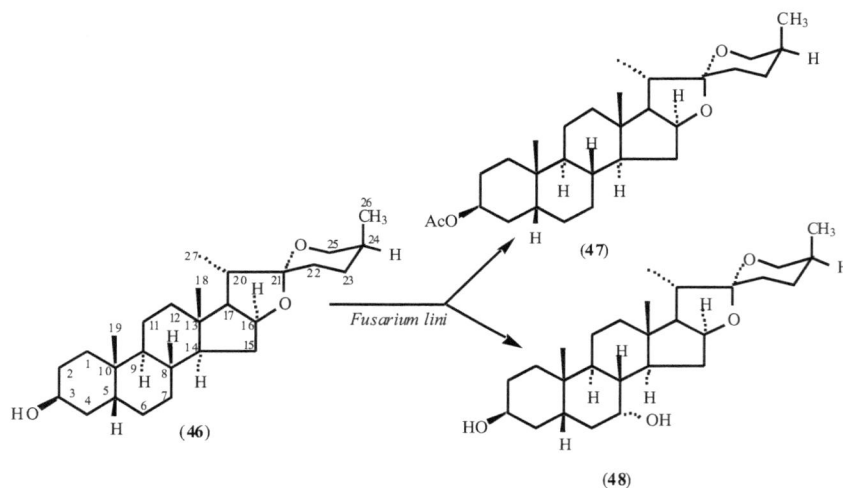

*Fusarium lini*

Scheme 10.

## 4. MICROBIAL TRANSFORMATION OF THE ALKALOID, VINDOLINE

Alkaloids are usually found in the seeds, roots, leaves and barks of the plants and generally occur as salts of various plant acids. They can be classified according to the structural types. The microbial transformation of alkaloids is a challenge because of its poor yields and poor solubility due to salt formation.

Vindoline (49) is an indole alkaloid isolated from *Catharanthus roseus* (Apocynaceae). It is a part of the structures of the anticancer bisindole alkaloids, vinblastine and vincristine. *Fusarium lini*, *Aspergillus niger* and *Fusarium monolinum* converted compound 49 into regioselective deacetylated product 50 [15] (Scheme 11).

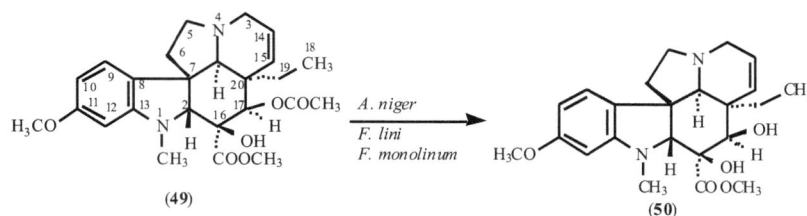

**Scheme 11.**

## 5. MICROBIAL TRANSFORMATION OF STEROIDAL DRUGS AND HORMONES

Steroids were the first group of natural products which were subjected to microbial transformations. Pioneering work in this field includes the conversion of progesterone into 11α-hydroxyprogesterone by *Rhizopus arhizus*. Widely available plant steroids, e.g. sitosterol, were incubated with a variety of fungal strains in order to synthesize various steroidal hormones and scale-up those reactions on an industrial level.

*E*-Guggulsterone (**51**) has been isolated from the gum resins of *Ailanthus grandis* and *Commiphora mukul*. The gum resin of *C. mukul* has been traditionally used in the treatment of epilepsy, ulcers, helminthus, rheumatoid arthritis, and hyperlipemia in the ancient Indian system of medicine. The gum extract of *C. mukul* called "guggulipid" has been found to be a safe and effective lipid-lowering agent comparable in efficacy to colifibrate. Compound **51** is one of the lead compounds isolated from *Commiphora mukul* and it is responsible for hypolipemic and hypocholestremic activity [19]. It also exhibited cytotoxic activity against the human cancer cell lines NCI-H-226. Microbial transformation of compound **51** led to the isolation of metabolites, 7β-hydroxy-*E*-guggulsterone (**53**), 7β-hydroxy-*Z*-guggulsterone (**55**), 7β-hydroxypregn-4-ene-3,16-dione (**56**), 15β, 7β-dihydroxypregn-4-ene-3,16-dione (**59**) by *Aspergillus niger* and the metabolites 11α-hydroxy-*E*-guggulsterone (**52**), 11α-hydroxy-*Z*-guggulsterone (**54**), 11α, 15β-dihydroxy-*E*-guggulsterone (**57**), 11α, 15β-dihydroxy-*Z*-guggulsterone (**58**) by *Cephalosporium aphidicola* (Scheme **12**). The metabolite **52** exhibited antibacterial activity against *Shigella boydii*, *Pseudomonas aeruginosa*, *Escherichia coli*, and *Corynebacterium diphtheriae*, although, interestingly, compound **55** lacks this activity [20].

Withaferin-A (**60**) is a withanolide (steroidal lactones) isolated from various *Withania* species. Incubation of compound **60** with *Aspergillus niger* yielded a regio- and chemoselactive product, 2,3-dihydrowithaferin-A (**61**) [21] (Scheme **13**).

(+)-Adrenosterone (**62**) is a tri-keto steroid, which was isolated from the cortical extracts by Reichstein. Fungal transformation of **62** was conducted by *Cephalosporium aphidicola*, which resulted in the formation of androsta-1,4-dien-3,11,17-trione (**63**), 17β-hydroxyandrost-4-en-3,11-dione (**64**), and 17β-hydroxyandrosta-1,4-dien-3,11-dione (**65**) (Scheme **14**). Broadly two types of transformations were observed: regioselective reduction of the C-17 keto group, and double bond formation between C-1/C-2 [22].

Androst-1,4-dien-3,17-dione (**66**) is commercially produced by the microbiological transformation of β-sitosterol and cholesterol. It is presently used in the industrial synthesis of estradiol or estrone. Compound **66** has been evaluated as an inhibitor of estrogen biosynthesis. Aromatse activity has a potential clinical application in controlling the estrogen mediated events such as ovulation and the growth of estrogen dependant tumors.

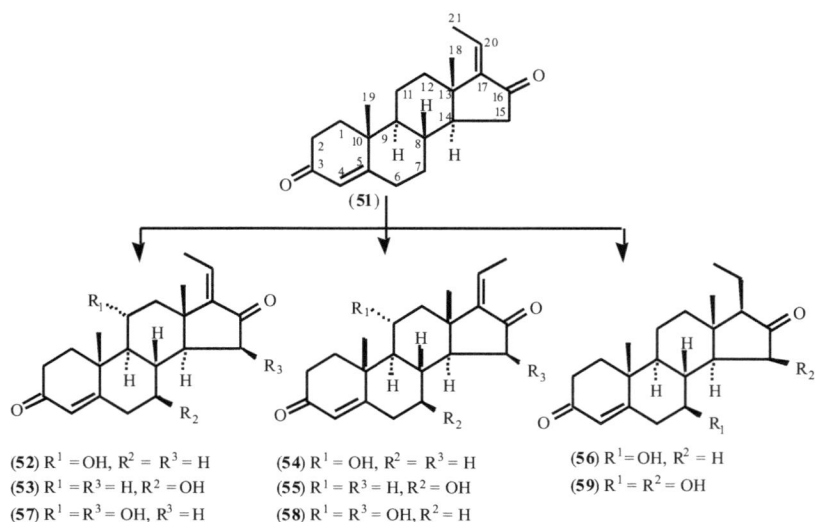

**(52)** R$^1$ = OH, R$^2$ = R$^3$ = H     **(54)** R$^1$ = OH, R$^2$ = R$^3$ = H     **(56)** R$^1$= OH, R$^2$ = H
**(53)** R$^1$ = R$^3$ = H, R$^2$ = OH     **(55)** R$^1$ = R$^3$ = H, R$^2$ = OH     **(59)** R$^1$ = R$^2$ = OH
**(57)** R$^1$ = R$^3$ = OH, R$^3$ = H     **(58)** R$^1$ = R$^3$ = OH, R$^2$ = H

**Scheme 12.**

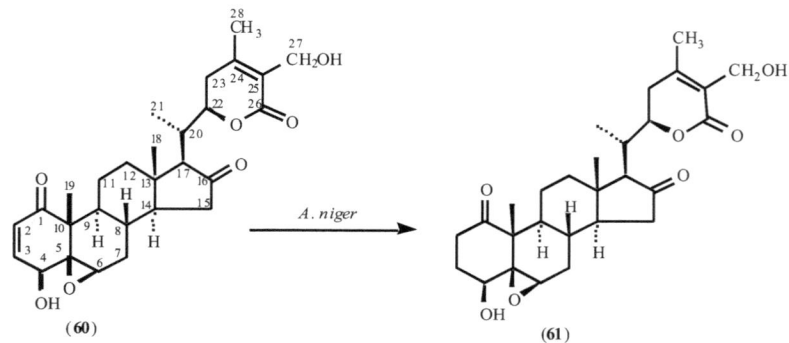

**Scheme 13.**

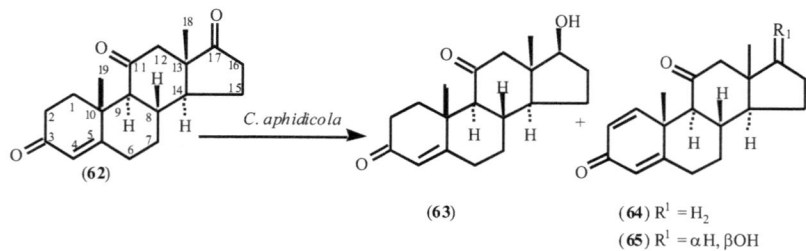

**(64)** R$^1$ = H$_2$
**(65)** R$^1$ = $\alpha$ H, $\beta$ OH

**Scheme 14.**

(+)-Androsta-1,4-dien-3,17-dione **(66)** was converted into six biotransformed products: androst-4-en-3,17-dione **(67)**, 17β-hydroxyandrosta-1,4-dien-3-one **(68)**, 11α-hydroxy-androsta-l,4-dien-3,17-dione **(69)**, 11α-hydroxyandrost-4-en-3,17-dione **(70)**, 17β,11αdihydroxyandrost-4-en-3-one (**71**) and 17β,11α-dihydroxyandrosta-1,4-dien-3-one (**72**) [23] (Scheme **15**).

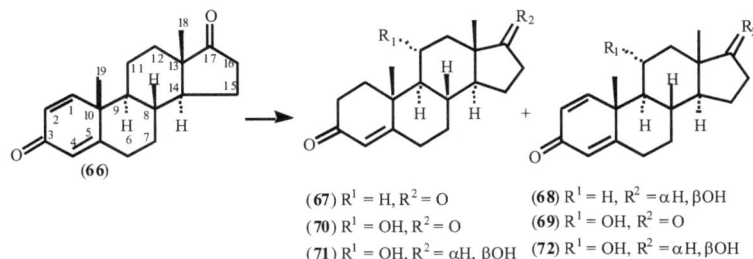

(**67**) R$^1$ = H, R$^2$ = O     (**68**) R$^1$ = H, R$^2$ = αH, βOH
(**70**) R$^1$ = OH, R$^2$ = O     (**69**) R$^1$ = OH, R$^2$ = O
(**71**) R$^1$ = OH, R$^2$ = αH, βOH     (**72**) R$^1$ = OH, R$^2$ = αH, βOH

**Scheme 15.**

Dehydroepiandrosterone (**73**) is the most dominant hormone in the body. It is the source of all sex and steroidal hormones and is known as the body's mother hormone. Transformation of dehydroepiandrosterone (DHEA) (**73**) was carried out by a plant pathogen *Rhizopus stolonifer,* which resulted in the production of seven metabolites. These metabolites were identified as 3β,17β-dihydroxyandrost-5-ene (**74**), 3β,17β-dihydroxy-androst-4-ene (**75**), 17β-hydroxyandrost-4-ene-3-one (**76**), 3β,11β-dihydroxyandrost-4-ene-17-one (**77**), 3β,7α-dihydroandrost-5-ene-17-one (**78**), 3β,7α,17β-trihydroxyandrost-5-ene (**79**) and 11β-hydroxyandrost-4,6-diene-3,17-dione (**80**) [24] (Scheme **16**). Incubation of compound **73** with *Cephalosporium aphidicola* afforded 3β-hydroandrost-5-ene-17-one (**81**) and 3β,7α-dihydroandrost-5-ene-17-one (**82**) [25].

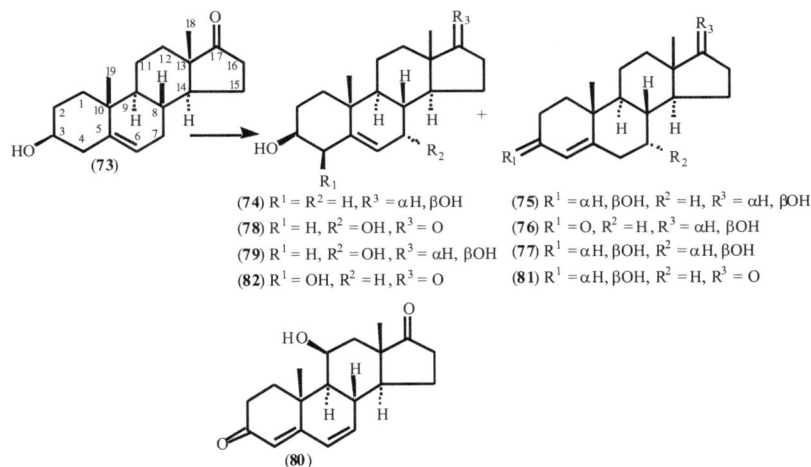

(**74**) R$^1$ = R$^2$ = H, R$^3$ = αH, βOH     (**75**) R$^1$ = αH, βOH, R$^2$ = H, R$^3$ = αH, βOH
(**78**) R$^1$ = H, R$^2$ = OH, R$^3$ = O     (**76**) R$^1$ = O, R$^2$ = H, R$^3$ = αH, βOH
(**79**) R$^1$ = H, R$^2$ = OH, R$^3$ = αH, βOH     (**77**) R$^1$ = αH, βOH, R$^2$ = αH, βOH
(**82**) R$^1$ = OH, R$^2$ = H, R$^3$ = O     (**81**) R$^1$ = αH, βOH, R$^2$ = H, R$^3$ = O

(**80**)

**Scheme 16.**

Norethisterone (17α-ethynyl-19-nortestestrone) (**83**) is a potent progestogen, widely used in oral contraceptive pills as an antifertility agent. Incubation of norethisterone (**83**) with *Cephalosporium aphidicola* afforded an oxidized metabolite, 17α-ethynylestradiol (**84**) [26] (Scheme **17**). Compound **84**, the first orally active well-known estrogen, has been known since 1938 and it is widely used as an oral contraceptive. Compound **84**, when incubated with *Cunninghamella elegans,* afforded several polar metabolites: 19-*nor*-17α-pregna-1,3,5 (10)-trien-20-yne-3,4,17β-triol (**85**), 19-*nor*-17α-pregna-1,3,5 (10)-trien-20-

yne-3,7α,17β-triol (**86**), 19-*nor*-17α-pregna-1,3,5 (10)-trien-20-yne-3,11α,17β-triol (**87**), 19-*nor*-17α-pregna-1,3,5 (10)-trien-20-yne-3,6β,17β-triol (**88**) and 19-*nor*-17α-pregna-1,3,5 (10)-trien-20-yne-3,17β-diol-6β-methoxy (**89**) [26] (Scheme **17**).

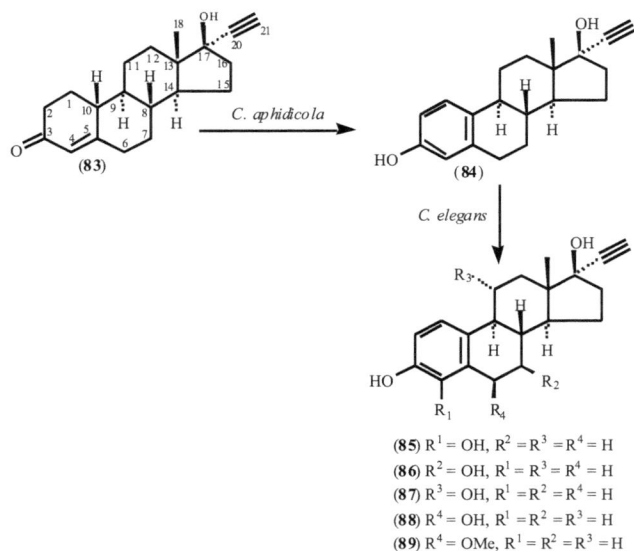

(**85**) R$^1$ = OH, R$^2$ = R$^3$ = R$^4$ = H
(**86**) R$^2$ = OH, R$^1$ = R$^3$ = R$^4$ = H
(**87**) R$^3$ = OH, R$^1$ = R$^2$ = R$^4$ = H
(**88**) R$^4$ = OH, R$^1$ = R$^2$ = R$^3$ = H
(**89**) R$^4$ = OMe, R$^1$ = R$^2$ = R$^3$ = H

**Scheme 17.**

Prednisone (**90**), 17α,21-dihydroxy-pregna-1,4-diene-3,11,20-trione, is commonly used in the treatment of severe asthma, rheumatic disorders, renal disorders and diseases of inflammatory bowel, skin, gastrointestinal tract. The microbial transformation of prednisone (**90**) by *Cunninghamella elegans* afforded two metabolites, 17α,21-dihydroxy-5α-pregn-1-ene-3,11,20-trione (**91**) and 17α,20S,21-trihydroxy-5α-pregn-1-ene-3,11-dione (**92**), while the fermentation of **90** with *Fusarium lini*, *Rhizopus stolonifer* and *Curvularia lunata* afforded a metabolite 1,4-pregnadiene-17α,20S,21-triol-3,11-dione (**93**) [27] (Scheme **18**).

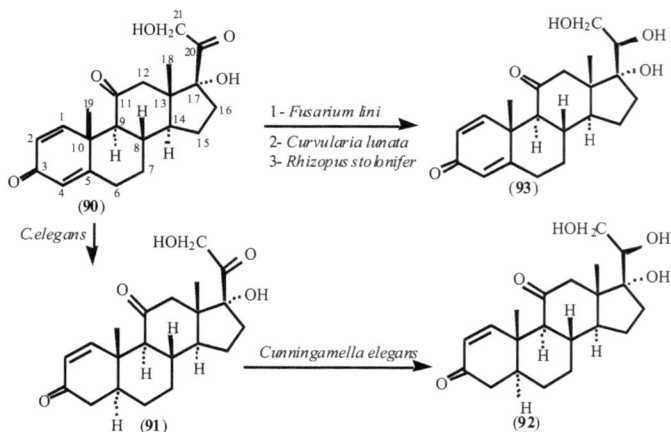

**Scheme 18.**

Testosterone (**94**) is a male sex hormone responsible for developing secondary characteristics. Microbial transformation of testosterone (**94**) with *Curvularia lunata* afforded 17-dehydrotestosterone (**95**), while incubation with *Pleurotus oestreatus* yielded 15β-hydroxytestosterone (**96**) [28] (Scheme **19**).

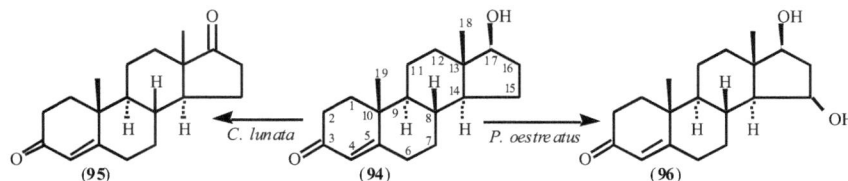

**Scheme 19.**

Cortisol (**97**) is an anabolic hormone used as an anti-inflammatory and antiallergic agent. Microbial transformation of compound **97** with *Gibberella fujikuruoi* yielded 11β-hydroxyandrost-4-en-3,17-dione (**98**), while fermentation of compound **97** with *Bacillus subtilis* and *Rhizopus stolonifer* yielded 11β, 17α, 20 (*S*), 21-tetrahydroxy-pregn-4-en-3-one (**99**). Metabolites 11β, 17α, 21-trihydroxy-5α-pregnan-3, 20-dione (**100**), 3β, 11β, 17α, 21-tetrahydroxy-pregnan-20-one (**101**) were obtained with *Bacillus cerus*. Compounds **98** and **100** showed significant inhibitory activity against prolyl endopeptidase (PEP) [29] (Scheme **20**).

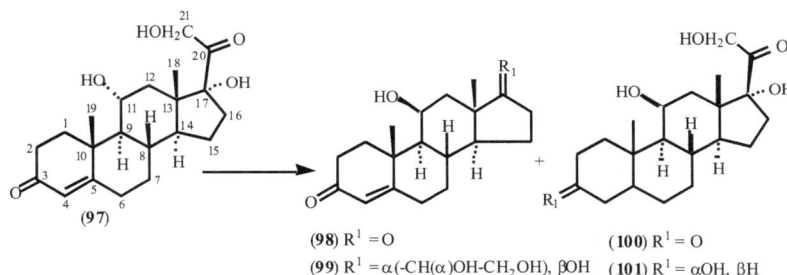

**Scheme 20.**

Danazol (**102**) is an orally effective, pituitary gonadotropin inhibitor devoid of estrogenic and progestational activities. It is effectively used in the treatment of endometriosis, benign fibrocystic mastitis, and precocious puberty. Microbial transformation of compound **102** showed the cleavage of oxazole ring and resulted in the formation of two metabolites: 17β-hydroxy-2-hydroxymethyl-17α-pregn-4-en-20-yne-3-one (**103**) and 17β-hydroxy-2-hydroxymethyl-17α-pregna-4-dien-20-yne-3-one (**104**) [30] (Scheme **21**).

## CONCLUSIONS

In the light of the above study we can conclude that microbial transformation can have wide applications in structural modifications of organic compounds. This procedure is widely used for the introduction of various functionalities in the molecule particularly at chemically inert positions in a stereospecific manner. Furthermore the use of microbial transformation procedures have led to the preparation of several new and novel derivatives of bioactive organic and synthetic compounds with improved biological and toxicological profiles. A large number of bioactive organic compounds remain to be subjected to

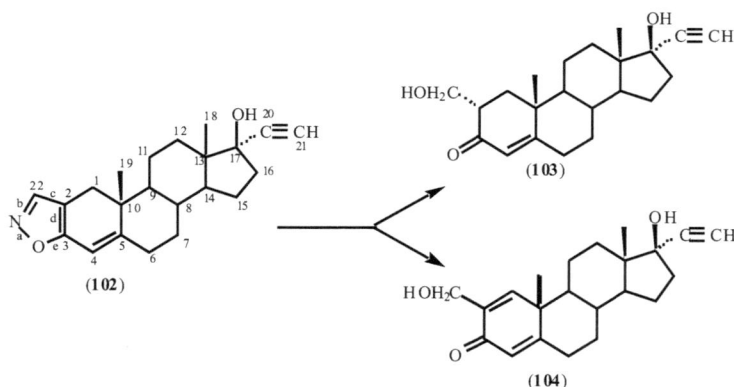

**Scheme 21.**

microbial transformation which can add into existing chemical diversity. It can also be used to synthesize libraries of structural analogues as effectively as synthetic combinatorial procedures.

## ACKNOWLEDGEMENTS

We wish to acknowledge here the hard work and commitment of following students and research collaborators, without whom this work would not have been possible. They are Dr. Farzana Shaheen, Dr. Athar Atta, Dr. Afgan Farooq, Dr. Syed Ghulam Musharraf, Mr. Faheem Asif, Mr. M. Yaqoob, Miss Sadia Sultan, Mr. Azizuddin, Mr. Adnan Ali Shah and Mr. Zafar Ali Sidiqqui.

## REFERENCES

[1]     Kieslich, K. General introduction to biocatalysis and screening. In Kieslich, K., van der Beck, C. P., de Bont, J. A. M. and van der Tweel W. J. J. (ed.), New Frontiers in Screening for Microbial Biocatalysis. Elsevier Science, Amsterdam, the Netherlands, **1998**, p: 3-11.

[2]     Chenevert, R., Caron, D. *Tetrahedron: Asymmetry* **2002**, *13*, 339.

[3]     Roberts, S. M., Turner, N. J., Willetts, A. J., Turner, M. K. Introduction to Biocalysis using Enzymes and Microorganisms. Cambridge University Press, Cambridge, **1995**.

[4]     Hanson, J. R. An Introduction to Biotransformation in Organic Chemistry. Oxford University Press, **1995**.

[5]     Belukha, U. K. *Med. Zh. Uzb.* **1969**, *10*, 23.

[6]     Atta-ur-Rahman, Yaqoob, M., Farooq, A., Anjum, S., Asif, F., Choudhary, M. I. *J. Nat. Prod.* **1998**, *61*, 1340.

[7]     Farooqa, A., Taharab, S., Choudhary, M. I., Atta-ur-Rahman, Ahmed, Z., Husnu Can Baser, K. and Demirci, F. *Z. Naturforsch C.* **2002**, *57*, 303.

[8]     Dolmazon, R., Albrand, M., Bessiere, J., Mahmout, Y., Wernerowska, D., Kolodziejczyk, K. *Phytochemistry* **1995**, *38*, 917.

[9]     Rodriguez, E., Towers, G. H. N., Mitchell, J. C. *Phytochemistry* **1976**, *15*, 1573.

[10]    Atta-ur-Rahman, Farooq, A., Choudhary, M. I. *J. Nat. Prod.* **1977**, *60*, 1038.

[11]    Choudhary, M. I., Musharraf, S. G., Atta-ur- Rahman, Sami, A. *Helv. Chim. Acta* **2004**, *87*, 2685.

[12]    Sohni, J. S., Rojatkar, S. R., Kulkarni, M. M., Dahneshawar, N. N., Tavale, S. S., Cururow, T. N., Nagasampagi, B. A. *J. Chem. Soc. Parkin Trans. I* **1988**, 1.

[13]    Atta-ur-Rahman, Choudhary, M. I., Atta, A., Alam, M., Farooq, A., Perveen, S., Shekhani, M. S., Ahmad, N. *J. Nat. Prod.* **1994**, *57*, 1251.

[14]    Farooq, A. "Structural Synthesis and Biotransformation Studies of Some Steroidal Alkaloids, Steroids and Sesquiterpenes", Ph. D. thesis, **1996**, p. 114, University of Karachi.

[15]    Atta-ur-Rahman, Choudhary, M. I., Shaheen, F., Rauf, A., Farooq, A. *Nat. Prod. Lett.* **1998**, *12*, 215.

[16]    Tanimoto, H., Oritani, T. *Tetrahedron* **1977**, *53*, 3527.

[17]    Choudhary, M. I., Musharraf, S. G., Khan, M. T. H., Abdelrahman, D., Parvaz, M., Atta-ur-Rahman, Shaheen, F. *Helv. Chim. Acta* **2003**, *86*, 3450.

[18]    Atta-ur-Rahman, Choudhary, M. I., Asif, F., Farooq, A., Yaqoob, M., Dar, A. *Phytochemistry* **1998**, *49*, 2341.

[19]    Bajaj, A. G., Dev. S. *Tetrahedron* **1982**, *38*, 2949,

[20]    Atta-ur-Rahman, Choudhary, M. I., Shaheen, F., Ashraf, M., Jahan, S. *J. Nat. Prod.* **1998**, *61*, 428.

[21]    Atta-ur-Rahman, Farooq, A., Anjum, S., Choudhary, M. I. *Curr. Org. Chem.* **1999**, *3*, 309.

[22]    Musharraf, S. G., Atta-ur-Rahman, Choudhary, M. I., Sultan, S. *Nat. Prod. Lett.* **2002**, *16*, 345.

[23]    Choudhary, M. I., Musharraf, S. G., Atta-ur-Rahman, Shaheen, F. *Nat. Prod. Lett.* **2002**, *16*, 417.

[24]    Choudhary, M. I., Shah, S. A. A., Musharraf, S. G., Atta-ur-Rahman, Shaheen, F. *Nat. Prod. Res.* **2003**, *17*, 215.

[25]    Atta-ur-Rahman, Choudhary, M. I., Asif, F., Farooq, A., Yaqoob, M. *Nat. Prod. Lett.* **2000**, *14*, 217.

[26]    Choudhary, M. I., Musharraf, S. G., Ali, R. A., Atta-ur-Rahman, Atif M. *Z. Naturforsch.* **2004**, *59b*, 323.

[27]    Choudhary, M. I., Sidiqqui, Z. A., Musharraf, S. G., Atta-ur-Rahman, Nawaz, S. A. *Nat. Prod. Res.* (in press).

[28]    Atta-ur-Rahman, Choudhary, M. I., Asif, F., Farooq, A., Yaqoob, M. *Nat. Prod. Lett.* **1998**,*12*, 225.

[29]    Choudhary, M. I., Sultan, S., Yaqoob, M., Musharraf, S. G., Yasin, A., Atta-ur-Rahman, Shaheen, F. *Nat. Prod. Res.* **2003**, *17*, 389.

[30]    Azizuddin, Atta-ur-Rahman, Choudhary, M. I. *Nat. Prod. Lett.* **2002**, *16*, 101.

# Mistletoe Lectins, Structure and Function

Wolfgang Voelter*, Roland Wacker, Stanka Stoeva, Rania Tsitsilonis and Christian Betzel

*Abteilung für Physikalische Biochemie des Physiologisch-chemischen Instituts der Universität Tübingen, Hoppe-Seyler-Str. 4, 72076 Tübingen, Germany*

**Abstract:** Based on isolation, sequence determination and X-ray studies, the primary and three-dimensional structure of the glycoprotein mistletoe lectin I (ML-I) are determined. ML-I is constituted of two chains (A chain: 254 amino acid residues; B chain: 264 amino acid residues) linked by a disulfide bridge. Three different structurally identified oligosaccharides (I, II, III) are attached to four N-type glycosylation sites ($N^{A112}$, $N^{B61}$, $N^{B96}$ and $N^{B136}$). According to these structural characterizations, ML-I is a member of ribosome inactivating proteins (RIP) of type II. The three-dimensional X-ray structure allows a clear-cut picture of the highly toxic effects of ML-I caused by its RNA-N-glycosidase activity, which is in contrast to its immunomodulating activity, applied for the treatment of cancer patients.

## INTRODUCTION

Mistletoe preparations have a long tradition as therapeutic drugs against various diseases. In addition, since the beginning of the 20th century, the use of mistletoe was extended to anti-cancer treatment. Nowadays, aqueous mistletoe extracts are widely used as immunomodulating agents in human cancer therapy.

In spite of the popularity and the medical application of these extracts, little information was available about the structure and the active principles of the ingredients few years ago. Several bioactive compounds could be identified in the past, i.e. flavonoids, biogenous amines, amino acids, alkaloids, polysaccharides, viscotonins and proteins [1-5]. The most important therapeutic application, the immunomodulatory effects of mistletoe extracts, was proven to be based on a group of glycoproteins [6]. These so-called mistletoe lectins are the representatives of the ribosome-inactivating proteins (RIP) of type II [7].

The first structurally determined member of this class of type II RIPs was ricin, an extremely toxic protein from the seeds of castor beans (*Ricinus communis*). Ricin consists of two different protein chains linked by an intermolecular disulfide bridge. The highly specific A-chain inactivates protein biosynthesis due to its RNA N-glycosidase activity. The B subunit binds, as a lectin, to target cell surface glycostructures and thereby facilitates penetration of the toxic A chain to the cytosol. All type II RIPs share this structural architecture.

The type II RIPs of mistletoe are further classified into three different isolectin species according to their different monosaccharide specificity of their B-chain and their molecular weight: Mistletoe lectin-1 (ML-I) is specifically binding to D-galactose, mistletoe lectin-3 (ML-III) to N-acetylgalactosamine and mistletoe lectin-2 (ML-II) to both monosaccharides [8-10].

---

*Corresponding author: E-mail: wolfgang.voelter@uni-tuebingen.de

The patient under mistletoe therapy is thought to benefit from an increase of the non-specific immune system. It was shown that non-toxic doses of ML-I cause a significant increase and activation of natural killer cells and T-cells [11-13]. The administration of ML-I enhances phagocytic activity of granulocytes, monocytes and the expression of receptors for interleukin-2 and B-cells [14-17]. Besides, an increase in the quality of life is discussed, caused by the observed rise of plasma levels of β-endorphin [18].

## PROTEIN ISOLATION

100 g of frozen mistletoe leaves and branches (host tree *populus*) were ground with a mincer and an aqueous suspension was obtained by mixing with water (130 ml). The mixture was homogenised for 1 hour and 113 g turbid extract sparated by aid of a tincture press. The extract was diluted 1:4 (v/v) with elution buffer (0.05 M $K_2HPO_4$, 0.5 M NaCl, pH 7.0) and clarified by centrigugation (20 min, 2000 x g), followed by sterile filtration (Sterivex GV, Millipore). The clear extract was loaded to a lactosyl-Sepharose 4B column (3 x 50 cm), equilibrated with elution buffer, and unbound proteins were eluted with buffer until absorption at 280 nm of the effluent decreased to 0.05 AUs. Elution was stopped and bound lectin was incubated with 5 % β-mercaptoethanol (v/v), based on column volume, over night. After reduction, the MLA-containing fractions were eluted using the elution buffer and as well as collected. The column-bound MLB was desorbed afterwards by adding 0.2 M lactose to the buffer. Both protein fractions were dialysed against water and lyophilised [19].

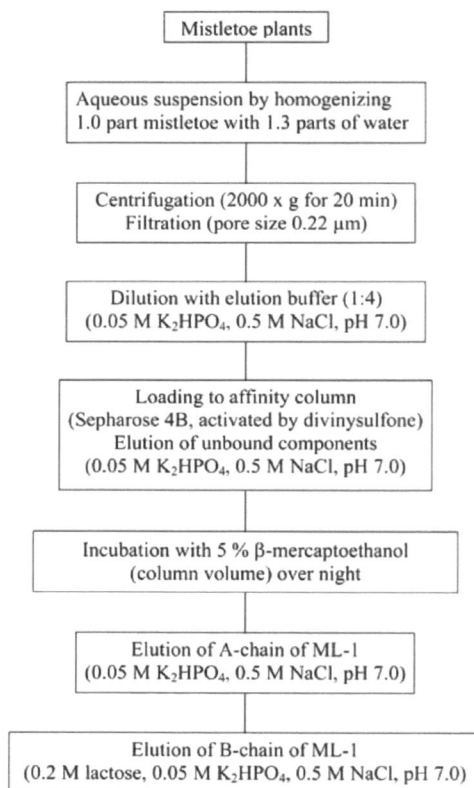

**Fig. (1).** Flow diagram for the isolation of mistletoe lectin A and B chains.

## SEQUENCE ANALYSIS OF ML-I

To achieve the sequence analysis of MLA, two different enzymatic cleavages with endoproteinase AspN and trypsin, respectively, were performed MLB was additionally digested with chymotrypsin. The resulting peptide fragments were isolated in each case via RP-HPLC on a Nucleosil C18 column (Fig. (2)) and lyophilised. Fractions containing cysteine residues were subjected to reduction with β-mercaptoethanol prior to sequence analysis, alkylated with 4-vinylpyridine and then recovered by RP-HPLC.

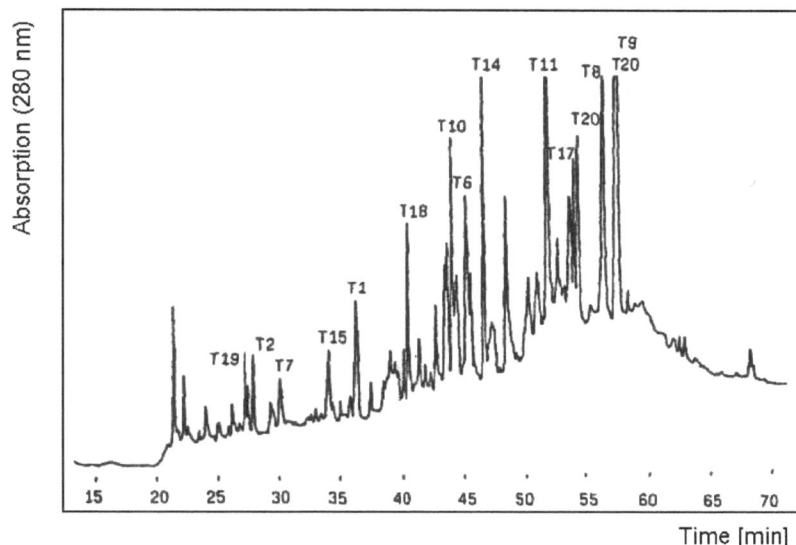

**Fig. (2).** Semi-preparative HPL chromatogram of the peptide mixture received after tryptic digestion of the soluble fraction (pH 4.8) of MLA. Column: Nucleosil $C_{18}$ (250 x 10 mm); eluents: A) 0.15 % TFA in $H_2O$, B) 0.10 % TFA, 80 % $CH_3CN$ in $H_2O$; gradient: 0-100 % B in 100 min; 1.0 ml/min; detection: UV, $\lambda$= 214 nm.

All cleaved peptide fractions were analysed by automated Edman degration sequence analysis (model 473A, Applied Biosystems) and sequence results confirmed by MALDI-mass spectrometry (Kratos Kompact MALDI, Shimadzu), as indicated in Table 1.

The complete sequence of ML-I could be determined from sequence data of overlapping peptides of the five enzymatically-cleaved peptide sets [19,20].

MLA consists of 254 amino acid residues. Based on sequence results, the molecular weight is calculated to be 28,480 Da. The presence of one potential N-type glycosylation site in MLA could be demonstrated ($Asn^{112}$-$Gly^{113}$-$Ser^{114}$). MLA comprises a single cysteine residue at position $Cys^{247}$, which is linked to the B-chain via a disulfide bridge (Fig. **3**).

Sequence comparison of ML-I with ricin (from the seeds of castor beans, Ricinus communis, PDB: 2AAI) and abrin (from jequirity bean, abrus precatorius, PDB: 1ABR) confirmed the high homology between different RIPs (Fig. (2)). For MLA, 143 amino acid residues are conserved (scoring matrix: BLOSUM 62) compared to RTA, resulting in an overall identity score of 36 % and a conservation score of 53 %, respectively. For all three sequences, the amino acid residues involved in the active site of type II RIPs (MLA: $Tyr^{76}$, $Tyr^{115}$, $Glu^{165}$, $Arg^{168}$ und $Trp^{199}$) are invariantly conserved.

**Table 1.** **HPLC-isolated Peptides from the Tryptic Digest of MLA (Glycosylation Site is Underlined; RT [min]: HPLC Retention Times, *: RT After Rechromatography).**

| Peptide | RT [min] | Position | Peptide sequence | Theoret. Mass [M, Da] | Experim. Mass [MH⁺, Da] |
|---|---|---|---|---|---|
| T1 | 25.78 | 1-3 | YER | 466.50 | 468.1 |
| T2 | 24.72 | 4-5 | LR | 287.36 | 288.2 |
| T3 | 24.72 | 6-7 | LR | 287.36 | 288.2 |
| T4 | 40.91 | 8-19 | VTHQTTGEEYFR | 1467.56 | 1468.5 |
| T3+T4 | 43.55 | 6-19 | LRVTHQTTGEEYFR | 1736.91 | 1737.8 |
| T5 | 51.45 | 20-25 | FITLLR | 761.97 | 763.1 |
| T6 | 53.66 | 26-41 | DYVSSGSFSNEIPLLR | 1783.96 | 1785.7 |
| T7 | 35.54 | 42-52 | QSTIPVSDAQR | 1201.31 | 1201.9 |
| T8 | 47.28* | 53-90 | FVLVELTNQGQDSVTAAIDVTNA YVVAYQAGDQSYFLR | 4167.61 | 4169.1 |
| T9 | 23.14 | 91-94 | DAPR | 457.49 | 460.2 |
| T10 | 41.77 | 95-106 | GAETHLFTGTTR | 1290.40 | 1289.6 |
| T11 | 45.66 | 107-120 | SSLPF<u>NGS</u>YPDLER | 1581.71 | 2754.7 |
| T12 | 26.16 | 121-125 | YAGHR | 602.65 | 603.0 |
| T12+T13+T14 | 42.00* | 121-150 | YAGHRDQIPLGIDQLIQSVTALRFP GGSTR | 3267.61 | 3268.7 |
| T15+T16 | 47.28* | 151-168 | TQARSILILIQMISEAAR | 2014.43 | 2016.6 |
| T17 | 53.66 | 169-177 | FNPILWR | 945.14 | 945.3 |
| T19 | 60.67 | 178-219 | QYINSGASFLPDVYMLELETSWG QQSTQVQHSTDGVFNNPIR | 4759.22 | 4760.3 |
| T20+T21 | 48.01* | 220-256 | LAIPPGNFVTLTNVRDVIASLAIML FVCGERPSSS | 3689.37 | 3689.8 |

For MLB, 264 amino acid residues and a molecular weight of 28,960 Da were determined. Sequence analysis of MLB revealed the existence of 7 cysteine residues and three potential N-glycosylation sites ($Asn^{61}$-$Gly^{62}$-$Ser^{63}$, $Asn^{96}$-$Gly^{97}$-$Thr^{98}$ and $Asn^{136}$-$Asp^{137}$-$Thr^{138}$) (Fig. (**4**)).

For the B-chain of ML-I, 199 conserved (75 %) and 165 identical (62 %) amino acid residues were determined in comparison with ricin (Fig. (**4**)). Aside from two in all three RIPs conserved N-glycosylation sites (MLB: $Asn^{96}$-$Gly^{97}$-$Thr^{98}$ and $Asn^{136}$-$Asp^{137}$-$Thr^{138}$), an additional potential glycosylation site was found for MLB($Asn^{61}$-$Gly^{62}$-$Ser^{63}$) due to mutation of a lysine ($Lys^{63}$) to a serine ($Ser^{63}$) residue. Two further mutations (($Cys^{21}$→

```
MLA  - - - - Y E R L R L R V T H Q T T G E E V F R F I T L L B D    26
RTA  I F P K Q Y P I I [N F T] T A G A T V Q S Y T N F I R A V R G  30
ABA  - - - - E D R P I K F S T E G A T S Q S Y K Q F I E A L R E   26

MLA  Y V S S G - S F S N E I P L L R Q S T I P V S D A Q R F V L    55
RTA  R L T T G A D V R H E I P V L P N R V G - L P I N Q R F I L    59
ABA  R L R G - - G L I H D I P V L P D P T T - L Q E R N R Y I T   53

MLA  V E L T N Q G Q D S T A A I D V T N A Y V V A Y Q A G D Q     85
RTA  V E L S N H A E L S V T L A L D V T N A Y V V G Y R A G N S   89
ABA  V E L S N S D T E S I E V G I D V T N A Y V V A Y R A G T Q   83

MLA  S Y F L R - - - D A P R G A E T H L F T G T T - R S S L P F  111
RTA  A Y F F H P D N Q E D A E A I T H L F T D V Q N R Y T F A F  119
ABA  S Y F L R - - - D A P S S A S D Y L F T G T D - Q H S L P F  109

MLA  [N G S V] P D L E R Y A G - H R D Q I P L G - - - I D Q L I Q  137
RTA  G G N Y D R L E Q L A G N L R E N I E L G N G P L E E A I S  149
ABA  Y G T V G D L E R W A H Q S R Q Q I P L G - - - L Q A L T H  136

MLA  S V T A L R F P G G S T R T Q A R S I L I L I Q M I S E A A  167
RTA  A L Y Y Y S T G G T Q L P T L A R S F I I C I Q M I S E A A  179
ABA  G I S F F R S G G N D N E E K A R T L I V I I Q M V A E A A  166

MLA  R F N P I L W R Y R Q Y I N S G A S F L P D V Y M L E L E T  197
RTA  R F Q Y I E G E M R T R I R Y N R R S A P D P S V I T L E N  209
ABA  R F R Y I S N R V R V S I Q T G T A F Q P D A A M I S L E N  196

MLA  S M G Q Q S T Q V Q H S T D G V F N N P I R L A I P P G N F  227
RTA  S W G R L S T A I Q E S N Q G A F A S P I Q L Q R R [N G S] K  239
ABA  N W D N L R G V Q E S V Q D T F P N Q Y T L T N I R N E P   226

MLA  V T L T N V R D - V T A S L A I M L F V C G E R P S S -      254
RTA  F S W Y D V S - I L I P I I A L M V Y R C A P P P S S Q F   267
ABA  V I V D S L S H P T V A V L A L M L F V C N - - P N - -    251
```

Fig. (3). Sequence alignment of the A chains of mistletoe lectin-I (MLA), ricin (RTA) and abrin (ABA). Conserved amino acid residues (scoring matrix: BLOSUM 62) are shaded in dark (100 %) and grey (66 %), respectively. Key residues of the active site are marked with asterisks and N-glycosylation sites are boxed.

| | | |
|---|---|---|
| MLB | | 25 |
| RTB | | 24 |
| ABB | | 29 |
| MLB | | 55 |
| RTB | | 54 |
| ABB | | 59 |
| MLB | | 85 |
| RTB | | 84 |
| ABB | | 89 |
| MLB | | 115 |
| RTB | | 114 |
| ABB | | 119 |
| MLB | | 145 |
| RTB | | 144 |
| ABB | | 149 |
| MLB | | 175 |
| RTB | | 173 |
| ABB | | 178 |
| MLB | | 205 |
| RTB | | 203 |
| ABB | | 208 |
| MLB | | 235 |
| RTB | | 233 |
| ABB | | 238 |
| MLB | | 264 |
| RTB | | 262 |
| ABB | | 267 |

**Fig. (4).** Sequence alignment of the B chains of mistletoe lectin-I (MLB), ricin (RTB) and abrin (ABB). Conserved amino acid residues (scoring matrix: BLOSUM 62) are shaded in dark (100 %) and grey (66 %), respectively. Key residues of the carbohydrate binding sites are marked with asterisks and N-glycosylation sites are boxed.

Arg$^{21}$) resp. (Cys$^{40}$→ Ser$^{40}$)) in the MLB chain causing the loss of one internal disulfide bridge compared to ricin.

In contrast, the positions of the remaining 7 cysteine residues of MLB are invariant compared to ricin. The N-terminal cysteine residue Cys$^5$ of MLB forms a disulfide bridge with Cys$^{247}$ of MLA. Based on homology considerations, the remaining cysteine residues of MLB can be assigned to three intramolecular disulfide bridges according to Fig. (5).

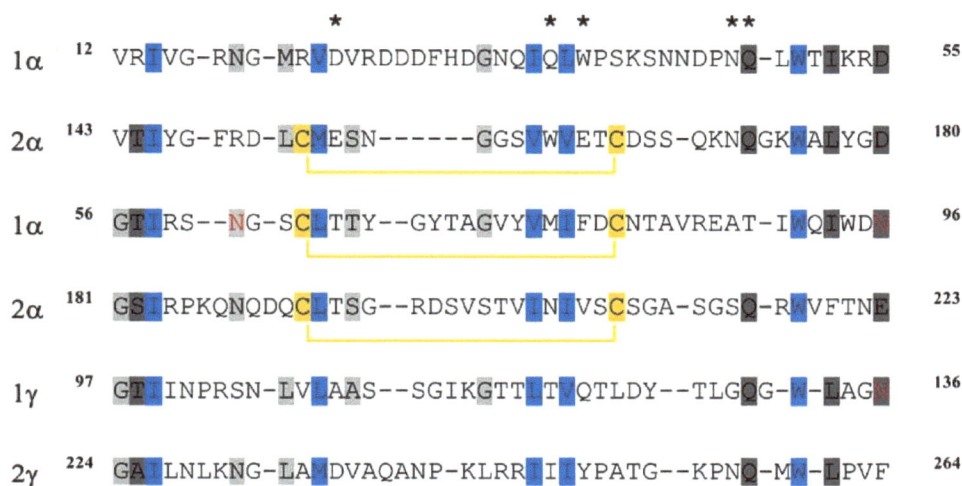

**Fig. (5).** Sequence alignment of the six homologous subdomains of ML-I. Conserved amino acid residues are shaded according to similarity scoring (dark (100 %), dark grey (83 %) and light grey (66 %), respectively). Cysteine residues and disulfide-bridges are marked by connecting lines. The positions of key residues of carbohydrate binding sites are marked with asterisks.

Like ricin, MLB is thought to be a product of a series of gene duplications of an ancestral galactose-binding peptide [21,22]. However, only two of these subdomains, 1α und 2γ, retained their ability to bind galactose. From sequence comparision with RTB it becomes obvious that the key residues of the carbohydrate binding sites of MLB in the subdomains 1α und 2γ are invariantly conserved.

## CRYSTAL STRUCTURE OF ML-I

With highly purified ML-I, X-ray-suitable crystals could be obtained by the hanging-drop vapour-diffusion method. Based on the results of the sequence analysis, the crystal structure of ML-I was solved by the molecular replacement technique using the coordinates of ricin (PDB: 2AAI) as search model. The results (PDB: 1CE7) are visualised in a cartoon plot, Fig. (6) [23].

MLA is a globular enzyme with extensive secondary structure and consists of three individual domains. The active site that is capable to excise a specific adenine base from a highly conserved loop region of 28S rRNA [24,25] is located in a prominent cleft at the interface of three domains. The N-glycosylation site at Asn$^{112}$ is located directly at the edge of this cleft, what is unique among Typ-II RIPs [26].

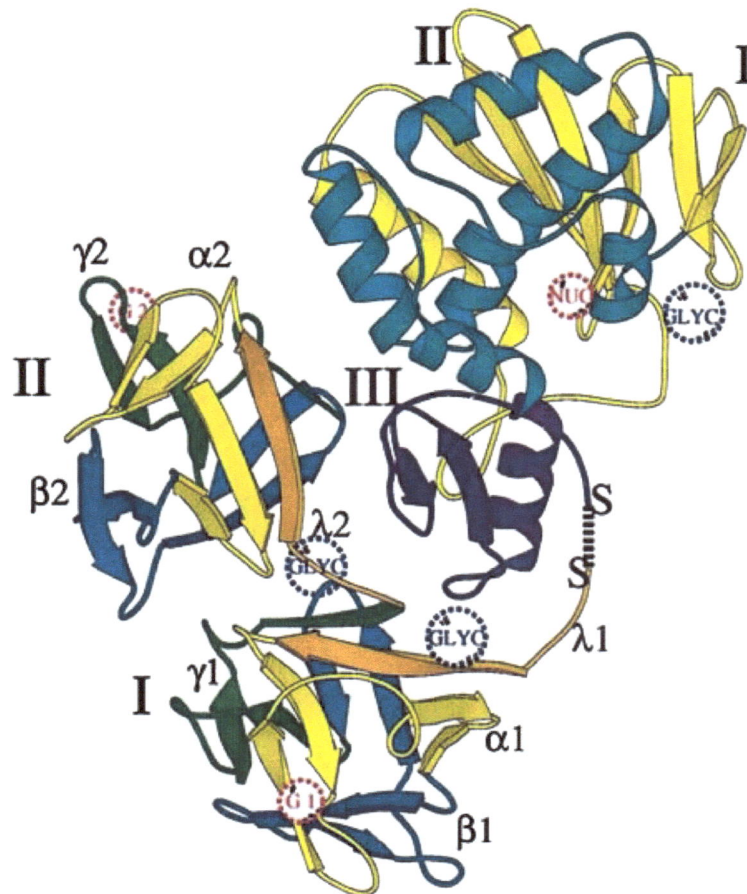

**Fig. (6).** Cartoon plot of the ML-I backbone [23]. The three domains for the A chain are labelled I, II, III and coloured yellow, turquoise and violet. For the B chain, domain I and II are coloured according to their subdomains: The linker regions λ1 and λ2 are shown in orange, the homologous subdomains α, β, γ are coloured yellow, blue and green. The disulfide bond connecting the two chains is shown in a bold dashed line. Dashed circles indicate the nucleotide binding site ("NUC") in chain A and the low ("G1") and high affinity ("G2") galactose binding sites in chain B.

MLB, for which only β-sheets were found, consists of two globular domains 1 and 2, each comprising homologous so–called linker subdomains. The subdomains are arranged along a pseudo threefold axis around a hydrophobic core, a motive classified as β-trefoil fold [27].

## THE RNA-N-GLYCOSIDASE ACTIVITY OF MLA

RIPs of type 1 and type 2 irreversibly damage the larger subunit of ribosomes, thereby preventing the ability to bind elongation factors. Consequently, protein synthesis of the ribosome is interrupted. The modification involves the removal of the first adenine base in a highly conserved rRNA loop sequence GAGA (A4324 in rat liver 28 S rRNA) [25,28]. For the rRNA-specific N-glycosidase activity of ricin, the key residues Tyr[80], Val[81], Gly[121],

Tyr[123], Glu[177] and Arg[180] were identified by X-ray structure, modelling and site-directed mutational analysis [29-37]. A model for the mechanism of the depurination has been proposed based on X-ray analysis of the interaction with substrate analogues [38].

According to this model, the adenine residue is arranged between the two ring planes of Tyr[80] (ML-I: Tyr[76]) and Tyr[123] (ML-I: Tyr[115]) by π-stacking [34], while a fine network of hydrogen bonds ensures the functional alignment of the substrate (ML-I: Gly[113]) and the catalytic active residues (ML-I: Arg[168] and Glu [165]; Fig. (7)).

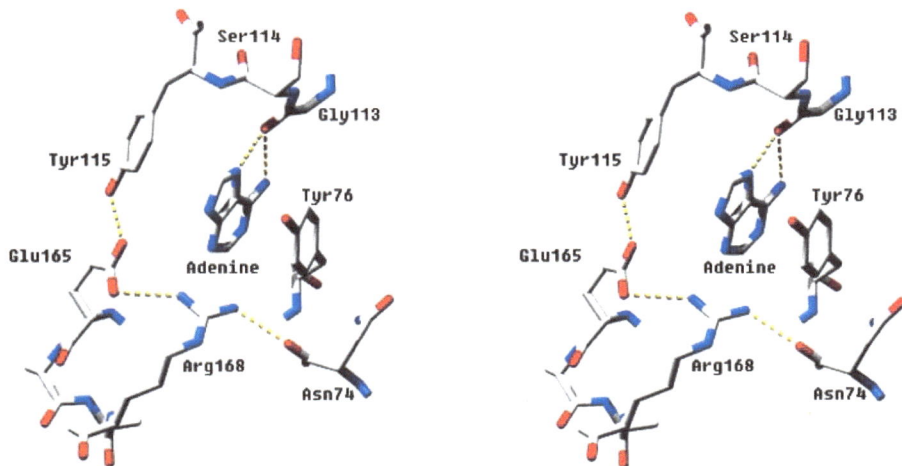

**Fig. (7).** Stereo plot of the active site of MLA in complex with adenine [40]. For details see text.

The main steps for the catalytic mechanism are activation of the leaving adenine residue and stabilisation of the forming oxocarbenium ion (Fig. (8)).

N3 of the adenine residue is likely to be protonated by the arginine residue, while the glutamic acid residue seems to stabilise the oxocarbenium ion (step A in Fig. (8)). A water molecule, activated in a trigonally-bonded transition state to adenine and arginine Arg[180], is supposed to attack the carbenium ion nucleophilic.

A different mechanism was supposed by Huang and co-workers [39], based on the crystal structures for the RIPs trichosanthin and α-momorcharin. Their model assumes that N7 of the adenine base is protonated by Asp[96] of RTA.

## CARBOHYDRATE BINDING SITES OF MLB

Before the endocytotic uptake of the toxic A chain the galactoside-specific B chain of ML-I has to interact with surface receptors of the cell in order to trigger the internalisation of MLA. As described above, the B chain contains two carbohydrate binding sites in the 1α and 2γ subdomains, respectively. With the exception of *Sambucus nigra* agglutinin [41], most type II RIPs are Gal- and / or GalNAc-specific lectins.

In ricin D, serving as a type II RIP- archetype, the binding site, located in subdomain 2γ ("high affinity site") is capable to bind galactose and N-acetylgalactosamine, while the other one, situated in the 1α ("low affity site") subdomain, is specifically binding galactose with reduced affinity [29]. In contrast, ML-I shows poor affinity to N-actylgalactosamine, indicating structural differences in, at least, the 2γ-subdomain, compared to ricin.

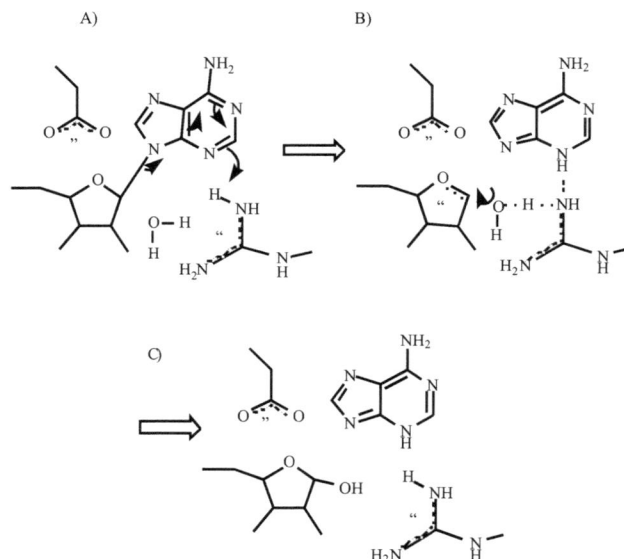

**Fig. (8).** Schematic illustration of the proposed mechanism of RNA-N-glycosidase activity of RTA (similar to [38]). For details see text.

The basic structure of the binding pocket is an aromatic side chain (Trp[38], Tyr[249]) providing stacking interactions with the galactose ring on top, a tripeptide kink loop forming the bottom (Asp[23]-Val[24]-Arg[25], Asp[235]-Val[236]-Ala[237]) and the side chain of a central asparagine residue (Asn[47], Asn[256]) interacting with the carbohydrate *via* hydrogen bonds.

Recently, the crystal structure of ML-I complexed with galactose (3 Å resolution) was published [26]. According to these results, the coordinates of both carbohydrate binding sites are visualized in figures **9** and **10**. The hydrogen bond network inside the low affinity carbohydrate binding site of ML-1 involves the amino acid residues Asp[23] (Oδ1 – 3-OH, Oδ2 – 4-OH), Asp[26] (N – 4-OH), Asp[27] (Oδ2 - 2-OH), Lys[41] (Nζ - 2-OH, Nζ - 3-OH) and Asn[47] (Nδ2 - 3-OH). In the high affinity site, Asp[235] (Oδ1 – 3-OH, Oδ2 – 4-OH), Asn[256] (Nδ2 - 3-OH) and Gln[238] (N – 4-OH) form hydrogen bonds to the galactose moiety.

The interactions of both binding sites with carbohydrates are based mainly on hydrogen bonds of Asp residues to C-3-OH and C-4-OH of the galactose moiety. The low affinity site of MLB cannot bind N-acetyl galactosamine due to steric hindrance caused by Asp[27] and Lys[41] with the 2-N-acetyl group. The reason for the lacking binding capacity of the high affinity site of MLB to GalNAc, which is in contrast to RTB, cannot be explained so far, and is a matter of speculations: Steric hindrance of the Lys[254] side chain with the N-acetyl group, or the missing hydrogen bond of the acetyl oxygen from GalNAc to the hydroxyl group of Ser[238], as observed in ricin, might be the possible explanations. In MLB an amino acid mutation of this serine to an alanine residue (ricin: Ser[238] → MLB: Ala[240]), prevents the hydrogen binding to GalNAc.

## GLYCOSYLATION OF ML-I

The structural characterization of the carbohydrate chains attached to ML-I was accomplished by Debray *et al.* [42] by a pronase digest of ML-I, followed by [1]H NMR analysis of the purified glycopeptides.

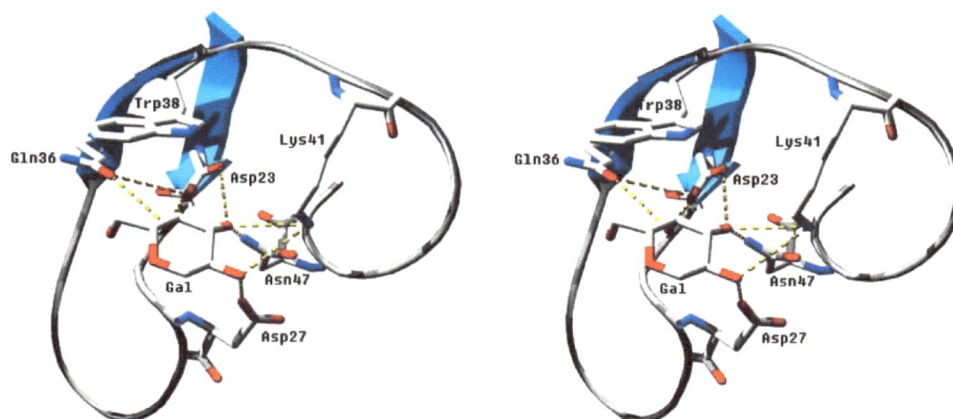

**Fig. (9).** Stereoplot of the low affinity galactose binding site of MLB complexed with galactose (similar to [26]). For details see text.

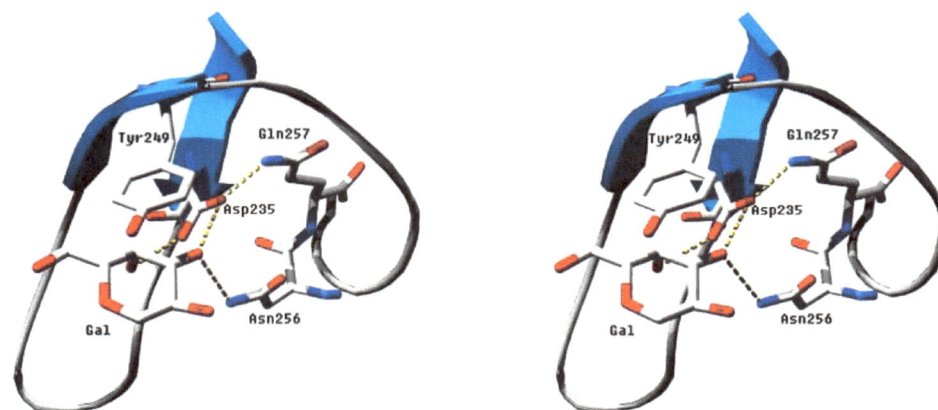

**Fig. (10).** Stereoplot of the high affinity galactose binding site of MLB complexed with galactose (similar to [26]). For details see text.

According to the authors, 3 different oligosaccharides could be identified (Fig. (**11**)).

Structure I, a fucosylated and xylosylated trimannosyl-heptasaccharide, is a common core structure of plant-derived glycoproteins. Furthermore, two oligomannoside-type glycans were identified to be attached to ML-I, composed of six (III) and five (II) mannose and two N-acetylglucosamine units, respectively, in a 4:1 ratio according to NMR data.

The assignment of the carbohydrate moieties to the four N-type glycosylation sites of ML-I could be solved by the comparison of MALDI-mass spectra of isolated glycopeptides with calculated mass values resulting from Edman degration sequencing of the corresponding glycopeptides [43].

As indicated in figure **11**, the solely glycosylation site of MLA ($N^{A112}$) is attached to carbohydrate moiety I. The same carbohydrate chain is found at $N^{B61}$ of the B chain. Oligosaccharide II is connected to the glycosylation sites $N^{B96}$ and $N^{B136}$ of MLB. Additionally, the oligosaccharide III could be identified at the glycosylation site $N^{B136}$.

**I**

Man α1
       ⟍6
        Man β1— 4 GlcNAc β1— 4 GlcNAc β1—Asn
       ⟋3  2                              3
Man α1     ⟍                              |
        Xyl β1                         Fuc α1

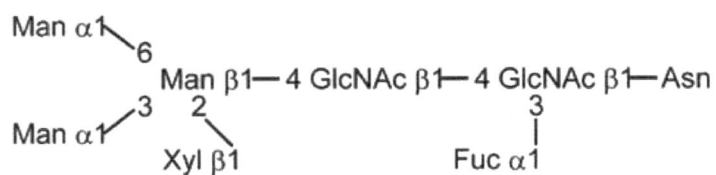

ML-IA 112-114 (Asn-Gly-Ser)

ML-IB 61-63(Asn-Gly-Ser)

**II**

Man α1
       ⟍6
        Man α1
       ⟋3     ⟍6
Man α1          Man β1— 4 GlcNAc β1— 4 GlcNAc β1—Asn
              ⟋3
        Man α1
       ⟋2
Man α1

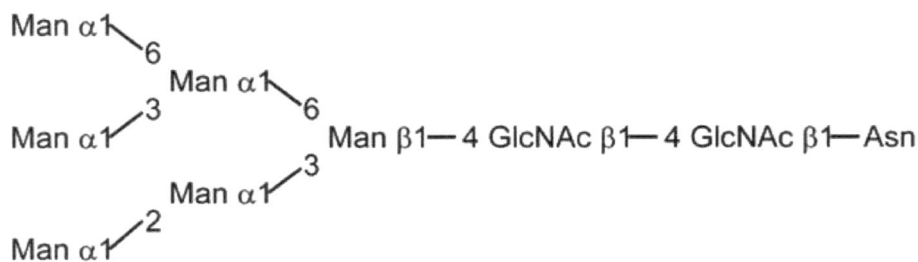

ML-IB 96-98 (Asn-Gly-Thr)

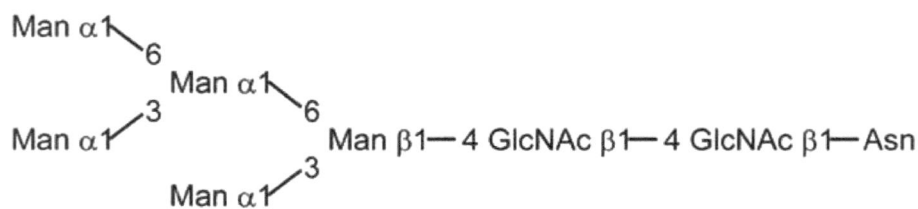

ML-IB 136-138 (Asn-Asp-Thr)

**III**

Man α1
       ⟍6
        Man α1
       ⟋3     ⟍6
Man α1          Man β1— 4 GlcNAc β1— 4 GlcNAc β1—Asn
              ⟋3
        Man α1

ML-IB 136-138 (Asn-Asp-Thr)

**Fig. (11).** Carbohydrate structures I-III of ML-I and their assignments to N-type glycosylation sites acccording to references [42,43].

## ABBREVIATIONS

| | | |
|---|---|---|
| ABA | = | Abrin A chain |
| ABB | = | Abrin B chain |
| MALDI-MS | = | Matrix-assisted laser desorption mass spectrometry |
| ML | = | Mistletoe lectin |
| MLA | = | Mistletoe lectin A chain |
| MLB | = | Mistletoe lectin B chain |
| PDB | = | PDB-accession code, URL: *http://www.rcsb.org/pdb/* |
| RIP | = | Ribosome-inactivating protein |
| RNA | = | Ribonucleic acid |
| RTA | = | Ricinus toxic agglutinin A chain |
| RTB | = | Ricinus toxic agglutinin B chain |

## REFERENCES

[1]     Voelter, W.; Soler, M.H.; Stoeva, S.; Betzel, C.; Eschenburg, S.; Krauspenhaar, R. *GIT Laboratory Journal, Int. Ed.*, **1997**, *1*, 32-34.

[2]     Voelter, W.; Wacker, R.; Franz, M.; Maier, T.; Stoeva, S. *J. Prakt. Chem.*, **2000**, *342*, 812-818.

[3]     Luther, P.; Becker, H.; Die Mistel: Botanik, Lektine, medizinische Anwendung, Springer-Verlag, **1987**.

[4]     Romagnoli, S.; Ugolini, R.; Fogolari, F; Schaller, G.; Urech, K.; Giannattasio, M.; Ragona, L.; Molinari, H. *Biochem. J.*, **2000**, *350*, 569-577.

[5]     Stoeva, S.; Franz, M.; Wacker, R.; Krauspenhaar, R.; Guthöhrlein, E.; Mikhailov, A.; Betzel, C.; Voelter, W. *Arch. Biochem. Biophys.*, **2001**, *392*, 23-31.

[6]     Beuth, J.; Ko, H.L.; Tunggal, L.; Buss, G.; Jeljaszewicz, J.; Steuer, M.K.; Pulverer, G. *Arzneim.-Forsch./Drug Res.*,**1994**, *44*, 1255-1258.

[7]     Barbieri, L.; Battelli, M.G.; Stirpe, F. *Biochim. Biophys. Acta*, **1993**, *1154*, 237-282.

[8]     Franz, H.; Ziska, P.; Kindt, A. *Biochem. J.*, **1981**, *195*, 481-484.

[9]     Samtleben, R.; Kiefer, M.; Luther, P. *Lectins: Biology, Biochemistry, Clinical Biochemistry*, **1985**, *4*, 617-626.

[10]    Eifler, R.; Pfüller, K.; Göckeritz, W.; Pfüller, U. *Lectins: Biology, Biochemistry, Clinical Biochemistry*, **1993**, *9*, 144-151.

[11]    Beuth, J.; Ko, H.L.; Gabius, H.-J.; Burrichter, H.; Oette, K.; Pulverer G. *Clin. Investig.*, **1992**, *70*, 658-661.

[12]    Beuth, J.; Ko, H.-L.; Tunggal, L.; Gabius, H.-J.; Steuer, M.; Uhlenbruck, G.; Pulverer G. *Med. Welt.*, **1993**, *44*, 217-220.

[13]    Beuth, J.; Ko, H.-L.; Tunggal, L.; Geisel, J.; Pulverer, G. *Arzneim.-Forsch./Drug Res.*, **1993**, *43*, 166-169.

[14]    Baxevanis, C.N.; Voutsas, I.F.; Soler, M.H.; Gritzapis, A.D.; Tsitsilonis, O.E.; Stoeva, S.; Voelter, W.; Arsenis, P.; Papamichail, M. *Immunopharm. Immunotox.*, **1998**, *20*, 355-372.

[15]    Hajto, T.; Hostanska, K.; Frei, K.; Rordorf, C.; Gabius, H.-J. *Cancer Res.*, **1990**, *50*, 3322-3326.

[16]    Beuth, J.; Stoffel, B.; Ko, H.-L.; Buss, G.; Pulverer, G. *Arzneim.-Forsch./Drug Res.*, **1995**, *45*, 505-507.

[17]    Beuth, J.; Ko, H.-L.; Tunggal, L.; Pulverer, G. *Dtsch. Zschr. Onkol.*, **1993**, *25*, 73-76.

[18]    Heiny, B.-M.; Beuth, J.; *Anticancer Res.*, **1994**, *14*, 1339-1342.

[19]    Soler, M.H.; Stoeva, S.; Schwarmborn, C.; Wilhelm, S.; Stiefel, T.; Voelter, W. *FEBS Let.*, **1996**, *399*, 153-157.

[20]    Soler, M.H.; Stoeva, S.; Voelter, W. *Biochem. Biophys. Res. Comm.*, **1998**, *246*, 596-601.

[21]    Villafranca, J.E.; Robertus, J.D. *J. Biol. Chem.*, **1981**, *256*, 554-556.

[22]    Rutenber, E.; Ready, M.; Robertus, J.D. *Nature*, **1987**, *326*, 624-626.

[23]    Krauspenhaar, R.; Eschenburg, S.; Perbandt, M.; Kornilov, V.; Konareva, N.; Mikailova, I.; Stoeva, S.; Wacker, R.; Maier, T.; Singh, T.; Mikhailov, M.; Voelter, W.; Betzel, C. *Biochem. Biophys. Res. Commun.*, **1999**, *257*, 418-424.

[24]    Eschenburg, S.; Krauspenhaar, R.; Mikhailov, A.; Stoeva, S.; Betzel, C.; Voelter, W. *Biochem. Biophys. Res. Comm.*, **1998**, *247*, 367-372.

[25]    Endo, Y.; Tsurugi, K.; Franz, H. *FEBS Lett.*, **1988**, *231*, 378-380.

[26]     Niwa, H.; Tonevitsky, A.G.; Agapov, I.I.; Saward, S.; Pfüller, U.; Palmer, R.A. *Eur. J. Biochem.*, **2003**, *270*, 2739-2749.

[27]     Sweeney, E.C.; Tonevitsky, A.G.; Palmer, R.A.; Niwa, H.; Pfueller, U.; Eck, J.; Lentzen, H.; Agapov, I.I.; Kirchpichnikov, M.P. *FEBS Lett.* **1998**, *431*, 367-370.

[28]     Endo, Y.; Mitsui, K.; Motizuki, M.; Tsurugi, K. *J. Biol. Chem.*, **1987**, *262*, 5908-5912.

[29]     Rutenber, E.; Robertus, J.D. *Proteins*, **1991**, *10*, 260-269.

[30]     Rutenber, E.; Katzin, B.J.; Ernst, S.; Collins, E.J.; Mlsna, D.; Ready, M.P.; Robertus, J.D. *Proteins*, **1991**, *10*, 240-250.

[31]     Day, P.J.; Ernst, S.R.; Frankel, A.E.; Monzingo, A.F.; Pascal, J.M.; Molina-Svinth, M.C., Robertus, J.D. *Biochemistry*, **1996**, *35*, 11098-11103.

[32]     Yan, X.; Hollis, T.; Svinth, M.; Day, P.; Monzingo, A.F.; Milne, G.W.A.; Robertus, J.D. *J. Mol. Biol.*, **1997**, *266*, 1043-1049.

[33]     Yan, X.; Day, P.; Hollis, T.; Monzingo, A.F.; Schelp, E.; Robertus, J.D.; Milne, G.W.A.; Wang, S. *Proteins*, **1998**, *31*, 33-41.

[34]     Chen, X.; Link, T.M.; Schramm, V.L. *Biochemistry*, **1998**, *37*, 11605-11613.

[35]     Kim, Y.; Robertus, J.D.; Protein Eng.; **1992**, *5*, 775-779.

[36]     Marsden, C.J.; Fülöp, V.; Day, P.J.; Lord, J.M. *Eur. J. Biochem.*, **2004**, *271*, 153-162.

[37]     Kitaoka, Y. *Eur. J. Biochem.*, **1998**, *257*, 255-262.

[38]     Monzingo, A.F.; Robertus, J.D. *J. Mol. Biol.*, **1992**, *227*, 1136-1145.

[39]     Huang, Q.; Liu, S.; Tang, Y; Jin, S.; Wang, Y. *Biochem. J.*, **1995**, *309*, 285-298.

[40]     Krauspenhaar, R.; Rypniewski, W.; Kalkura, N.; Moore, K.; DeLucas, L.; Stoeva, S.; Mikhailov, A.; Voelter, W.; Betzel, C. *Acta Cryst.*, **2002**, *D58*, 1704-1707.

[41]     Van Damme, E.J.M.; Barre, A.; Rougé, P.; Van Leuven, F.; Peumans, W.J. *Eur. J. Biochem.*, **1996**, *235*, 128-137.

[42]     Debray, H.; Wieruszeski, J.M.; Strecker, G.; Franz, H. *Carbohydr. Res.*, **1992**, *236*, 135-143.

[43]     Stoeva, S.; Maier, T.; Soler, M.H.; Voelter, W. *Polish J. Chem.*, **1999**, *73*, 125-133.

Atta-ur-Rahman/Choudhary/Khan (Eds.) *Frontiers in Natural Product Chemistry, Vol. 1*     163

# Polyacetylenes and Sterols from the Aerial Parts of *Chrysanthemum coronarium* L. (Garland)

M.-Ch. Song[a], D.-H. Kim[a], Y.-H. Hong[a], H.-J. Yang[a], I.-S. Chung[a], S.-H. Kim[b], B.-M. Kwon[c], D.-K. Kim[d], M.-H. Park[e] and N.-I. Baek[a,*]

[a]*Graduate School of Biotechnology & Plant Metabolism Research Center; KyungHee University, Suwon, 449-701,* [b]*Department of Pharmacy, Woosuk University, Jeunbuk, 565-701,* [c]*Graduate School of East-West Medical Science, KungHee University, Suwon, 449-701,* [d]*Erom Life Co. Ltd., Seoul, 135-825,* [e]*Korea Research Institute of Bioscience and Biotechnology, K/S1; Taejon, 305-333, Korea*

**Abstract:** The aerial parts of *Chrysanthemum coronarium* were extracted in MeOH, and the extract was partitioned using EtOAc, *n*-BuOH and $H_2O$. The repeated column chromatography of EtOAc fraction gave four sterols, whose chemical structures were identified as stigmast-4-en-6β-ol-3-one (**1**), stigmast-4-en-6α-ol-3-one (**2**), which have been so far reported only in the aquatic plants and were isolated for the first time from the land plants, β-sitosterol (**3**) and daucosterol (**4**) based on several spectral data including gCOSY, gHSQC, gHMBC and comparison of the data with those of literature. And the repeated column chromatography of EtOAc and *n*-BuOH fractions gave nine polyacetylens, which were identified as 2-[(1Z,4Z)-5-methylsulfinyl-2-pentyn-4-enyliden]-1,6-dioxaspiro[4,4]non-3-ene (**5**), 2-[(1E,4Z)-5-methylsulfinyl-2-pentyn-4-enyliden]-1,6-dioxaspiro[4,4]non-3-ene (**6**), 2-[1Z-2,4-dipentyn-6-methyliden]-1,6-dioxaspiro[4,4]non-3-ene (**7**), 2-[1E-2,4-dipentyn-6-methyliden]-1,6-ioxaspiro[4,4]non-3-ene (**8**), 2-[1E-2,4-dipentyn-6-methyliden]-1,6-dioxaspiro[4,5]non-3-ene (**9**), 2-[1Z-2,4-dipentyn-6-methylidene]-1,6-dioxaspiro[4,4]non-3,7-dien-9α-ol (**10**), 2-[1E-2,4-dipentyn-6-methyliden]-1,6-dioxaspiro[4,4]non-3,7-dien-9β-ol (**11**), 2-[1E-2,4-dipentyn-6-methyliden]-1,6-dioxaspiro[4,4] non-3,7-dien-9α-ol (**12**) and 2-[1Z-2,4-dipentyn-6-methyliden ]-1,6-dioxaspiro[4,4]non-3,7-dien-9β-ol (**13**). Some of them showed the inhibitory effect on the activity of ACAT (Acyl-CoA: cholesterol acyltransferase), the catalyzing enzymes of the intracellular esterification of cholesterol, and FPTase (Farnesyl-protein transferase), the farnesylation enzymes for Ras protein in charge of cancer promotion, PLT aggregation, and the growth of HUVEC (Human umbilical vascular endothelial cell) or A549 cells.

**Key Words:** *Chrysanthemum coronarium,* sterone, anticancer, polyacetylene, HUVEC, A549, ACAT, FPTase, PLT aggregation.

## INTRODUCTION

During the course of evaluating edible plants for biological activity, authors have reported the isolation of secondary metabolites with biological functionality from several plants such as sweet potato [1], pumpkin leaves [2], a wild garlic [3,4] and lettuce [5].

---

*Corresponding author: Tel: +82-31-201-2661; Fax: +82-31-204-8116; E-mail: nibaek@khu.ac.kr

*Chrysanthemum coronarium* L. (Garland, Compositae) is an annual herb, which has been favorably ingested in the Korean diet because of its fragrant taste as well as abundance in nutrition. Moreover, the aerial parts of *C. coronarium* have been used for the protection or remedy of several diseases in oriental medicinal systems [6]. Although several constituents like essential oil [7], flavonoids [8], sesquiterpenes lactones [9], have been isolated from *C. coronarium,* the relationship between biological activity and the constituents has not been reported so far. Therefore, phytochemical and pharmacological study on the plant was carried out.

This paper deals with not only the isolation and structure determination of some sterols and polyacetylenes from the aerial parts of *Chrysanthemum coronarium* but also evaluation of their pharmacological activities like inhibitory effect on ACAT activity, PLT aggregation, FPTase activity and the growth of HUVEC or A549 cells.

## MATERIALS & METHODS

### Plant Materials

*C. coronarium* L. was purchased from a farm located in Yangju-Si, Korea in December, 2002. A voucher specimen (KHU020809) was reserved at the Laboratory of Natural Products Chemistry, KyungHee University, Suwon, Korea.

### Isolation of Compounds

The fresh aerial parts of *C. coronarium* (80 kg) were extracted at room temperature with MeOH (40L x 3) for 24 hr. The filtrate was concentrated *in vacuo* at 40 °C to render the MeOH extracts. The extracts were partitioned with water (2 L), EtOAc (2 L x 3) and *n*-BuOH (2L x 3), successively, to yield the EtOAc (168 g), *n*-BuOH (126 g) and water (512 g) extracts. The EtOAc extract (168 g) was applied to silica gel (1500 g) column chromatography (CHCl$_3$-MeOH = 10:1→8:1→6:1→4:1→2:1→1:1) monitoring by thin layer chromatography (TLC) to produce twenty fractions (NCE1~NCE20). From the third, fifth and thirteenth fractions, polyacetylene and steroid compounds were isolated using repeated silica gel and ODS column chromatography.

Compound **1 (stigmast-4-en-6β-ol-3-one)**; [1]H-NMR (400 MHz, CDCl$_3$, δ) : 5.78 (lH, br. s, H-4), 4.31 (lH, br. s, H-6), 1.34 (3H, s, H-19), 0.89 (3H, d, *J*=6.4 Hz, H-21), 0.81 (3H, t, *J*=7.6 Hz, H-29), 0.80 (3H, d, *J*=6.9 Hz, H-27), 0.78 (3H, d, *J*=6.8 Hz, H-26), 0.71 (3H, s, H-18), [13]C- NMR (100 MHz, CDCl$_3$, δ) : 200.40 (C-3), 168.53 (C-5), 126.17 (C-4), 73.19 (C-6), 56.04 (C-14), 55.87 (C-17), 53.61 (C-9), 45.82 (C-24), 42.52 (C-13), 39.61 (C-12), 38.57 (C-7), 38.02 (C-10), 37.10 (C-1), 36.15 (C-20), 34.29 (C-22), 33.91 (C-2), 29.75 (C-8), 29.16 (C-25), 28.23 (C-16), 26.10 (C-23), 24.20 (C-15), 23.10 (C-28), 21.02 (C-11), 19.88 (C-26), 19.55 (C-19), 19.08 (C-27), 18.78 (C-21), 12.08 (C-29), 12.04 (C-18).

Compound **2 (stigmast-4-en-6α-ol-3-one)**; [1]H-NMR (400 MHz, CDCl$_3$, δ) : 6.17 (lH, d, *J*=1.6 Hz, H-4), 4.32 (lH, ddd, *J*=12.0, 5.6,1.6 Hz, H-6), 1.17 (3H, s, H-19), 0.92 (3H, d, *J*=6.8 Hz, H-21), 0.86 (3H, t, *J*=7.6 Hz, H-29), 0.85 (3H, d, *J*=6.8 Hz, H-26), 0.82 (3H, d, *J*=6.9 Hz, H-27), 0.71 (3H, s, H-18), [13]C-NMR (100 MHz, CDCl$_3$, δ) : 199.50 (C-3), 171.71 (C-5), 119.52 (C-4), 68.66 (C-6), 55.94 (C-14), 55.55 (C-17), 53.74 (C-9), 45.81 (C-24), 42.46 (C-13), 41.46 (C-7), 41.46 (C-12), 39.46 (C-10), 36.27 (C-1), 36.12 (C-20), 34.17 (C-22), 33.82 (C-2), 29.75 (C-8), 29.15 (C-25), 28.19 (C-16), 26.06 (C-23), 24.23 (C-15), 23.10 (C-28), 21.07 (C-11), 19.87 (C-26), 19.07 (C-19), 18.75 (C-27), 18.33 (C-21), 12.04 (C-29), 12.00 (C-18).

Compound **5** (**2-[(lZ,4Z)-5-methylsulfinyl-2-pentyn-4-enyliden]-1,6-dioxaspiro[4,4] non-3-ene**); [1]H-NMR(400 MHz, CDCl$_3$, δ) : 6.73 (lH, dd, $J$=6.0, 4.0 Hz, H-8), 6.50 (lH, d, $J$=10.0 Hz, H-2), 6.27 (lH, ddd, $J$=6.0, 2.0, 1.2 Hz, H-9), 6.22 (lH, dd, $J$=10.0, 4.0 Hz, H-3), 5.03 (lH, dd, $J$=2.0, 1.2 Hz, H-6), 4.17 (lH, m, H-13a), 3.98 (lH, m, H-13b), 2.70 (3H, d, $J$=1.6 Hz, H-1), 2.24 (H, m, H-12a), 2.22 (2H, m, H-11a), 2.06 (2H, m, H-11b, 12b), [13]C-NMR (100 MHz, CDCl$_3$, δ): 168.33 (C-7), 142.90 (C-2), 136.75 (C-9), 125.98 (C-8), 121.14 (C-10), 118.59 (C-3), 99.60 (C-5), 85.87 (C-4), 79.84 (C-6), 69.87 (C-13), 40.32 (C-1), 35.58 (C-11), 24.51 (C-12).

Compound **6** (**2-[(1E,4Z)-5-methylsulfinyl-2-pentyn-4-enyliden]-1,6-dioxaspiro [4,4] non-3-ene**); [1]H-NMR(400 MHz, CDCl$_3$, δ) : 6.56 (lH, d, $J$=10.0 Hz, H-2), 6.31 (lH, dd, $J$=6.0, 2.0 Hz, H-8), 6.28 (lH, d, $J$=6.0 Hz, H-9), 6.28 (lH, dd, $J$=10.0, 2.4 Hz, H-3), 4.77 (lH, dd, $J$=2.0, 2.4 Hz, H-6), 4.23 (1H, m, H-13a), 4.02 (lH, m, H-13b), 2.78 (3H, d, $J$=1.6 Hz, H-1), 2.32 (H, m, H-12a), 2.25 (H, m, H-11a), 2.12 (2H, m, H-11b, 12b), [13]C-NMR (100 MHz, CDCl$_3$, δ) : 166.38 (C-7), 144.53 (C-2), 136.14 (C-9), 127.16 (C-8), 120.99 (C-10), 117.76 (C-3), 98.61 (C-5), 87.97 (C-4), 78.51 (C-6), 69.67 (C-13), 40.06 (C-1), 35.55 (C-11), 24.35 (C-12).

Compound **7** (**2-[lZ-2,4-dipentyn-6-methyliden]-1,6-dioxaspiro[4,4]non-3-ene**); [1]H-NMR (400 MHz, CDCl$_3$, δ) : 6.57 (lH, d, $J$=5.6 Hz, H-8), 6.14 (lH, dd, $J$=5.6, 1.6 Hz, H-9), 4.80 (lH, dd, $J$=2.0, 1.2 Hz, H-6), 4.05 (lH, m, H-13a), 3.87 (lH, m, H-13b), 1.94-2.15 (4H, m, H-11a/11b, 12a/12b), 1.88 (3H, d, $J$=1.6 Hz, H-1), [13]C-NMR (100 MHz, CDCl$_3$, δ) : 168.46 (C-7), 135.75 (C-9), 125.30 (C-8), 120.54 (C-10), 79.40 (C-2), 79.25 (C-6), 76.07 (C-4), 71.14 (C-5), 69.38 (C-13), 64.71 (C-3), 35.23 (C-11), 24.26 (C-12), 4.35 (C-1).

Compound **8** (**2-[lE-2,4-dipentyn-6-methyliden]-1,6-ioxaspiro[4,4]non-3-ene**); [1]H-NMR(400 MHz, CDCl$_3$, δ) : 6.20 (lH, d, $J$=5.6 Hz, H-8), 6.12 (lH, dd, $J$=5.6, 1.2 Hz, H-9), 4.55 (lH, dd, $J$=1.2 Hz, H-6), 4.20(lH, m, H-13a), 3.95 (lH, m, H-13b), 2.13-2.32 (2H, m, H-lla, 12a), 1.95-2.07 (2H, m, H-11b, 12b), 1.95 (3H, d, $J$=1.6 Hz, H-1), [13]C-NMR (100 MHz, CDCl$_3$, δ): 166.96 (C-7), 135.13 (C-9), 127.26 (C-8), 120.90 (C-10), 80.55 (C-2), 78.75 (C-4), 78.62 (C-6), 70.66 (C-5), 69.61 (C-13), 65.07 (C-3), 35.56 (C-11), 24.47 (C-12), 4.77 (C-1).

Compound **9** (**2-[1E-2,4-dipentyn-6-methyliden]-1,6-dioxaspiro[4,5]non-3-ene**); [1]H-NMR (400 MHz, CDCl$_3$, δ) : 6.21 (1H, d, $J$=5.6 Hz, H-8), 6.13 (1H, dd, $J$=5.6, 0.8 Hz, H-9), 4.57 (1H, dd, $J$=0.8 Hz, H-6), 4.21(1H, m, H-14a), 3.94 (1H, m, H-14b), 2.18-2.31 (2H, m, H-lla, 12a), 2.05-2.08 (4H, m, H-llb, 12b, 13a/b), 1.96 (3H, d, $J$=1.2 Hz, H-1), [13]C-NMR (100 MHz, CDC$_3$, δ) : 166.98 (C-7), 135.13 (C-9), 127.33 (C-8), 120.93 (C-10), 80.58 (C-2), 78.82 (C-4), 78.74 (C-6), 70.70 (C-5), 69.66 (C-14), 65.13 (C-3), 35.62 (C-11), 29.73 (C-13), 24.51 (C-12), 4.84 (C-l).

Compound **10** (**2-[1Z-2,4-dipentyn-6-methyliden]-1,6-dioxaspiro[4,4]non-3,7-dien-9α-ol**); [1]H-NMR(400 MHz, CDCl$_3$, δ) : 6.79 (1H, d, $J$=5.6 Hz, H-8), 6.46 (1H, m, H-13), 6.29 (1H, dd, $J$=5.6, 1.6 Hz, H-9), 5.25 (1H, m, H-12), 5.14 (1H, d, $J$=0.8 Hz, H-6), 4.91 (1H, hr. s., H-11), 1.97 (3H, d, $J$=0.8 Hz, H-1), [13]C-NMR (100 MHz, CDCl$_3$, δ) : 168.16 (C-7), 146.31 (C-13), 133.40 (C-9), 126.89 (C-8), 117.74 (C-10), 105.78 (C-12), 82.96 (C-6), 80.47 (C-2), 77.50 (C-4), 76.23 (C-11), 70.02 (C-5), 64.66 (C-3), 4.77 (C-l).

Compound **11** (**2-[1E-2,4-dipentyn-6-methyliden]-1,6-dioxaspiro[4,4]non-3,7-dien-9β-ol**); [1]H-NMR(400 MHz, CDCl$_3$, δ) : 6.59 (1H, dd, $J$=3.2, 1.6, H-13), 6.34 (1H, d, $J$=6.0 Hz, H-8), 6.28 (1H, dd, $J$=6.0, 0.8 Hz, H-9), 5.63 (1H, dd, $J$=2.4, 1.6, H-ll), 5.19 (1H, dd, $J$=3.2, 2.4, H- 12), 4.76 (1H, hr. s., H-6), 1.96(3H, d, $J$=0.8 Hz, H-l), [13]C-NMR (100 MHz, CDC1$_3$, δ) : 166.90 (C-7), 148.70 (C-13), 133.16 (C-9), 126.90 (C-8), 117.07 (C-10), 100.07

(C-12), 82.99 (C-2), 82.13 (C-6), 75.08 (C-4), 75.02 (C-11), 69.28 (C-5), 64.93 (C-3), 4.83 (C-l).

Compound 12 (2-[1E-2,4-dipentyn-6-methyliden]-1,6-dioxaspiro[4,4]non-3,7-dien-9α-ol); $^1$H-NMR(400 MHz, CDCl$_3$, δ) : 6.75 (1H, d, *J*=5.6 Hz, H-8), 6.57 (1H, dd, *J*=2.8, 1.6, H-13), 6.28 (1H, dd, *J*=5.6, 0.8 Hz, H-9), 5.68 (1H, dd, *J*=2.0, 1.6, H-11), 5.18 (1H, dd, *J*=2.8, 2.0, H- 12), 5.12 (1H, hr. s., H-6), 1.97 (3H, d, *J*=0.8 Hz, H-l), $^{13}$C-NMR (100 MHz, CDCl$_3$, δ) : 168.58 (C-7), 148.35 (C-13), 133.51 (C-9), 125.86 (C-8), 117.08 (C-10), 100.62 (C-12), 82.99 (C-6), 80.37 (C-2), 77.15 (C-4), 75.07 (C-11), 70.11 (C-5), 64.68 (C-3), 4.79 (C-l).

Compound 13 (2-[1Z-2,4-dipentyn-6-methyliden]-1,6-dioxaspiro[4,4]non-3,7-dien-9β-ol); $^1$H-NMR(400 MHz, CD3OD, δ) : 6.77 (1H, d, *J*=6.0 Hz, H-8), 6.50 (1H, dd, *J*=3.2, 2.4, H-13), 6.47 (1H, dd, *J*=6.0, 1.6 Hz, H-9), 5.23 (1H, dd, *J*=3.2, 2.4, H-12), 5.09 (1H, br. s., H-6), 4.88 (lH, d, *J* =2.4, H-11), 1.95 (3H, d, *J*=0.8 Hz, H-1), $^{13}$C-NMR (100 MHz, CD$_3$OD, δ) : 170.54 (C-7), 147.06 (C-13), 136.58 (C-9), 126.75 (C-8), 119.56 (C-10), 106.50 (C-12), 81.90 (C-6), 80.64 (C-2), 77.86 (C-4), 76.45 (C-11), 71.19 (C-5), 65.38 (C-3), 4.04 (C-1).

### Cytotoxicity and Proliferation Test *In Vitro*

MTT bioassay method [10] was used for evaluation of cytotoxicity and proliferation inhibitory activity on A549 (non small cell lung adenocarcinoma) and HUVEC (Human umbilical vascular endothelial cell) cells.

### ACAT Inhibitory Activity Assay

ACAT was measured according to Gillies and cowordkers [11]. The microsomes were first activated by an Ih incubation at 37°C in the presence of deactivated plasma (15-20 µg of microsomal proteins for 20 µg plasma cholesterol). Two minutes later, the enzymatic reaction was initiated by addition of 30 µM of $^{14}$C-oleyl-CoA (1.96 GBq/mmol) and incubated for 90 min at 37°C. The reaction was stopped by addition of Folch solvent [12]. The organic phase containing $^{14}$C-labeled lipids was collected. $^{14}$C-Oleyl cholesterol was separated by TLC (silica gel G25-merck) using diethylether/petroleum ether/acetic acid (10:90:1 v/v). The radioactivity of the samples was measured by liquid scintillation (Dynagel 10ml, on Packard counter 1900Ca). Each measurement was carried out four times at each concentration. The final enzymatic activity was expressed as the followings; % inhibition of ACAT activity = [1-(T-C2) / (Cl-B)] x 100, CPM(T): sample and enzyme, CPM(Cl): without sample and with enzyme, CPM(C2): with sample and without enzyme, CPM(B): without sample and enzyme, $^*$CPM : count per minute

### *In Vitro* Enzyme Assay of FPTase

FPTase assays were done with use of a scintillation proximity assay(SPA)kit following the protocol described by the manufacturer [13] except that a biotinylated substrate peptide containing the Ki-Ras carboxyl-terminal sequence was used. The C-terminal peptide of Ki-Ras (Biotin-KKKSKTKCVIM) was synthesized by solid-phase peptide synthesis. FPTase activity was determined by measuring transfer of $^3$H-farnesyl pyrophosphate to Biotin-KKKSKTKCVIM. The inhibitory activity was expressed as the followings; % inhibition of FPTase = [1-(Sample-B2) / (C-B1) ] x 100, Blank 1 (B1) : without sample and enzyme, Blank 2 (B2) : with sample and without enzyme, Control (C) : without sample and with enzyme.

## Platelet Aggregation Inhibition Assay [14]

A fresh platelet concentrate obtained from 400 mL of whole human blood was purchased from the Red Cross Blood Center and Ajou University Medical School. The platelet concentrate was centrifuged at room temperature and the platelet-rich plasma (PRP) was decanted. Platelet-poor plasma (PPP) was prepared from the remaining platelet solution by centrifugation at 1000 g for 10 min. PRP was diluted to 300000 platelets per ≠1 with PPP. PRP(300 ≠1) plus 10 ≠1 of either sample in appropriate vehicle of vehicle alone was incubated for 3 min in a dual aggregometer (Chrono-Log, USA) at 37°C. Light transmittance was recorded after initiation of platelet aggregation by adding B 16BL6 melanoma cells ($2 \times 10^5$, 200 ≠1) as an agonist. The inhibition of platelet aggregation was measured at the maximum aggregation response.

## RESULTS & DISCUSSION

In order to search for biologically active materials from edible plants, the aerial parts of *C. coronarium* was extracted in MeOH and the extracts were partitioned with EtOAc, *n*-BuOH and water. Repeated silical gel or ODS column chromatography of EtOAc and n-BuOH fractions led to the isolation of nine polyacetylenes and four sterols. Their chemical structures were determined based on several spectral data including gCOSY, gHSQC, gHMBC and comparison of the data with those of literature.

Among four sterols, two ones were identified as β-sitosterol (**3**) and its 3-0-β-O-glucopyranoside, daucosterol (**4**). Other two ones, which might be formed from (3-sitosterol through oxidative reactions, were identified as stigmast-4-en-6f3-01-3-one (**1**), stigmast-4-en-6β-01-3-one (**2**). The stereochemical structure of C-6 were determined from the coupling patterns (**1** : br. s. ; **2** : ddd, *J*=12.0, 5.6, 1.6 Hz) of each H-6 proton signals. Both sterones, compounds **3** and **4,** have been so far reported only in the aquatic plants [15] and were isolated for the first time from the land plants.

Sulphur containing polyacetylenes, compounds **5** and **6**, which were geometric isomers each other, were identified as 2-[(lZ,4Z)-5-methylsulfinyl-2-pentyn-4-enyliden]-1,6-dioxa spiro[4,4]non-3-ene and 2-[lE,4Z)-5-methylsulfinyl-2-pentyn-4-enyliden]-1,6-dioxaspiro [4,4]non-3-ene, respectively. Compounds **7** and **8**, which are also geometric isomers each other, were identified as 2-[1Z-2,4-dipentyn-6-methyliden]-1,6-dioxaspiro[4,4]non-3-ene, 2-[1E-2,4-dipentyn-6-methyliden]-1,6-dioxaspiro[4,4]non-3-ene, respectively. Compound **9** was identified as 2-[1E-2,4-dipentyn-6-methyliden]-1,6-dioxaspiro[4,5]non-3-ene, which was very similar to compound **7** exception with the presence of pyran ring instead of furan ring. Compounds **10-13** were identified as 2-[1Z-2,4-dipentyn-6-methylidene]-1,6-dioxaspiro[4,4]non-3,7-dien-9β-ol, 2-[1E-2,4-dipentyn-6-methyliden]-1,6-dioxaspiro[4, 4]non-3, 7-dien-9{3-ol,2-[lE-2, 4-dipentyn-6-methyliden]-1, 6-dioxaspiro[4,4]non-3, 7-dien-9α-ol and 2-[lZ-2,4-dipentyn-6-methyliden]-1,6-dioxaspiro[4,4]non-3,7-dien-9β-ol, respectively. Even though they were stereochemical isomers with very similar structure, they were successfully separated each other just using open column chromatography.

All of the isolated compounds were evaluated for the pharmacological activity relating to anticancer or anti-hypercholesterolemia.

In order to evaluate inhibitory activity of the compounds on angiogenesis, the cytotoxicity for cancer cell and inhibitory activity for proliferation of HUVEC cell were tested. One of the polyacetylenes showed 64 % and 60 % inhibitory activity for HUVEC and A549 cell lines, respectively, at 20 and 50 μg/ml.

Acyl-CoA: Cholesterol Acyltransferase (ACAT) is a key enzyme responsible for cholesteryl ester formation in atherogenesis and in cholesterol absorption from the intestines [16]. In addition under pathological conditions, formation and accumulation of cholesteryl ester as lipid droplets by ACAT within macrophages constitute a characteristic feature of early lesions of atherosclerotic plaques. ACAT inhibitors are expected to be effective for treatment of atherosclerosis and hypercholesterolemia. ACAT inhibitors of natural origin have been rarely reported. One of polyacetylenes showed 64.6 % inhibitory effect on ACAT at 100 μg/ml.

Ras induced-gene is relating with the growth of cancer cell. The Ras Protein, the product of Ras-induced gene, is activated by binding to cell membrane. FPTase (Farnesyl-protein Transferase) is a key enzyme in charge of membrane binding of Ras protein. In other words FPTase catalyzed a key step in the post-translational modification of different kind of proteins implicated in cell proliferation. Therefore, the regulation of FPTase leads to inhibition of cancer promotion [13]. Two sterols and two polyacetylenes showed the inhibitory effects with 53.2, 96.6, 92.5, 76.0 %, respectively at 50 ug/ml.

Platelet aggregation in the blood vessel has a role to accelerate transference of cancer induced-factor between the cell wall [14]. Therefore, It's efficient on the inhibition of growth and transference of cancer cell, to inhibit aggregation of platelet. And one of sterol compounds showed the inhibitory activity for the platelet aggregation with 20 % at 50 μg/ml. This result suggests that tumor cell-induced platelet aggregation (TCIPA) is suppressed by the compound.

## ACKNOWLEDGEMENTS

This study was supported by the BioGreen 21 Program from Rural Development Administration, Republic of Korea, and by a grant from the Korea Science & Technology Foundation through Plant Metabolism Research Center, KyungHee University.

## REFERENCES

[1]     Baek, N.-I., Ahn, E. M., Bang, M. H. and Kim, H. Y. *J. Korean Soc. Agric. Chem. Biotechnol.* **1997**, *40*, 583-587.

[2]     Han, J. T., Ahn, E. M. and Baek, N.-I. *J. Korean Soc. Agric. Chem. Biotechnol.* **1999**, *42*, 267-270.

[3]     Ahn, E. M., Jang, T. H. and Baek, N.-I. *J. Korean Soc. Agric. Chem. Biotechnol.* **2000**, *43*, 314-316.

[4]     Baek, N.-I., Ahn, E. M., Kim, H. Y., Park, Y. D., Chang, Y. J. and Kim S. Y. *Korean J. Life Sci.* **2001**, *11*, 93-96.

[5]     Jang, T. O., Bang, M. H., Song, M. C., Hong, Y. H., Kim, J. Y., Chung, D. K., Pai, T. K., Kwon, B. M., Kim, Y. K., Lee, H. S., Kim, I. H. and Baek, N.-I. *J. Korean Soc. Agric. Chern. Biotechnol.* **2003**, *42*, 267-270.

[6]     Jung, E. B. and Shin, M. K. In *'Hyang Yak Dae Sa Jun',* Young Lim Sa(3rd ed.), Seoul, Korea **1990**.

[7]     Kameoka, H., Kitagawa, C. and Husebe, Y. *J. Agri. Chern. Soc. Japan* **1975**, *49*, 652-657.

[8]     Anyos, T. and Steel ink, C. *Arch. Biochem. Biophys.* **1960**, *90*, 63-67.

[9]     EI-Masry, S., Abou-Dania, A. H. A., Darwish, F. A., Abou-Karum, M. A., Grenz, M. and Bohlmann, F. *Phytochem.* **1984**, *23*, 2953-2954.

[10]    Skehan, P., Storeng, R., Scudiero, D., Monks, A., McMahon, J., Vistica, D., Warren, J.T., Bokesch, H., Kenney, S. and Boyd, M.R. *J. Natl. Canceer Inst.* **1990**, *82*, 1107-1112.

[11]    Gillies, P.J., Rathbert, K.A., Perri, M.A., Robinson, C.S. *Exp. Mol. Pathol.* **1986**, *44*, 329-339

[12]    Folch J, Lees M, Sloane-Stanley. *J. Biol. Chem.* **1957**, *226*, 497-509

[13]    Lee, S-H., Kim, H.-K., Seo, J.-M., Kang, H.-M., Kim, J. H., Son, K.-H., Lee, H. and Kwon, B.-M. *J. Org. Chem.*, **2002**, *67*, 7670-7675.

[14]    Saiki, 1., Murata, J., lida, J. *et al. Br. J. Cancer* **1989**, *60*, 722-728.

[15]    Greca, M. D., Monaco, P. and Previtera, L. *J. Nat. Prod.* **1990**, *53*, 1430-1435.

[16]    Bocan, T. M. A., Mueller, S. B., Brown, E. Q., Lee, P., Bocan, M. J., Rea, T. and Pape, M. E. *Atherosclerosis* **1998**, *139*, 21-30.

Atta-ur-Rahman/Choudhary/Khan (Eds.) *Frontiers in Natural Product Chemistry, Vol. 1*     169

# Cyclitols: Conduritols Aminoconduritols and Quercitols

Metin Balci[a,*], Murat Çelik[a,b], Emine Demir[a], Murat Ertas[a], Serdar M. Gultekin[a,b], Nihal Ozturk[a], Yunus Kara[b] and Nurhan Horasan-Kishali[b]

*[a]Department of Chemistry, Middle East Technical University, 06531, Ankara-Turkey,*
*[b]Department of Chemistry, Ataturk University, 25240 Erzurum-Turkey*

**Abstract**: All of the possible conduritol isomers have already been synthesized starting from completely different materials and their biological importance studied. Conduritols are useful precursors in the preparation of cyclitols such as *myo*-inositols phosphates, and pseudo-sugars, some of which are important mediators in many cellular processes. The synthesis of conduritpls, quercitols and the development of new synthetic methods are discussed in this paper.

## INTRODUCTION

Conduritol was first isolated in 1908 by Kübler from the bark of the vine *Marsdenia condurango* [1]. It was optically inactive and apparently of unsaturated cyclic constitution. Its constitution and configuration were later established by Dangshat and Fischer [2] to be conduritol-A. To avoid ambiguity, the diastereisomers have been labelled A, B, C, D, E, and F.

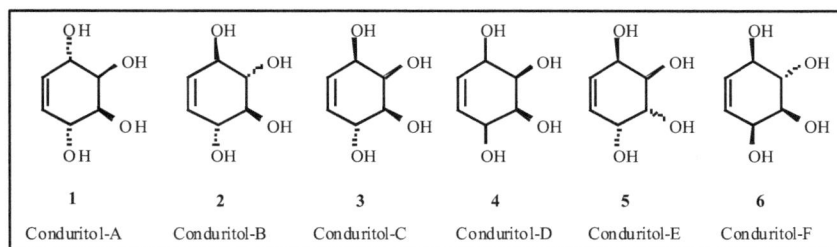

| 1 | 2 | 3 | 4 | 5 | 6 |
|---|---|---|---|---|---|
| Conduritol-A | Conduritol-B | Conduritol-C | Conduritol-D | Conduritol-E | Conduritol-F |

Conduritols are a very important class of compounds in view of their synthetic applications and biological activities. Various syntheses of all the possible cnduritol isomers have already been reported in the literature [3]. Biological activities of conduritol derivatives are also well studied [4]. For example, conduritol epoxides and aminoconduritols act as inhibitors of glycosidases and cyclophellitols and they have proven to be potent inhibitors of human immunodeficiency virus (HIV), gylosidases, and the conduritol-A analogues modulate the release of insulin [5]. A number of conduritol derivatives have also been found to possess antifeedant, antibiotic, antileukaemia, and growth-regulating activity.

Inhibitors of glycosidase enzymes have a potential for the treatment of various disorders, and diseases such as diabetes, cancer, and AIDS [6]. Phosphorylated inositols, for instance,

*Corresponding author: Tel: 90-312 210 5140; Fax: 90-312 210 1280; E-mail: mbalci@metu.edu.tr

have been shown to be regulators of a number of cellular processes [7]. After observation by Berridge and Irvine that the inositol 1,4,5-triphosphate (IP$_3$) was the missing second messenger, a fundamental cell-signal transduction mechanism was elucidated [8]. After recognizing the important biological roles of inositols and their derivatives, interest was then directed toward the synthesis of chiral cyclitol derivatives in particular and has dramatically increased.

## CONDURITOLS

As aforementioned in the introduction section, conduritol-A is a natural product and was first isolated by Kübler in 1908 [1]. The first successful and non-stereospecific synthesis of conduritol-A was carried out by Nakajima *et al.* [9] starting from *trans*-benzenediol.

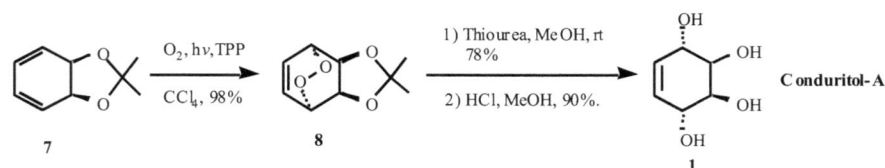

**Fig. (1).** Synthesis of Conduritol-A.

Our synthetic strategy was based on the introduction of two oxygen functionalities at the C$_1$ and C$_4$ positions by way of photooxygenation of the diene **7**, followed by the cleavage of the peroxide-linkage in **8** by the thiourea and subsequent hydrolysis [10] (Figure **1**).

The occurrence in nature of only two conduritols, namely conduritol-A and conduritol-F has been established. In 1962 Plouvier [11] discovered a new optically active conduritol derivative from *Crysanthemum Leucanthemitol* that was an isomer with conduritol-A and he named this new conduritol, L-Leucanthemitol (Conduritol-F). Conduritol-F **6** can be detected, at least in traces, in nearly green plants. We have developed two new stereospecific syntheses for the racemic conduritol-F [12]. The photooxygenation of the known *trans*-benzenediacetate **9** provided the bicyclic endoperoxide **10** as a single isomer in a 56% yield. Selective reduction of the peroxide linkage in **10** followed by deacetylation exclusively produced the (±)-conduritol-F **6**, which was also obtained via the photooxygenation of the benzeneoxide-oxepine system **11**. The endoperoxide **12** was easily transferred into the epoxydiol **13** whose ring-opening and hydrolysis smoothly provided the conduritol-F. However, the acid-catalyzed ring-opening reaction of epoxydiacetate **14** produced a mixture consisting of conduritol-B and conduritol-F tetraacetates **15** and **16** in a ratio of 1:2 (Figure **2**). For the formation of the conduritol-B, the involvement of the neighbouring acetoxy group on the course of epoxide-opening was suggested.

Furthermore, the stereospecific synthesis of racemic (±)-conduritol-F **6** was achieved by the cycloaddition of singlet oxygen to cyclohexadiene ketal **7** followed by the reductive extrusion of one of the oxygen atoms. The obtained allylic monoepoxide **17** was smoothly opened to conduritol-F in the presence of acid [13] (Figure **3**). Furthermore, trietyhyl phosphite deoxygenation of endoperoxide **8** gave rise to a single monoepoxide **17** in a 55% yield. Opening of the epoxide ring by NH$_3$ in methanol followed by deketalization provided the corresponding conduramine-F$_4$ **18** in a high yield.

The first synthesis of conduritol-C was reported by McCasland and Nakajima *et al.* starting from *epi*-inositol or benzenediols [9,14]. We have synthesized the racemic conduritol-C starting from the known dibromodiacetate **19** which can be synthesized in two

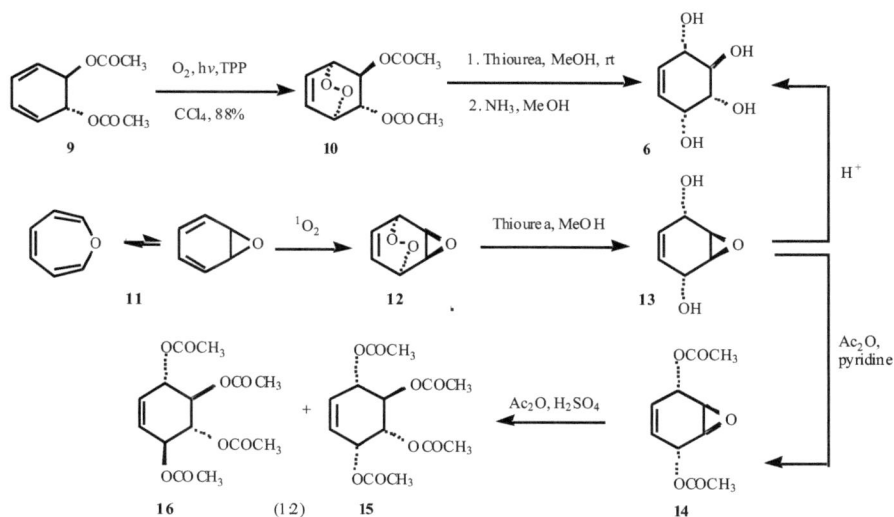

**Fig. (2).** Synthesis of conduritol-F and conduritol-B.

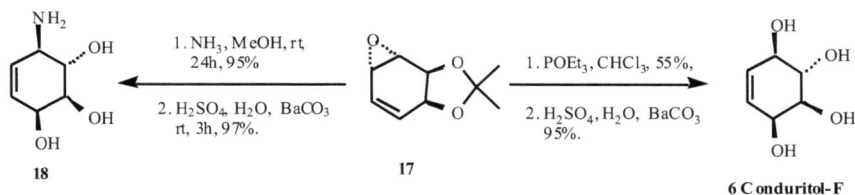

**Fig. (3).** Synthesis of conduritol-F and conduramine-F.

steps from *p*-benzoquinone. *Cis*-Hydroxylation of **19** led to the diol **20a** as the sole isomer. The tetraacetate **20b** provided upon reaction with zinc-DMSO the unsaturated tetraacetate from which the free tetrol, conduritol-C (**3**) was obtained by ammonolysis [15] (Figure **4**).

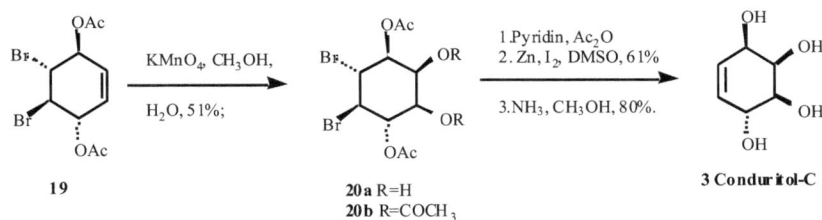

**Fig. (4).** Synthesis of conduritol-C.

Recently, we developed a simple synthesis for conduritol-E [15] starting from the known epoxydiol **22** [16]. Acid-catalyzed ring opening reaction of **22** resulted exclusively in the formation of a tetrol that was readily converted into di-O-isopropylidene derivative **23**. The cyclic ketal **23** was converted to conduritol-E **5** by reacting with zinc and the subsequent hydrolysis (Figure **5**).

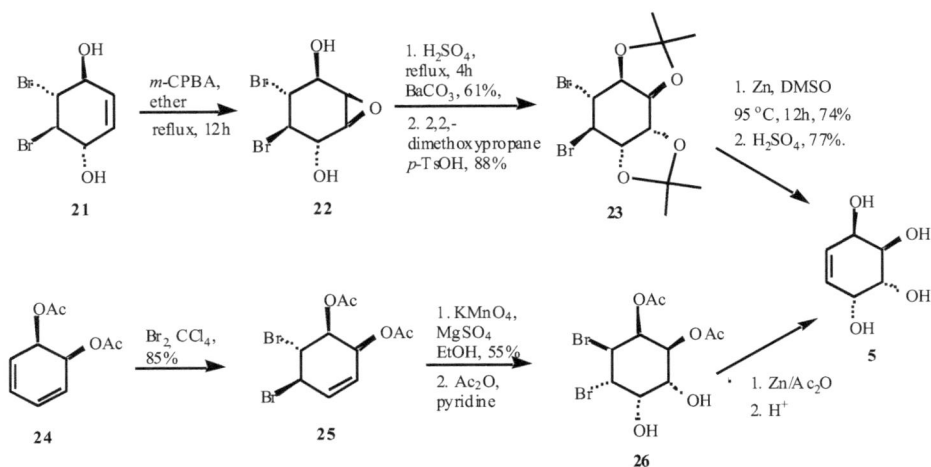

**Fig. (5).** Synthesis of conduritol-E.

Furthermore, the bromination of the *cis*-diacetate followed by *cis*-hydroxylation gave **26**. Zn-elimination of **26** and hydrolysis also afforded conduritol-E. The least accessible of the conduritol isomers was conduritol-D having all *cis* stereochemistry. The first synthesis of conduritol-D (**4**) was achieved from suitably substituted inositols [17]. Osmylation of 1,3-cyclic dienes has received more attention in the synthesis of polyhydroxylated compounds in the last two decades.

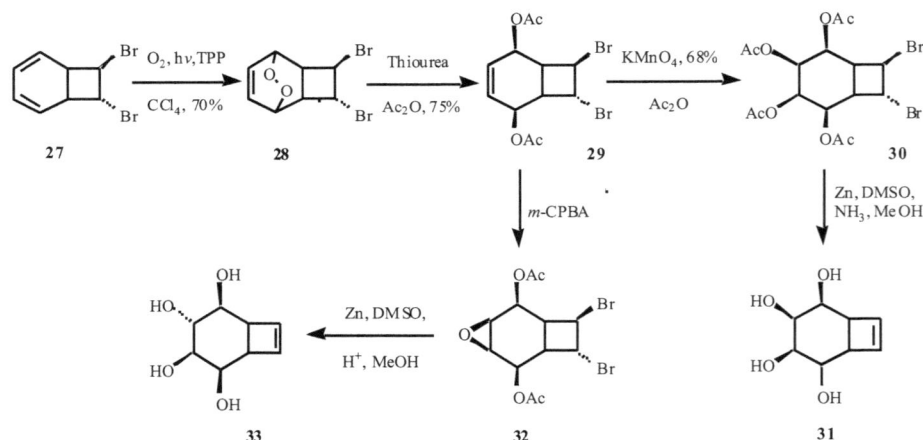

**Fig. (6).** Synthesis of *bis*-homoconduritol-D and conduritol-F.

Recently, we succeeded in the synthesis of a new class of compounds, *bis*-homoconduritol-D **31** and *bis*-homoconduritol-F **33**, starting from **27** [18]. Photooxygenation of the diene **27** followed by thiourea reduction gave the diol that was converted into diacetate **29**. KMnO$_4$ oxidation of **29** followed by acetylation that exclusively led to **30** (Figure **6**). The exact configuration of the acetate groups was determined by X-ray analysis. Removal of the bromine atoms by the zinc-dust elimination provided the *bis*-

homoconduritol-D **31**. Epoxidation of the double bond in **29** and hydrolysis followed by elimination and the epoxide-opening gave the corresponding conduritol-F analogue **33**. The application of the similar synthetic methodology to *trans*-7,8-acetyloxybicyclo[4.2.0]octa-2,4-diene produced new *bis*-homoinositol derivatives [19].

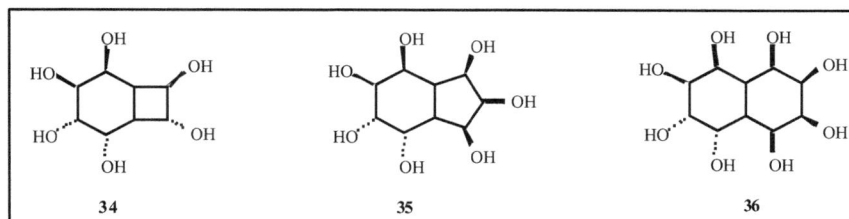

Mehta and Ramesh [20] also designed a new family of polyhydroxylated polycyclic systems **35** and **36**. An isomer of the hybrid of conduritol-A and conduritol-E was found to exhibit significant and selective α-glucosidase activity.

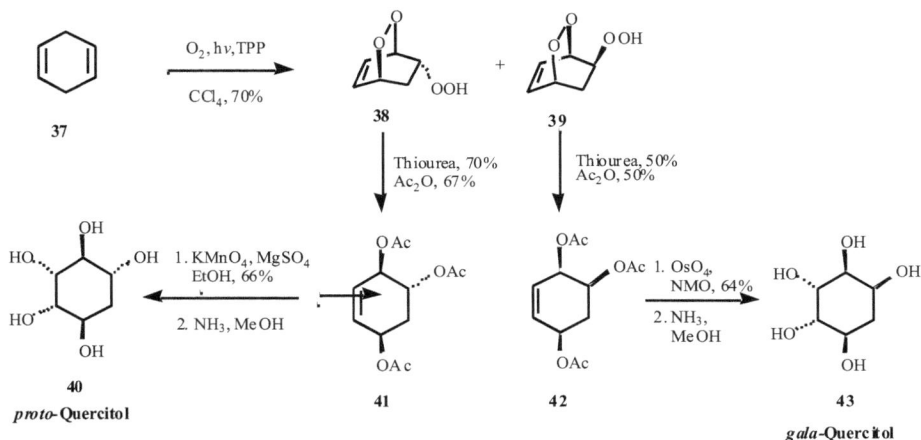

**Fig. (7).** Synthesis of quercitols.

For the first time we applied the singlet oxygen ene-reaction combined with the singlet oxygen (2+4) cycloaddition [21] to the synthesis of racemic *proto*-quercitol **40** [22]. The photooxygenation of **37** resulted in the formation of hydroperoxy endoperoxides **38** and **39** (Figure **7**). The reduction of the hydroperoxy endoperoxides **38** and **39** followed by KMnO$_4$ oxidation of the double bond produced *proto*- **40** and *gala*-quercitol **43**, respectively.

Recently, we have developed new synthetic strategies leading to the synthesis of aminocyclitols containing an ester group which can be easily converted to a –CH$_2$OH functional group that is frequently observed in the natural products. The cycloadduct **44** was the starting material. Desymmetrisation of the anhydride functionality, Curtius rearrange-ment and the ring-opening reaction of the oxa-bridge resuted in the formation of **49** [23], Fig. (**8**).

The application of the similar reaction sequences to the anhydride **50** resulted in the formation **55** [24], Fig. (**9**). Further functionalisation of **55** is currently under investigation.

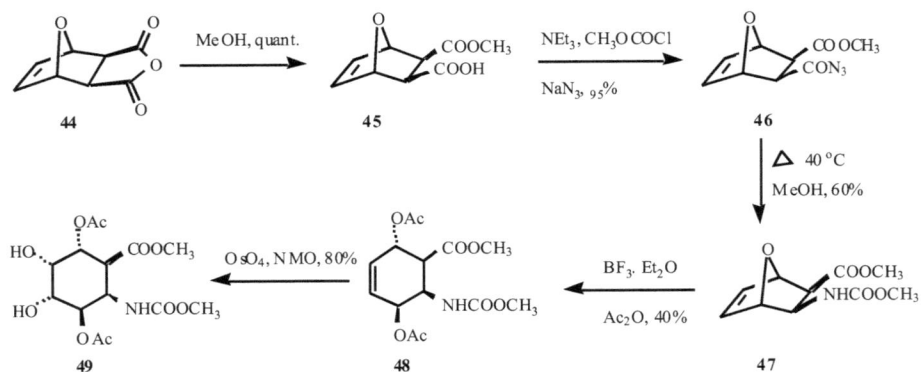

**Fig. (8).** Synthesis of aminocyclitols starting from the oxaborbornane derivative.

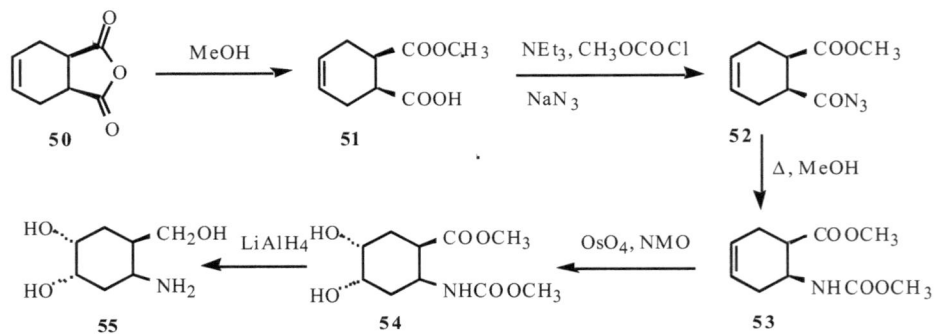

**Fig. (9).** Synthesis of aminotriols.

More recently, we have used the ketene adduct as the starting material to develop new synthetic methodology leading to aminocyclitols., [25], Fig. (**10**).

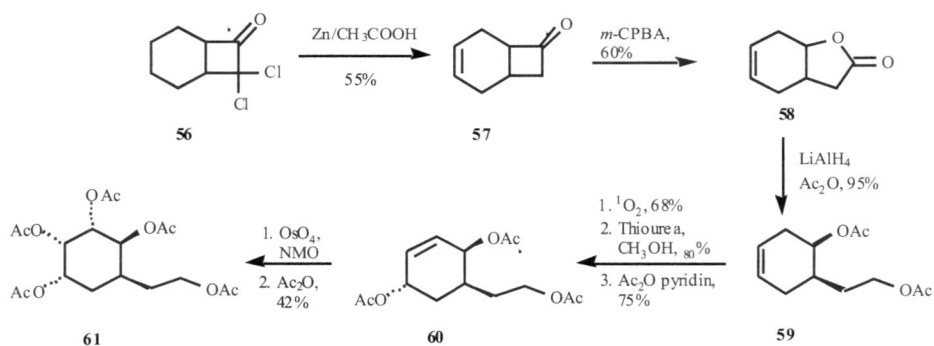

**Fig.(10).** Synthesis of cylitols containing a –CH$_2$CH$_2$OH unit.

## ACKNOWLEDGEMENTS

The authors greatly acknowledge the Departments of Chemistry (Middle East Technical University and Atatürk University), the State Planning Organization of Turkey (DPT-2002K 120540-18) as well as the Turkish Academy of Sciences (TUBA) for their financial support of this work. Furthermore, M.S.G. would like to thank The Scientific and Technical Research Council of Turkey (TUBITAK) for a post-doctoral grant.

## REFERENCES

[1] Kübler, K. *Arch. Pharm.,* **1908**, *346*, 620.
[2] (a) Dangshat, G.; Fischer, H. O. L. *Naturwissenschaften,* **1939**, *27*, 756.
[3] For reviews on conduritols see: (a) Balci, M. *Pure Appl. Chem.,* **1997**, *69*, 97. (b) Hudlicky, T.; Entwistle, D. A.; Pitzer, K. K.; Thorpe, A. J. *Chem. Rev.,* **1996**, *96*, 1195. (c) Carless, H. A. J. *Tetrahedron: Asymmetry,* **1992**, *3*, 795. (d) Balci, M.; Sütbeyaz, Y.; Secen, H. *Tetrahedron,* **1990**, *46*, 3715.
[4] For recent reviews see: (a) Bols, M. *Acc. Chem. Res.,* **1998**, *31*, 1. (b) Ganem, B. *Acc. Chem. Res.,* **1996**, *29*, 340.
[5] (a) Billington, D.C.; Perron-Sierra, F.; Beaubras, S.; Duhault, J.; Espinal, J.; Challal, S. *Bioorg. Med. Chem. Lett.* **1994**, *4*, 2307. (b) Billington, D.C.; Perron-Sierra, F.; Picard, I.; Beaubras, S.; Duhault, J.; Espinal, J.; Challal, S. In *Carbohydrate Mimics – Concepts, and Methods;* Chapleur, Y. Ed.; Wiley-VCH: Weinheim, **1998**; p 433.
[6] Stütz, A. E., Ed. Iminosugars as Glycosidase Inhibitors: Nojirimycin and Beyond, Wiley-VCH, Weinheim, **1999**.
[7] Gültekin, M.S., Çelik, M.; Balci, M. *Curr. Org. Chem.* **2004**, *8*, 1159.
[8] Berridge, M. J.; Irvine, R. F. *Nature,* **1984**, *341*, 197.
[9] Nakajima, M.; Tomida, I.; Takei, S. *Chem. Ber.* **1957**, *90*, 246.
[10] Sütbeyaz, Y.; Secen, H.; Balci, M. *J. Chem. Soc. Chem. Commun.* **1988**, 1331.
[11] Plouvier, V. *Cr. Hebd. Acad. Sci.* **1962**, *225*, 360.
[12] Secen, H.; Sütbeyaz, Y.; Balci, M. *Tetrahedron Lett.* **1990**, *31*, 1323.
[13] Secen, H.; Gültekin, S.; Sütbeyaz, Y.; Balci, M. *Synth. Commun.* **1994**, *24*, 2103.
[14] McCasland, G. E.; Reeves, J. M. *J. Am. Chem. Soc.* **1955**, *77*, 1812.
[15] Secen, H.; Maras, A.; Sütbeyaz, Y.; Balci, M. *Synth. Commun.* **1992**, *22*, 2613.
[16] Altenbach, H.-J.; Stegelmeier, H.;Vogel, E. *Tetrahedron Lett.,* **1978**, *36*, 3333.
[17] Angyal, S. J.; Gilham, P. T. *J. Chem. Soc.,* **1955**, 375
[18] Kara, Y.; Balci, M.; Bourne, S. A.; Watson, W. H. *Tetrahedron Lett.,* **1994**, *35*, 3349.
[19] Kara, Y.; Balci, M. *Tetrahedron,* **2003**, *59*, 2063.
[20] Mehta, G.; Ramesh, S. S. *Chem. Commun.* **2000**, 2429.
[21] For the application of singlet oxygen cycloaddition reaction to the synthesis of dihydroconduritols see: (a) Akbulut, N.; Balci, M. *Turk. J. Chem.* **1987**, *11*, 47. (b) Akbulut, N.; Balci, M. *J. Org. Chem.* **1988**, *53*, 3338.
[22] (a) Secen, H.; Salamci, E.; Sütbeyaz, Y.; Balci, M. *Synlett,* **1993**, 609. (b) Salamci, E.; Secen, H.; Sütbeyaz, Y.; Balci, M. *J. Org. Chem.,* **1997**, *62*, 2453. (c) Adam, W.; Balci, M.; Kilic, H. *J. Org. Chem.,* **2000**, *65*, 5926. (d) Salamci, E.; Secen, H.; Sütbeyaz, Y.; Balci, M. *Synth. Commun.* **1997**, *27*, 2223. (e) Gültekin, M. S.; Çelik, M.; Turkut, E.; Tanyeli, C.; Balci, M. *Tetrahedron-Asymmetry,* **2004**, *15*, 453. f) Gültekin, M. S.; Salamci, E.; Balci, M. *Carbohyd. Res.* **2003**, *338*, 1615. g) Baran, A.; Secen, H.; Balci, M. *Synthesis,* **2003**, 1500. h) Maras, A.; Secen, H.; Sütbeyaz, Y.; Balci, M. *J. Org. Chem.* **1998**, *63*, 2039.
[23] Demir, E.; Celik, M.; Gultekin, S. M.; Balci, M. unpublished results.
[24] Ozturk, N.; Gultekin, S. M.; Celik, M.; Balci, M. unpublished results.
[25] Ertas, M..; Horasan-Kishali, N.; Kara, Y.; Balci, M. unpublished results.

Atta-ur-Rahman/Choudhary/Khan (Eds.) *Frontiers in Natural Product Chemistry, Vol. 1*

# Efficient HPLC Procedures for Natural Product Isolation: Application to Phenolics from Timber

Ibtisam Abdul Wahab[a,*], Noel F. Thomas[b], Jean-Frédéric F. Weber[a], Khalijah Awang[b], A. Hamid A. Hadi[b] and Pascal Richomme[c]

[a] *Faculty of Pharmacy, Universiti Teknologi MARA, 40450 Shah Alam, Malaysia,* [b]*Department of Chemistry, Faculty of Sciences Universiti Malaya 59100 Kuala Lumpur, Malaysia,* [c]*Faculté des Sciences, Université d'Angers, 2, boulevard Lavoisier, 49045 Angers, France*

**Abstract:** We undertook the (re-)investigations of the chemical composition of the phenolic contents of Malaysian timber species. In order to efficiently isolate these constituents, we developed semi-automated separation procedures. It includes the extensive use of HPLC systems, operated at low or high pressure, in conjunction with automatic injection and automatic fraction collection. The efficiency of this procedure is demonstrated by the isolation of an array of oligostilbenoids from the heartwood of chengal (*Neobalanocarpus heimii*, Dipterocarpaceae), when only a single compound was isolated by the previous investigators.

## INTRODUCTION

Malaysia is blessed with a rich biodiversity including a large array of timber trees. Most of them belong to the Dipterocarpaceae family, and are traded under the vernacular names of balau, chengal, meranti, merawan *etc*. More than 1/3 of the world species is found in Malaysia (155 out of 510) belonging to 9 of the 16 genera [1]. Timber trees also include non-dipterocarps from various families such as Leguminosae, Moraceae, Guttiferae and Rhizophoraceae [2]. The just concern for the protection of the biodiversity led the Malaysian government to implement sustainable forest management policies. However, there is also a need to generate higher revenue from logging activities. This could be achieved by raising the commercial values of the waste generated from the milling process, which represent an average of 40% of a tree. The resistance to decay of these timber trees is thought to be largely related to their phenolic content [3]. So far, only in the case of a few dipterocarps species, have detailed investigations of the phenolic content of these trees been carried out. They are characterised by a rather uncommon type of phenolic, the oligostilbenoids [4-6]. Meanwhile, the traditional medicinal uses of dipterocarps are supported by some biological activities such as antimicrobial, antifungal, antiulcer and/or antioxidant properties [6-8]. With this in mind, we embarked on a long-term study, the objective of which was the examination of the chemistry and the biological/pharmacological properties of the phenolic content of Malaysian timber trees with special emphasis on dipterocarps. We concluded that we needed to develop an efficient isolation procedure for rapid and reproducible isolation of these compounds, based on as much automation as possible. We thought that the phenolic extract of chengal (*Neobalanocarpus heimii*, Dipterocarpaceae), which had been studied previously, [9-10] would be a material of choice to test the technique.

*Corresponding author: ibtisam@salam.uitm.edu.my

## MATERIALS AND METHODS

### Samples

A heartwood sample of *Neobalanocarpus heimii* was provided by the Forest Research Institute of Malaysia (FRIM) in plank form, after proper identification.

### General Precautions

All experiments were conducted at temperatures not exceeding 35°C and in the dark (wrapping of all glassware, vials and rotary evaporator with aluminium foils). When not in use, all extracts, fractions, residues and pure compounds were stored either in a refrigerator (+4°C) for short-term storage or in a freezer (-18°C) for long-term storage.

### Extraction

The wood was first converted into powder. The powder was delipidated with hexane (maceration for 20 hours, lixiviation with fresh solvent for 4 hours). After removal of hexane, the samples were extracted with a mixture water/acetone 30:70 (maceration for 20 hours, lixiviation with fresh solvent for 8 hours). The combined extracts were evaporated under reduced pressure. The residues were then partitioned between water and ethyl acetate. The ethyl acetate solutions were concentrated to dryness under reduced pressure. In this account, the residue will be referred to as *Residue P*.

### Fractionation of Chengal Residue P

Fractionation of 4 grams of chengal *Residue P* on Sephadex® LH-20 was performed by using a Büchi® medium pressure liquid chromatography system. A gradient mobile phase consisting of methanol/water 50:50 to 100% methanol was used. The eluent was collected in 15-ml tubes. They were combined into 46 fractions according to the UV chromatogram and concentrated to dryness under reduced pressure. Each fraction was analysed by TLC.

### HPLC Isolation and Purification of Chengal Residue P Constituents

Pure compounds were obtained from the various fractions by repetitive semi-preparative high performance liquid chromatography (HPLC) after establishing analytical conditions. The HPLC system used in this work consists of two pumps (Gilson® 305 and 307), able to deliver a binary gradient. Solvent mixing was achieved with a simple T connector without excessive pressure pulses. Auto-injector cum fraction collector (Gilson® 233 XL fitted with a Gilson® 402 syringe pump and a Rheodyne® 7025 injection port, loop 700 µl) and a dual wavelength UV detector (Gilson® 155) were used. The whole system is controlled by Gilson® Unipoint™ version 2.1 on a PC. This software allows to inject from any pre-determined tube from the 233 XL and to collect in predetermined tubes on the same platform.

The system was fitted with 2 columns, one analytical (250 x 4.6 mm I.D.) and one semi-preparative (250 x 10 mm I.D.) filled with 5 µm ODS (Genesis®). The column was protected with guard cartridges, packed with the same material (10 x 4.0 mm I.D.) in an integrated holder (all from Jones Chromatography®, Mid-Glamorgan, United Kingdom). Samples were filtered through Whatman® 0.2 µm membrane syringe filters prior to injections.

The isolation and purification process of the components of the crude extract was carried out by taking advantage of the possibilities offered by the HPLC system. This process can be consisted of 3 stages:

### Stage 1: Fraction Analysis

Each fraction is analysed on the analytical column and the chromatographic conditions are adapted so that:

- peaks of interest are separated well enough from the impurities;
- retention times remain acceptable (less that 15 minutes); and
- the separation is achieved on isocratic mode, whenever possible.

As a result, seven methods (P1-P7, Table 1) were developed for the purification of the components of the 46 fractions.

**Table 1.    HPLC Procedures for the Isolation of Oligostilbenoids from Chengal.**

| Fraction | Preparative procedure[a] | | Compound | Analytical procedure[a] | |
|---|---|---|---|---|---|
| 13 | P$_1$: | MeOH/H$_2$O: 23:77 | heimiol A **10** | A$_1$: | MeCN/H$_2$O: 23:77 |
| | | | ampelopsin A **9** | | |
| 15 & 16 | | | balanocarpol **8** | A$_2$: | MeCN/H$_2$O: 20-22% in 30 min |
| 18 | P$_2$: | MeOH/H$_2$O: 23:30% in 45 min | copalliferol A **5** | A$_3$: | MeCN/H$_2$O: 23:77 |
| | | | hopeaphenol **1** | A$_4$: | MeCN/H$_2$O: 26-27% in 30 min |
| 19 | P$_3$: | MeCN/H$_2$O: 22-30% in 32 min | hopeaphenol **1** | A$_5$: | MeCN/H$_2$O: 22-30% in 32 min |
| 21 &22 | P$_4$: | MeCN/H$_2$O: 30:70% in 10 min | vaticanol A **6** | A$_6$: | MeCN/H$_2$O: 30:70 |
| 24 | P$_5$: | MeCN/H$_2$O: 22-30% in 30 min | heimiol C[b] **12** | | |
| 25 & 26 | P$_6$: | MeCN/H$_2$O: 22-30% in 30 min | vaticanol E **7** | A$_7$: | MeCN/H$_2$O: 22-29% in 32 min |
| | | | hemsleyanol D **4** | | |
| 29 | P$_7$: | MeCN/H$_2$O: 25-32% in 27 min | hemsleyanol C **3** | A$_8$: | MeCN/H$_2$O: 25-32% in 27 min |
| 30 & 31 | | | vaticaphenol A **2** | | |

[a] All solvents were added with 0.01% TFA. [b] Structure to be confirmed, see text below.

### Stage 2: Scale Up Operations

The semi-preparative column is then connected to the system. Since, it is packed with the same material and has the same length as the analytical column, it can be anticipated that the quality of the separation can be maintained if the mobile phase velocity is kept constant by applying the following relationship (1);

$$\text{Semi-prep flow rate} = \frac{\text{analytical flow rate} \times D_{prep}^2}{D_{anal}^2} \qquad (1)$$

where $D_{prep}$ is the internal diameter of the semi-preparative column, and $D_{anal}$ is the internal diameter of the analytical column

In our case, the flow rate of the semi-preparative column was rounded at 5 ml/min. The column load was adjusted for every fraction. If the peak of interest was well resolved, then up to 80 mg per injection of the fraction were loaded. Conversely, only 20 mg per injection of poorly resolved peaks were loaded. The system was programmed to run automatically as many times as required to exhaust the fraction. The eluting compounds were colleted only when the UV signal exceeded the threshold set at 115% of the baseline noise.

### Stage 3: Re-analysis

Each tube containing the eluted material was then re-analysed on the analytical column using a slightly faster eluting conditions (method A1-A7, 1 ml/min, **Table 1**) and the purity of the separated compound was checked. Pure fractions are pooled and taken to dryness. This procedure allowed us to isolate a pure form of **12** compounds in a relatively short time, in a highly reproducible manner.

Direct injection of chengal *Residue P* on the semi-preparative column was performed by an isocratic procedure (MeCN/H$_2$O: 18:82, both solvents added with 0.01% TFA). It yielded an additional minor compound, heimiol B **12** compounds, along with the other constituents.

## Spectroscopic Analysis

The optical rotations were measured using a Polartronic D, Schmidt + Haench digital polarimeter. UV spectra were recorded on a Shimadzu UV-300 spectrophotometer and IR spectra (KBr pellet) were run on a Perkin-Elmer 683.

Mass data were collected either from a MALDI-TOF BIFLEX$^{TM}$ III Bruker or from a LCQ Finnigan MAT LCMS interfaced to a Waters 600-MS HPLC system. A mass spectrum from LC-MS-MS was also obtained by this system.

$^1$H- and $^{13}$C- spectra were recorded either in CD$_3$COCD$_3$ or CD$_3$OD on BRUKER DRX spectrometer, 500 and 125 MHz respectively. Preliminary $^1$H-NMR data were collected by using JEOL spectrometer, 400 MHz. Two-dimensional and inverse experiments were performed on BRUKER DRX 500 MHz spectrometer.

## RESULTS AND DISCUSSION

The extraction of 468g of chengal wood powder yielded as much as 90.0g of *Residue P*, *i.e.* 19.2% dry weight.

This *Residue P* gave a significant response to the FeCl$_3$ test, showing that it had a high content of phenolic hydroxyl groups. Sephadex$^®$ LH-20 was used to fractionate this phenolic-rich residue as it is known to provide a satisfactory alternative to standard silica [11]. The fractions were combined according to the UV profile, as shown in Figure 1. This demonstrated the presence of a number of compounds in the heartwood of chengal, in contrast with previously published work, where only one compound from chengal heartwood had been reported [10].

Acidic properties of standard silica gel can promote the oxidation of phenolic derivatives [12]. Therefore, we developed an isolation procedure based on the automated HPLC set up described in the materials and methods section and used a reverse phase technique on ODS.

An example of the quality of the results obtained through this procedure is given by the purification of the main component of the chengal fraction F18. First, an efficient analytical method was established for F18. Then, the chromatographic conditions were transposed to semi-preparative scale. Compound **A** appeared as a single, sharp, and symmetrical peak at 36.5 minutes [Fig. (**2**)]. Just next to it is minor compound **B**, at 37.9 minutes. Appropriate

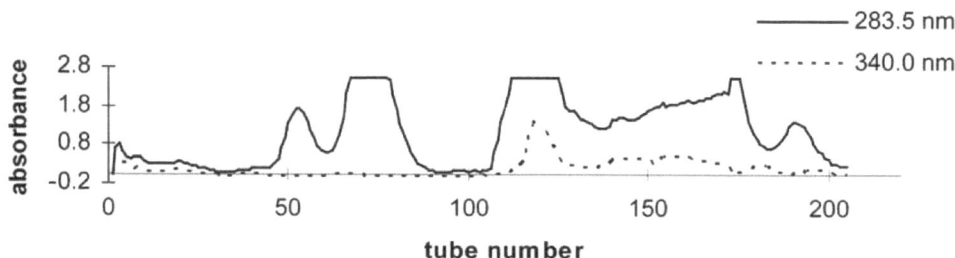

Fig. (1). Fractionation of chengal Residue P on Sephadex® LH-20.

setting of the parameters governing the fraction collector (*e.g.* eluent volume per tube, lower absorbance limit for collection) combined with repetitive automated injections of the same sample (F18) allowed the isolation of both pure **A** and **B**.

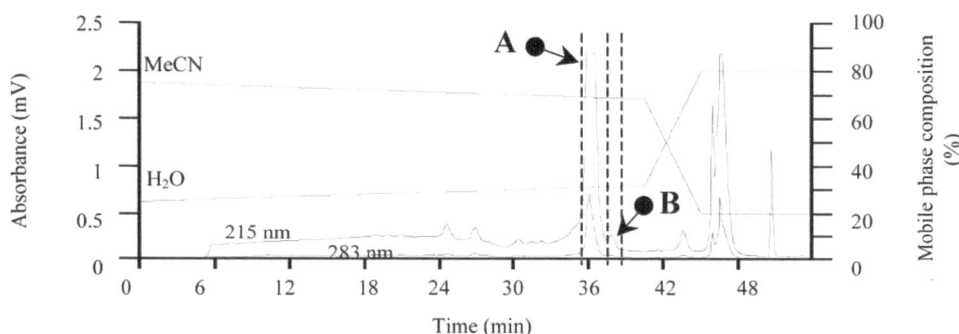

Fig. (2). Chromatogram from chengal fraction F18.

This method was applied to all chengal fractions from and allowed the isolation of twelve pure compounds [fig. (**3**)]. Nine compounds are known (hopeaphenol **1**, vaticaphenol A **2**, hemsleyanol C **3**, hemsleyanol D **4**, copalliferol A (= vaticanol G) **5** vaticanol A **6**, vaticanol E **7**, balanocarpol **8** and ampelopsin A **9**), one is a new compound, heimiol A **10** [13], while the structures of the remaining two compounds **11** and **12** have just been tentatively postulated [14].

We also found out that, by moving away from the traditional two-stage procedure (fractionation followed by purification), we could i) save time; ii) isolate minor compounds which might be lost along the long fractionation procedure; iii) maintain the resolution of the separation and the purity of the isolated compounds; iv) no significant loss performance of the column after more than 50 injections with standard column care (regular flushing, regular change of the guard column).

## CONCLUSION

Our results showed that our semi-automated HPLC preparative technique is able to isolate efficiently sensitive compounds from a complex matrix. Simultaneously, the composition of *N. heimii* was shown to be much more complex than it had been previously reported. We shall apply this technique to a large number of Malaysian timber trees and medicinal plants.

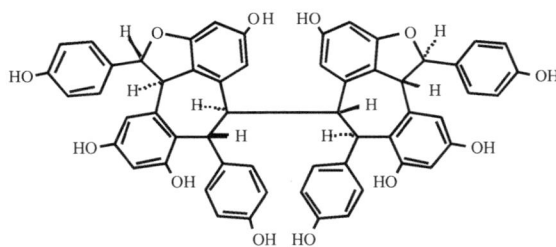

**1**: Hopeaphenol

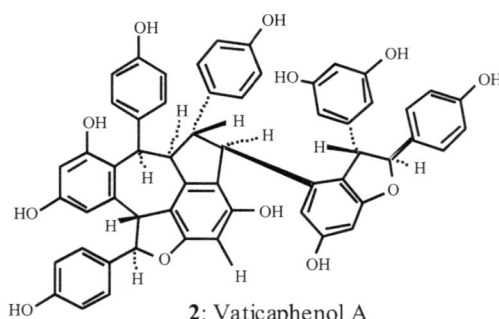

**2**: Vaticaphenol A

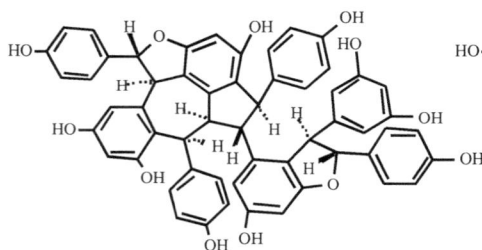

**3**: Hemsleyanol C

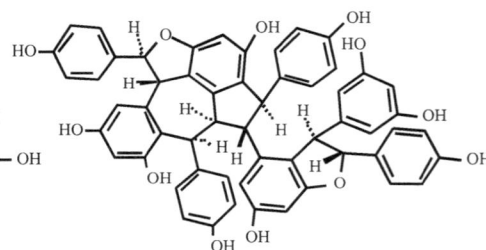

**4**: Hemsleyanol D

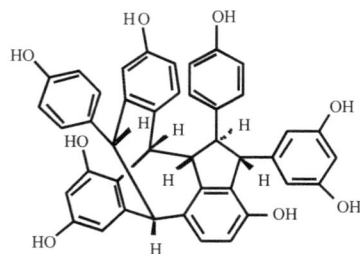

**5**: Copalliferol A (= vaticanol G)

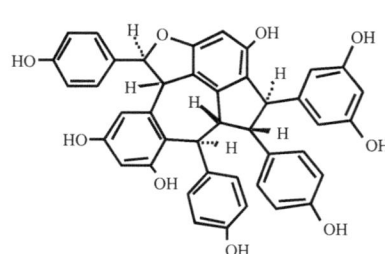

**6**: Vaticanol A

(Fig. 3. Contd....)

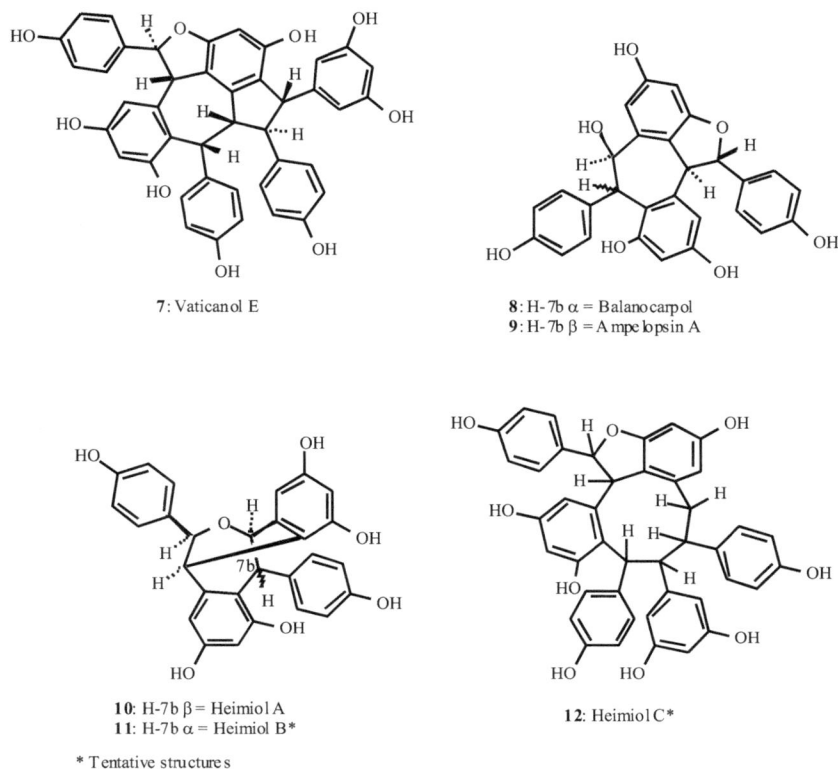

7: Vaticanol E

8: H-7b α = Balanocarpol
9: H-7b β = Ampelopsin A

10: H-7b β = Heimiol A
11: H-7b α = Heimiol B *

12: Heimiol C *

* Tentative structures

**Fig. (3).** Oligostilbenoids isolated from chengal *(Neobalanocarpus heimii)*.

## ACKNOWLEDGEMENTS

We would also like to thank the Malaysian Ministry of Science, Technology and Environment and Ministry of Education for the award of an IRPA grant (09-02-02-0037), as well as the French Government for financial support for one of us (IAW).

## REFERENCES

[1]     Ashton, P. *Flora Malesiana I*, **1987**, *9*, 237-552.
[2]     Hsuan Keng *Order and Family of Malayan Seed Plants*, 1ˢᵗ edn, Singapore University Press, **1983**.
[3]     Rhodes, M.J.C. In *Polyphenols 96*, Vercauteren, J.; Chèze, C.; Triaud, J. Eds, INRA Éditions, Paris, **1998**, pp. 13-30.
[4]     Saraswathy, A.; Purushothaman, K.K.; Patra, A.; Dey, A.K.; Kundu, A.B. *Phytochemistry*, **1992**, *31*, 2561-2562.
[5]     Sotheeswaran, S.; Pasupathy, V. *Phytochemistry*, **1993**, *32*, 1083-1092.
[6]     Dai, J.R.; Hallock, Y.F.; Cardellina II, J.H.; Boyd, M.R. *J. Nat. Prod.*, **1998**, *61*, 351-3.
[7]     Oshima, Y. *Experentia*, **1995**, *51*, 63-66.
[8]     Kulanthaivel, P.; Janzen, W.P.; Ballas, L.M.; Jiang, J.B.; Hu, C.Q.; Darges, J.W.; Seldin, J.C.; Cofield, D.J.; Adams, L.M. *Planta Med.*, **1995**, *61*, 41-44.
[9]     Bate-Smith, E.C.; Whitmore, T.C. *Nature*, **1959**, *184*, 795-796.
[10]    Coggon, P.; King, T.J.; Wallwork, S.C. *Chem. Commun.*, **1966**, 439-440.
[11]    Cattell, D. J.; Nursten, H. E. *Phytochemistry*, **1976**, *15*, 1967-1970.

[12]    Hart, J.H. *Ann. Rev. Phytopathology*, **1981**, *19*, 437-458.
[13]    Weber, J.F.F.; Abd. Wahab, I.; Marzuki, A.; Thomas, N.F.; Abd. Kadir, A.; A. Hadi, A.H.; Awang, K.; Abd. Latiff, A.; Rashwan, H.; Richomme, P.; Delaunay, J. *Tetrahedron Lett.*, **2001**, *42*, 4895-4897.
[14]    Abd. Wahab, I. PhD. Thesis, Universiti Kebangsaan Malaysia, Malaysia, **2003**.

Atta-ur-Rahman/Choudhary/Khan (Eds.) *Frontiers in Natural Product Chemistry, Vol. 1*  185

# Chemical Investigation on *Zingiber zerumbet* Sm

Mir Ezharul Hossain\*, Sreebash Chandra Bhattacharjee and
M.D. Enayetul Islam

*Department of Medicinal Chemistry, BCSIR Laboratories Chittagong, Chittagong-
4220, Bangladesh*

**Abstract:** Essential oil (0.51%) has been isolated from the rhizomes of *Zingiber zerumbet* from which a white crystalline fraction-A (m.p.62$^0$C) has been separated and purified. Another fraction-B (m.p. 66$^0$C) has been isolated from petroleum ether (40-60$^0$C) extract. The fraction-A & B have been analyzed by, IR, GC/MS. From the above observation it appears that the major constituent of fraction-A & B is same and the structure is possibly 2,6,10- cycloundecatriene-1-one 2,6,9,9-tetramethyl.

## INTRODUCTION

*Zingiber zerumbet* Sm. (Beng.-Zongli Ada) is widely cultivated in tropical Asia. The rhizome is used in the diseases of heart and a hot remedy for coughs, asthma, worms, leprosy and other skin diseases. In Madagascar, the boiled rhizome is given in pulmonary affections. In Comboia, the rhizome is given internally as an aromatic tonic, externally it is applied to boils and enlarged glands. In China and Malaya, the rhizome is largely used as a condiment and in domestic medicine. It is prescribed as an adjunct to many tonic and stimulating remedies. Dry ginger enters as an ingredient into several combinations in the Indian Pharmacopoeia [1].

The essential oil from the rhizomes of *Zingiber zerumbet* has been the subject of several previous investigations [2-6]. The isolation of several monoterpenes, humulene and zerumbone has been reported and the structure of zerumbone is elucidated. But there is no report from Bangladesh on this plant. So, an attempt has been taken to find out new compound/s from the essential oil and pet-ether extract of *Z.zerumbet* rhizome.

## EXPERIMENTAL

1 Kg of dried rhizome powder has been subjected to steam distillation. The aqueous portion is allowed to stand for one hour in a separating funnel. The lower portion has been discarded and the oil has been separated. The oil thus obtained, has been dried over anhydrous sodium sulphate and filtered. It is kept in the freeze and a white crystalline fraction was separated out and named as fraction-A.

After steam distillation, the dried meal of *Zingiber zerumbet* (800 gm) has been charged with pet-ether (40-60$^0$C). After 24 hours the solvent has been removed with the help of rotary evaporator. Simultaneously, the meal powder again charged for five consecutive days. Different concentrated portions have been tested by TLC. It has been observed that almost all the fractions having same Rf value. Thus all the fractions were mixed and distilled in a rotary evaporator. The concentrated portion was kept in refrigerator for 72 hours. From it, a square planner white crystalline compound has been separated out and

\*Corresponding author: ctglab@spnetctg.com

named as fraction-B. The purity of the fraction-B examined by TLC using n-hexane and ethyl acetate mixture (4:1) as running solvent and vaniline-$H_2SO_4$ mixture as spraying reagent. The melting point of the fraction is $66\,^0C$. It showed that the Rf value of the isolated fraction is 0.71. Both the fractions have been analysed by IR & GC-MS.

GC-MS analysis was conducted by election impact ionisation (EI) method on GC-17A gas chromatograph (Shimadzu, Japan) coupled to a GCMS-QP5050A mass spectrometer (Shimadzu); fused silica capillary column, 30m x 0.25mm i.d., coated with DB-I (J & W), 0.25µm film thickness; column temperature $60\,^0C$ to $185\,^0C$ at the rate of $3\,^0C$/min., injection port temperature was $170\,^0C$, constant pressure of carrier gas helium was 90 KPa, acquisition parameters full scan; scan range 40 to 450 amu, sample was soluble in n-Pentane.

## RESULTS AND DISCUSSION

From the elemental analysis of the fractions-A and B, it appears that the percentage of C and H are 86.36, 9.56 and 86.72, 11.92 respectively. IR spectra of fraction-A and B are same and showed carbonyl group at 1654 cm-1 and the methyl group at 2950 cm-1. GC/MS analysis of fraction-A showed four components (Table-1). Among them the major compound is 2,6,10-Cycloundecatrien-1-one, 2,6,9,9-tetramethyl, - (E, E, E)-having M. W. 218 and M. F. $C_{15}H_{22}O$, which appears to be 82.21% of the total fraction.

**Table 1.    Percentage of Different Components with M.W. and  M.F. Present in Fraction-A.**

| PK NO. | % TOTAL | NAME | M.W. | M.F |
|--------|---------|------|------|-----|
| 1 | 16.77 | Benzene, 1,2-dimethyl | 106 | $C_8H_{10}$ |
| 2 | 0.85 | alpha.- Caryophyllene | 204 | $C_{15}H_{24}$ |
| 3 | 82.21 | 2,6,10-Cycloundecatrien-1-one, 2,6,9,9-tetramethyl,-(E,E,E)- | 218 | $C_{15}H_{22}O$ |
| 4 | 0.17 | 1,3-Bis (bromomethyl)cyclohexane. | 268 | $C_8H_{14}Br_2$ |

The GC/MS analysis of fraction-B showed seven components (Table-2). From the Table, it clearly indicates that the major compound of fraction-B is 2,6,10-cycloundecatrien-1-one, 2,6,9,9-tetramethyl, -(E, E, E)- resolved 84.94% and M.W. and M.F. are 218 and $C_{15}H_{22}O$ respectively.

**Table 2.    Percentage of Different Components with M.W. & M.F. Present in Fraction-B.**

| PK NO. | % TOTAL | NAME | M.W. | M.F |
|--------|---------|------|------|-----|
| 1 | 11.50 | 1,3,5- Triazine-2,4-diamine, 6-chloro-N-propyl.- | 187 | $C_6H_{10}CIN_5$ |
| 2 | 0.41 | alpha.- Caryophyllene | 204 | $C_{15}H_{24}$ |
| 3 | 0.37 | [-]-Neoclovene-(11),dihydro- | 206 | $C_{15}H_{26}$ |
| 4 | 0.23 | 3-Penten-2-one,4-(2,6,6-trimethyl-2 -cyclohexene-1-yl)- | 206 | $C_{14}H_{22}O$ |
| 5 | 0.47 | Cyclopentane,1-acetoxymethyl-3-isopropenyl-2-methyl | 196 | $C_{12}H_{20}O_2$ |
| 6 | 84.94 | 2,6,10-Cycloundecatrien-1-one, 2,6,9,9-tetramethyl,-(E,E,E)- | 218 | $C_{15}H_{22}O$ |
| 7 | 2.08 | cis-Z-, alpha.-Bisabolene epoxide. | 220 | $C_{15}H_{24}O$ |

From the result it appears that the major components of Fraction-A and Fraction-B have the same M.W and M.F. the structure of the major compound of both the fractions is also same (Fig.-1). Zakaria and Ibrahim detected five phenolic compounds in Z. zerumbet rhizome through TLC [6].

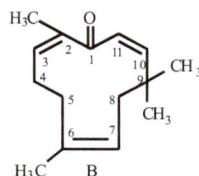

**Fig. (1).** 2,6,10- cycloundecatrien-1-one 2,6,9,9-tetramethyl, - (E, E, E).

Merh, Daniel and Sabnis Isolated and detected Cyanidin, Rosinidin, Syringic acid, Ferolic acid and P-OH Benzoic acid, Alkaloids and saponins in different parts of Z. zerumbet [5].

## ACKNOWLEDGEMENTS

The authors wishe sincere thanks to the Chairman, BCSIR, Prof. Dr. Md. Amzad Hossain for his valuable advice and guidance. Thanks also to Dr. Mozzaffar Hossain, SO and Mr. Md. Shahidul Islam, SSO of Analytical Research Division, BCSIR, Dhaka for doing elemental analysis, IR and GC-MS.

## REFERENCES

[1]    Kirtikar K. R. and Basu, B. D. *Indian Medicinal Plants*, **1918,** *IV*, 2439-2441.
[2]    Varier, N. S. *Proc. Indian Acad. Sci.*, **1944,** *20A*, 257-260.
[3]    Dev, S. *Tetrahedran*, **1960,** *8*, 171-180.
[4]    Chhabra, B. R., Dhillon, R. S., Wadia, M. S. and Kalsi, P. S. *Indian J. Chem.*, **1975,** *30*, 222-224.
[5]    Merh, P. S., Daniel, M. and Sabnis, S. D. *Curr. Sci.*, **1986,** *55*(17), 835-839.
[6]    Zakaria, M. B. and Ibrahim, H. *Malaysian J. Sci.*, **1986,** *8*, 125-128.

Atta-ur-Rahman/Choudhary/Khan (Eds.) *Frontiers in Natural Product Chemistry, Vol. 1*

# Bioflavonoids as Bioactive Natural Products from Plants

Evangeline C. Amor*

*Institute of Chemistry, College of Science, University of the Philippines, Diliman 1101 Quezon City, Philippines*

**Abstract:** Bioflavonoids were once known as vitamin P and are also considered semi-essential nutrients that are responsible for the color of fruits and flowers. They are used in the treatment or prevention of various diseases. There are four categories and these are the proanthocyanidins, quercetin, the citrus flavonoids and green tea polyphenols. The major sources of these bioflavonoids are from plants. The bioflavonoids are known for their antioxidant activity but a great number of other bioactivities are also attributed to them. Some of these bioactivities will be presented as well as the bioactivities of the rare flavonoids isolated from *Syzygium samarangense* (Blume) Merr. & L.M. Perry. Plant natural products, arguably, will still play a major role in providing the world with an alternative and a more effective health care.

## INTRODUCTION

Bioflavonoids or bioactive flavonoids were once considered secondary and non-essential dietary factors [1]. However, because of recent studies enumerating the various bioactivities of flavonoids [1-5], they are now viewed as potential therapeutics that can be used in the treatment or prevention of various diseases with their low toxicity as an added advantage. Bioactivities include their ability to extend the activity of vitamin C, anti-inflammatory, anti-feedant, antioxidant, antiallergic, hepatoprotective, antithrombotic, antimicrobial, antiviral, anticarcinogenic and antitumor activities.

Bioflavonoids, responsible for the color of fruits and flowers, were once known as vitamin P because of their beneficial effects in capillary permeability [5]. There are four categories, Table **1**, and these are generally known as the proanthocyanidins, quercetin, citrus flavonoids and green tea polyphenols [6]. The major sources of these bioflavonoids are from plants. Examples of commonly used herbs that contain significant amount of flavonoids are chamomile, dandelion, ginkgo, green tea, hawthorn, licorice, passionflower, milk thistle and thyme [7,8]. The major component of *Ginkgo biloba*, which is used primarily in the management of vascular insufficiency dementia, is flavonoid that is present as glycosides of kaempferol and quercetin [9]. The uses and flavonoid content of the other common herbs are summarized in Table **2**.

In the Philippines, the use of herbs as alternative medicines is gaining popularity. Examples of Philippine herbs and plants that contain bioflavonoids are sambong (*Blumea balsamifera* L.), tamarind (*Tamarindus indicus* L.) and oregano (*Origanum vulgare* L.). Their flavonoid content and uses are given in Table **2**.

In a recent phytochemical investigation of a Philippine plant locally known as makopa (*Syzygium samarangense* (Blume) Merr. & L.M. Perry), a number of flavonoids, Fig. (**1**),

---

*Corresponding author: E-mail: evangeline.amor@up.edu.ph

**Table 1.    Representative Chemical Classes of Flavonoids [6].**

| Class | Examples | Sources |
|---|---|---|
| Flavonols | Catechins | Grape seeds, pine bark, green tea |
| Proanthocyanidins | Oligomeric catechins | Ginkgo, grape seeds, pine bark |
| Flavones and flavonols | Quercetin, kaempferol | Ginkgo, grape skins, green tea, apples |
| Flavanones | Hesperidin, naringin | Citrus peels |

**Table 2.    Some Commonly Used Herbs and Plants and their Flavonoid Content.**

| Herb/Plant | Part(s) used | Uses/Activity | Flavonoid Content |
|---|---|---|---|
| Chamomile [8] (*Matricaria chamomilla* L.) | Flowering herb | Intestinal disorders, wound healing, inflammations, anxiety, antispasmodic | Apigenin, luteolin |
| Ginkgo [8] (*Ginkgo biloba* L.) | leaves | Dementia, cognitive decline, mental fatigue | flavonol (quercetin and kaempferol) glycosides, flavones (luteolin), biflavones (ginkgetin, bilobetin), catechins |
| Green Tea [4] (*Camella sinensis* L.) | leaves | Hepatoprotective effect | (+)-catechin, gallocatechin, epicatechin, epigalocatechin, epicatechin gallate, epigallocatechin gallate |
| St. John's wort [8] (*Hypericum perforatum* L.) | shoots | Mild and moderate depression, epilepsy | flavonol glycosides (quercetin, quercetrin, rutin) |
| Milk thistle [8] (*Silybum marianum gaertn.*) | Ripe seeds | Liver disorders, lactation problems | Flavonolignans, apigenin, chrysoeriol, quercetin, taxifolin |
| Licorice [4,10] (*Glycyrrhiza glabra* L.) | Root bark | Expectorant, anti-inflammatory, thirst quenching, spasmolytic effect | Liquiritin, liquiritigenin, kumatakenin, licoricone, glabrol, chalcones |
| Black cohosh [8,10] (*Cimicifuga racemosa* Nutt.) | Root | Premenstrual symptoms, dysmenorrhea | Isoflavones |
| Hawthorn [11] (*Crataegus laevigata* (Poiret) DC) | Leaves with flowers and/or fruits | Heart and cardiovascular ailments | PCOs, quercetin, rutin, vitexin |

(Table 2. Contd....)

| Herb/Plant | Part(s) used | Uses/Activity | Flavonoid Content |
|---|---|---|---|
| Passion flower [12] (*Passiflora incarnata* L.) | | Analgesic, antispasmodic, anxiolytic, hypotensive activity | Chrysin (5,7-dihydroflavone) |
| Thyme [12] (*Thymus vulgaris* L.) | | Antispasmodic, carminative, expectorant | polyphenols, flavones |
| Tamarind [13] (*Tamarindus indica* L.) | Seed coat | Antioxidant | PCO |
| Sambong [14] (*Blumea balsamifera* L.) | Leaves | Liver injury | Blu (5,3',5'-trihydroxy-7-methoxy-dihydroflavone) |

were isolated [15]. These were identified as 2',4'-dihydroxy-6'-methoxy-3'-methylchalcone (**1**), 2'-hydroxy-4',6'-dimethoxy-3'-methylchalcone (**2**), 2',4'-dihydroxy-6'-methoxy-3',5'-dimethylchalcone (**3**), 2',4'-dihydroxy-6'-methoxy-3'-methyldihydrochalcone (**4**) and 7-hydroxy-5-methoxy-6,8-dimethylflavanone (**5**). These flavonoids were tested for enzyme inhibitory activity against serine proteases (prolyl endopeptidase (EC 3.4.21.26), trypsin (3.4.21.4) and thrombin (EC 3.4.21.5)) and cholinesterases (acetylcholinesterase (EC 3.1.1.7) and butyrylcholinesterase (EC 3.1.1.8)). Prolyl endopeptidase and cholinesterase inhibitors are implicated in neurodegenerative disorders such as Alzheimer's disease [16,17]. Table 3 summarizes the inhibitory activities of compounds **1-5** against the serine proteases mentioned above. Compounds **1** and **4** show more potent activity against prolyl endopeptidase than bacitracin, the positive control. Both compounds did not inhibit the other two serine proteases, tyrpsin and thrombin. None of the compounds exhibited inhibitory activity against the cholinesterases.

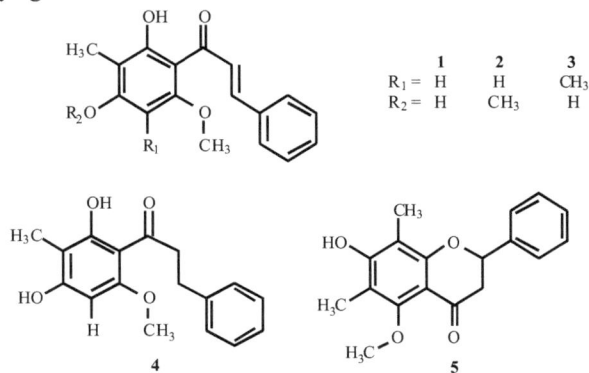

**Fig. (1).** Structures of compounds **1-5**.

It is evident from the foregoing discussion that flavonoids exhibit a wide spectrum of biological activity, which may offer an alternative cure to various illnesses. Various numbers of plants provide significant amounts of flavonoids. Hence, plant natural products will remain to play a major role in providing the world with an alternative and effective health care.

**Table 3.** **Inhibitory Activities of the Compounds from *S. samarangense* Against Serine Proteases (Prolyl Endopeptidase, Trypsin, Thrombin).**

| Compound | % Inhibition (concentration [$m$M]) | | $IC_{50}$ [$\mu$M] |
|---|---|---|---|
| | Trypsin | Thrombin | PEP |
| 1 | 5.6 (0.125 mM) | NA[b] (0.125 mM) | 37.5 ± 1.0 |
| 2 | 15.8 (0.25 mM) | 30.7 (0.25 mM) | > 200 |
| 3 | NA[c] (0.25 mM) | 1.8 (0.25 mM) | 149.8 ± 7.1 |
| 4 | 31.9 (0.25 mM) | 14.9 (0.25 mM) | 12.5 ± 0.2 |
| 5 | 7.4 (0.1 mM) | NA[c] (0.1 mM) | [a] 13.9 % |
| Bacitracin (PEP positive control) | - | - | 129.26 ± 3.28 |
| Leupeptin (Trypsin positive control) | 0.026 ± 0.001 [c] | - | - |
| Leupeptin (Thrombin positive control) | - | 0.045 ± 0.003 [c] | - |

- Not performed in this assay.
[a] % Inhibition at 0.5 mM.
[b] NA = no activity.
[c] $IC_{50}$ in $\mu$M.

# REFERENCES

[1] Middleton, E. Jr.; Kandaswami, C.; Theoharides, T.C. *Pharmacol. Rev.*, **2000**, *52*, 673-751.
[2] Narayana, K.R.; Reddy, M.S.; Chaluvadi, M.R.; Krishna, D.R. *Indian J. Pharm.*, **2001**, *33*, 2-16.
[3] Cowan, M.M. *Clinical Microbiological Reviews*, **1999**, *12*, 564-582.
[4] Luper, S. *Altern. Med. Rev.*, **1999**, *4*, 178-189.
[5] Cody, V.; Middleton, E. Jr.; Harborne, J.B.; Beretz, A. Eds. *Plant Flavonoids in Biology and Medicine II. Biochemical, Cellular and Medicinal Properties.* New York, Alan R. Liss, Inc., **1988**.
[6] Wincor, M.Z.; *Bioflavonoids. Continuing Education Module.* University of Southern California, **1999**.
[7] Craig, W.J. *Am. J. Clin. Nutr.*, **1999**, *70*(suppl.), 491S-499S.
[8] Raskin, I.; Ribnicky, D.M.; Komarnytsky, S.; Ilec, N.; Poulev, A.; Borisjuk, N.; Brinker, A.; Moreno, D. A.; Ripoll, C.; Yakoby, N.; O'Neal, J.M.; Cornwell, T.; Pastor, I.; Fridlender, B. *Trends in Biotechnology*, **2002**, *20*, 522-531.
[9] Briskin, D.P. *Plant Physiology*, **2000**, *124*, 507-514.
[10] Mayo, J.L. *Applied Nutritonal Science Reports*, **1999**, *5*(7), 1-8.
[11] *HerbalGram*, American Botanical Council, **1990**, *22*, 19.
[12] *HerbalGram*, American Botanical Council, **1997**, *39*, 19.
[13] Tsuda, T.; Mizuno, K.; Ohshima, K.; Kawakishi, S.; Osawa, T. *Journal of Agricultural and Food Chemistry*, **1995**, *43*(11), 2803-2806.
[14] Xu, S.B.; Chen, W.F.; Liang, H.Q.; Lin, Y.C.; Deng, Y.J.; Long, K.H. *Zhongguo Yao Li Xue Bao*, **1993**, *14*(4), 376-8.
[15] Amor, E.C.; Villaseñor, I.M.; Yasin, A.; Choudhary, M.I. *Z. Naturforschung C*, **2004**, *59*, 86-92.
[16] Gauthier, S.; Emre, M.; Farlow, M.R.; Bullock, R.; Grossberg, G.T.; Potkin, S.G. *Curr. Med. Res. Opin.*, **2003**, *19*(8), 707-714.
[17] De Nanteuil, G.; Portevin, B.; Lepagnol, J. *Drugs of the Future*, **1998**, *23*, 167-179.

Atta-ur-Rahman/Choudhary/Khan (Eds.) *Frontiers in Natural Product Chemistry, Vol. 1*     **193**
© 2005 Bentham Science Publishers Ltd. All rights reserved

# Search for Biologically Active Compounds from Sri Lankan Plants

U.L.B. Jayasinghe[1,*] and Y. Fujimoto[2]

*[1]Institute of Fundamental Studies, Hantana Road, Kandy, Sri Lanka, [2]Department of Chemistry and Materials Science, Tokyo Institute of Technology, Meguro, Tokyo 152-8551, Japan*

**Abstract**: In a continuation of our studies towards the discovery of biologically active compounds from Sri Lankan plants, recently we have chemically investigated the various parts of *Diploclisia glaucescens* (Menispermaceae), *Filicium decipiens*, *Pometia eximia* (Sapindaceae), *Artocarpus nobilis* (Moraceae) and *Bridelia retusa* (Euphorbiaceae). These work led to the isolation of a number of ecdysones, triterpenes, saponins, chalcones, stilbenes, flavonoids including over twenty-five new natural products. Some of these compounds showed high molluscicidal, insecticidal, antifungal activities and radical scavenging properties towards DPPH.

## INTRODUCTION

The flora of Sri Lanka comprises about 3500 flowering plants of which about 850 species are endemic to the island [1]. Among these, approximately 750 species are claimed to have use in the indigenous system of medicine [2]. In a continuation of our studies towards the discovery of biologically active substances from Sri Lankan plants, recently we have chemically investigated the various parts of *Diploclisia glaucescens* (Menispermaceae), *Filicium decipiens*, *Pometia eximia* (Sapindaceae), *Artocarpus nobilis* (Moraceae) and *Bridelia retusa* (Euphorbiaceae). These works led to the isolation of a number of ecdysteroids, triterpenes, saponins, chalcones, stilbenes, flavonoids including over twenty-five new natural products. Some of these compounds showed high molluscicidal, insecticidal, antifungal and antioxidant activities.

*Diploclisia glaucescens* (Bl.) Diels (=*Cocculus macrocarpus* W. & A.) is a liana of the family Menispermaceae, growing in the mid-country regions of South India and Sri Lanka. The leaves have been used in the treatment of biliousness and venereal diseases [3]. Earlier studies on the seeds of this plant described the isolation of a principle ecdysteroid, 20-hydroxyecdysone (ecdysterone) (**1**) (0.46% from seeds) along with four additional ecdysteroids, which were active to larvae of the European corn borer, *Ostrinia nubialis* [4]. 20-Hydroxyecdysone (0.5% from roots) was isolated also from the roots of *D. glaucescens* [5]. Our previous studies on the stem of this plant furnished 20-hydroxyecdysone in 3% yield, which is the highest recorded for the isolation of **1** from plants [6], together with a proaporphine alkaloid stepharine [7] and triterpenoids serjanic acid (**2**), phytolaccagenic acid (**3**) and a series of their glycosides [8-11].

Recently we have carried out detailed analysis on the constituents of the fruits and leaves of *D. glaucescens*. Chromatographic separation of the methanol extract of the fruits of *D.*

*Corresponding author: Fax: 0094-81-2232131; E-mail: lalith@ifs.ac.lk

*glaucescens* furnished a new ecdysteroid, 2-deoxy-5β,20-dihydroxyecdysone (**4**) together with 3-deoxy-1β,20-dihydroxyecdysone (**5**), 2-deoxy-20-hydroxyecdysone (**6**), 24-ethyl-20-hydroxyecdysone (makisterone C) (**7**) [12], bidesmosidic triterpenoidal saponins, 3-*O*-β-D-glucopyranosylphytolaccagenic acid 28-*O*-β-D-glucopyranosyl ester (**8**), 3-O-[β-D-glucopyranosyl-(1→3)-β-D-glucopyranosyl]phytolaccagenic acid 28-*O*-β-D-glucopyranosyl ester (**9**), 3 - *O* - [α - L - rhamnopyranosyl - (1 → 2) - β - D - glucopyranosyl - (1→2) - β-D-glucopyranosyl]phytolaccagenic acid 28-β-D-glucopyranosyl ester (**10**), 3-*O*-[α-L-rhamnopyranosyl-(1→2)-β-D-glucopyranosyl-(1→2)-β-D-glucopyranosyl]serjanic acid 28-*O*-β-D-glucopyranosyl ester (**11**) [13], 3-*O*-[β-D-glucopyranosyl-(1→2)-β-D-gluco-pyranosyl]serjanic acid 28-*O*-β-D-glucopyranosyl ester (**12**), 3-*O*-[β-D-xylopyranosyl-(1→2)-β-D-glucopyranosyl-(1→2)-β-D-glucopyranosyl]serjanic acid 28-*O*-β-D-glucopy-ranosyl ester (**13**), 3-*O*-β-D-glucopyranosyl-20-hydroxyecdysone (**14**) [14], and phenyl glycosides 4-[β-D-xylopyranosyl-(1→6)-β-D-glucopyranosyloxy]benzonitrile (**15**) and 4-(2-nitroethyl)phenyl β-D-xylopyranosyl -(1→6)-β-D-glucopyranoside (**16**) [15]. Chromato-graphic separation of the methanol extract of the leaves of *D. glaucescens* furnished a new ecdysteroid 3-deoxy-1β,20-dihydroxyecdysone (**5**) [16] together with makisterone A (**17**), dihydrorubrosterone (**18**), *epi*-pterosterone (**19**) [17] and four oleanane glycosides 3-*O*-[β-D-glucopyranosyl-(1→3)-β-D-glucopyranosyl]oleanolic acid 28-*O*-β-D-glucopyranosyl ester (**20**), 3-*O*-[β-D-xylopyranosyl-(1→2)-β-D-glucopyranosyl]oleanolic acid 28-*O*-β-D-glucopyranosyl ester (**21**) [18], 3-*O*-{β-D-glucopyranosyl-(1→2)-[β-D-glucopyranosyl-(1→3)]-β-D-glucopyranosyl}oleanolic acid 28-*O*-β-D-glucopyranosyl ester (**22**) and 3-*O*-{β-D-glucopyranosyl-(1→3)-[β-D-xylopyranosyl-(1→2)]-β-D-glucopyranosyl} oleanolic acid 28-*O*-β-D-glucopyranosyl ester (**23**) [17]. The new ecdysteroid (**5**) showed 40% potency of 20-hydroxyecdysone in the spiracle index assay using the fourth instar larvae of the silkworm *Bombyx mori* [16]. Chromatographic separation of the non-quaternary alkaloidal fraction of the methanol extract of *D. glaucescens* furnished a novel pyridine ring-containing ecdysteroid, named diploclidine (**24**) [19].

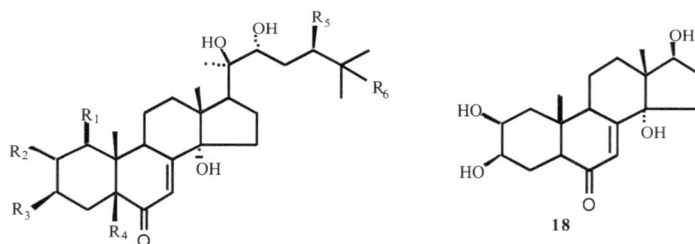

| | $R_1$ | $R_2$ | $R_3$ | $R_4$ | $R_5$ | $R_6$ |
|---|---|---|---|---|---|---|
| **1** | H | OH | OH | H | H | OH |
| **4** | H | H | OH | OH | H | OH |
| **5** | OH | OH | H | H | H | OH |
| **6** | H | H | OH | H | H | OH |
| **7** | H | OH | OH | H | $C_2H_5$ | OH |
| **14** | H | OH | glc-O | H | H | OH |
| **17** | H | OH | OH | H | $CH_3$ | OH |
| **19** | H | OH | OH | H | OH | H |

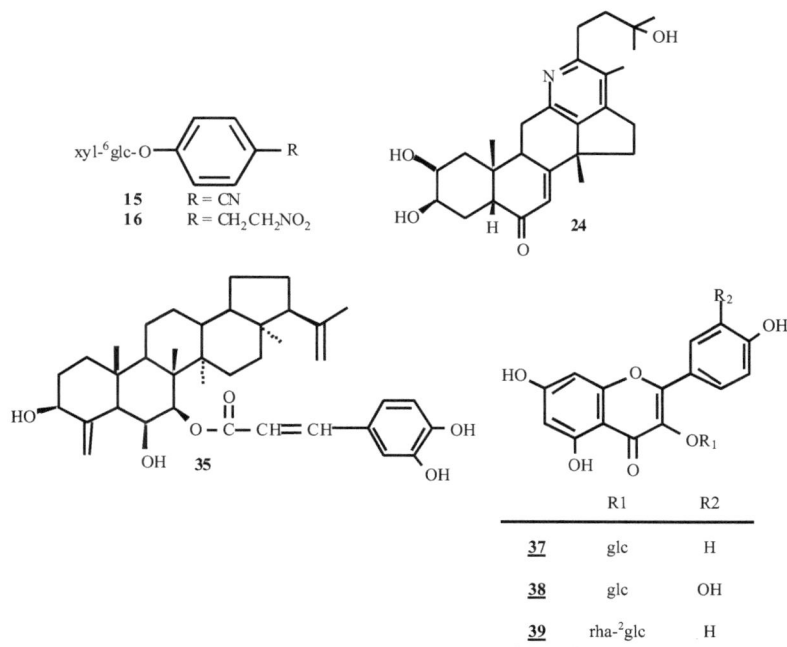

xyl-⁶glc-O— R

**15**  R = CN
**16**  R = CH₂CH₂NO₂

| | R1 | R2 |
|---|---|---|
| **37** | glc | H |
| **38** | glc | OH |
| **39** | rha-²glc | H |

*Pometia eximia* Hook f. of the family Sapindaceae is a tree of moderate size growing in Sri Lanka. Preliminary studies of the methanol extract of the stem of the plant showed strong molluscicidal and larvicidal activities. At a minimum concentration of 15 ppm, the methanol extract caused 100% mortality of *Biomphalaria glabrata* snails, one of the intermediate hosts of *Schistosoma* parasite. At a 300 ppm, the methanol extract caused 84% mortality of *Aedes albopictus* larvae within 24 hours. No antileukaemic activity was observed against L-1210 cells *in vitro*. The methanol extract also showed highly positive froth test indicating the presence of saponins. Chromatographic separation of the methanol extract furnished hederagenin (**25**) and nine hederagenin glycosides: 3-*O*-α-L-arabinopyranosyl (**26**), 3-*O*-β-D-xylopyranosyl-(1→3)-α-L-arabinopyranosyl (**27**), 28-*O*-β-D-apiosyl-(1→2)-β-D-glucopyranosyl (**28**), 3-*O*-α-L-arabinofuranosyl-(1→3)-[α-L-rhamnopyranosyl-(1→2)]-β-D-xylopyranosyl (**29**), 3-*O*-β-D-apiosyl-(1→3)-[α-L-rhamnopyranosyl-(1→2)]-β-D-glucopyranosyl (**30**), 3-*O*-α-L-arabinofuranosyl-(1→3)-[α-L-rhamnopyranosyl-(1→2)]-β-L-arabinopyranosyl (**31**), 3-*O*-β-D-xylopyranosyl-(1→3)-[α-L-rhamnopyranosyl-(1→2)]-α-L-arabinopyranosyl (**32**), 3-*O*-β-D-xylopyranosyl-(1→3)-[α-L-rhamnopyranosyl-(1→2)]-β-D-glucopyranosyl (**33**), 3-*O*-β-D-galactopyranosyl-(1→3)-[α-L-rhamno pyranosyl-(1→2)]-β-D-glucopyranosyl (**34**). Saponins **28 – 34** are new natural products [20]. The saponins **26, 27, 29, 31** and **32** which contain arabinose showed strong molluscicidal activity at a concentration of 40 ppm, 40 ppm, 10 ppm, 2.5 ppm and 5 ppm, respectively, whereas the saponins **28, 30, 33** and **34** which contain glucose did not show any molluscicidal activity [21]. However, the presence of arabinose moieties and the absence of the glucose does not seems to be a prerequisite for molluscicidal activity, since certain saponins of *D. glaucescens* containing glucose showed activity against the same snails *B. glabrata* [10]. The saponin **31** showed strong insecticidal activity against the brown rice planthopper *Nilaparvata lugens* [22].

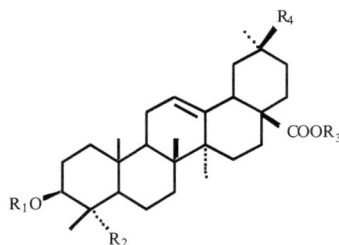

| | $R_1$ | $R_2$ | $R_3$ | $R_4$ |
|---|---|---|---|---|
| 2 | H | $CH_3$ | H | $COOCH_3$ |
| 3 | H | $CH_2OH$ | H | $COOCH_3$ |
| 8 | glc | $CH_2OH$ | glc | $COOCH_3$ |
| 9 | glc-$^3$glc- | $CH_2OH$ | glc | $COOCH_3$ |
| 10 | rha-$^2$glc-$^2$glc- | $CH_2OH$ | glc | $COOCH_3$ |
| 11 | rha-$^2$glc-$^2$glc- | $CH_3$ | glc | $COOCH_3$ |
| 12 | glc-$^2$glc- | $CH_3$ | glc | $COOCH_3$ |
| 13 | xyl-$^2$glc-$^2$glc- | $CH_3$ | glc | $COOCH_3$ |
| 20 | glc-$^3$glc- | $CH_3$ | glc | $CH_3$ |
| 21 | xyl-$^2$glc- | $CH_3$ | glc | $CH_3$ |
| 22 | glc-$^3$glc$_2$-<br>&#124;<br>glc | $CH_3$ | glc | $CH_3$ |
| 23 | glc-$^3$glc$_2$-<br>&#124;<br>xyl | $CH_3$ | glc | $CH_3$ |
| 25 | H | $CH_2OH$ | H | $CH_3$ |
| 26 | ara- | $CH_2OH$ | H | $CH_3$ |
| 27 | xyl-$^3$ara- | $CH_2OH$ | H | $CH_3$ |
| 28 | H | $CH_2OH$ | api-$^2$glc- | $CH_3$ |
| 29 | rha-$^2$xyl$_3$-<br>&#124;<br>ara(*f*) | $CH_2OH$ | H | $CH_3$ |
| 30 | rha-$^2$glc$_3$-<br>&#124;<br>api | $CH_2OH$ | H | $CH_3$ |
| 31 | rha-$^2$ara$_3$*-<br>&#124;<br>ara(*f*) | $CH_2OH$ | H | $CH_3$ |

Table Contd....

| | | | | |
|---|---|---|---|---|
| 32 | rha-²ara₃-<br>\|<br>xyl | CH₂OH | H | CH₃ |
| 33 | rha-²glc₃-<br>\|<br>xyl | CH₂OH | H | CH₃ |
| 34 | rha-²glc₃-<br>\|<br>gal | CH₂OH | H | CH₃ |

| | |
|---|---|
| api = β-D-apiofuranosyl | ara = α-L-arabinopyranosyl |
| ara* = β-L-arabinopyranosyl | ara(f) = α-L-arabinofuranosyl |
| gal = β-D-galactopyranosyl | glc = β-D-glucopyranosyl |
| rha = α-L-rhamnopyranosyl | xyl = β-D-xylopyranosyl |

*Filicium decipiens* (Wight et Arn.) Thw. of the family Sapindaceae is a tree of moderate size growing in wet and intermediate zones of Sri Lanka. Preliminary investigations of the dichloromethane, methanol and n-butanol fraction of the methanol extract from the leaves and the stem showed a variety of biological activities, *e.g.,* antifungal, antibacterial and molluscicidal activities [23]. Chromatographic separation of the dichloromethane extract of the stem furnished a new natural product 24-norneohopa-4(23),22(29)-diene-3β,6β,7β-triol 7-caffeate (**35**) [24] and the *n*-butanol extract from the methanol extract of the leaves furnished sitosterol β-D-glucoside (**36**), 3-*O*-β-D-glucopyranosylkaempferol (**37**), 3-*O*-β-D-glucopyranosylquercetin (**38**) and 3-*O*-[α-L-rhamnopyranosyl-(1→2)-β-D-glucopyranosyl] kaempferol (**39**) [25].

*Bridelia retusa* (L.) Spreng. of the family Euphorbiaceae is a tree of moderate size growing in Sri Lanka. Roots and stem bark of this plant used in the indigenous system of medicine for the treatment of rheumatism and as an astringent [26]. Antifungal activity guided fractionation of dichloromethane, ethyl acetate and methanol extracts of the stem bark of *B. retusa* furnished new bisabolane sesquiterpenes, (*E*)-4-(1,5-dimethyl-3-oxo-1-hexenyl)benzoic acid (**40**), (*E*)-4-(1,5-dimethyl-3-oxo-1,4-hexadienyl)benzoic acid (**41**), (*R*)-4-(1,5-dimethyl-3-oxo-4-hexenyl)benzoic acid (**42**) and (-)-isochaminic acid (**44**), together with the known (*R*)-4-(1,5-dimethyl-3-oxohexyl)benzoic acid (ar-todomatuic acid) (**43**), 5-allyl-1,2,3-trimethoxybenzene (elemicin) (**45**), (+)-sesamin (**46**) and 4-isopropyl-benzoic acid (cumic acid) (**47**) [27]. Antifungal bioassay on TLC bioautography method [28] revealed that the minimum amount of compounds needed to inhibit the growth of *Cladosporium cladosporioides* were **40** (50 μg/spot), **41** (25 μg/spot), **42** (5 μg/spot), **43** (25 μg/spot), **44** (10 μg/spot), **45** (No activity), **46** (25 μg/spot), **47** (10 μg/spot). Compound **42** showed the most potent antifungal activity [27].

*Artocarpus nobilis* Thw. is an endemic tree of the family Moraceae growing in mid country regions of Sri Lanka. This is the only endemic species of the genus *Artocarpus* in Sri Lanka. Several pyranodihydrobenzoxanthones, chromenoflavonoids, triterpenes have been reported from the bark of the plant [29]. Antifungal activity-guided fractionation of the *n*-butanol extract from the methanol extract of the stem bark of *A. nobilis* with a combination of chromatographic separation furnished two stilbene derivatives, *(E)*-4-isopentenyl-3,5,2',4'-tetrahydroxystilbene (**48**) and *(E)*-4-(3-methyl-*E*-but-1-enyl)3,5,2',4'-tetrahydroxystilbene (**49**). Both compounds showed strong antifungal activity at 10 μg/spot against *C. cladosporioides* when assayed by TLC bio-autography method. Antioxidant properties of **48** and **49** were evaluated against the DPPH radical by TLC bio-autography method, in which both compounds were active at 1 μg/spot [30].

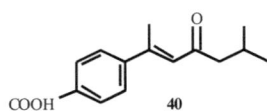
**40**

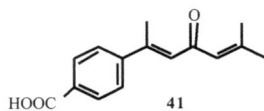
**41**

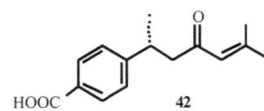
**42**

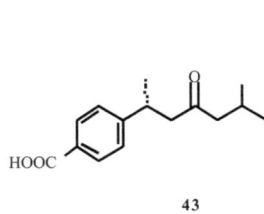
**43**

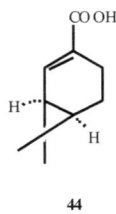
**44**

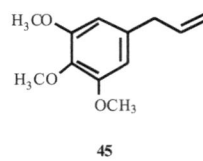
**45**

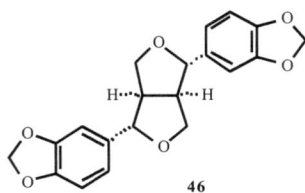
**46**

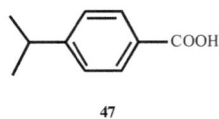
**47**

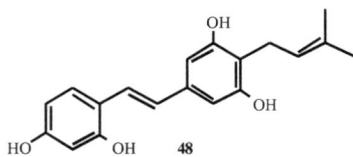
**48**

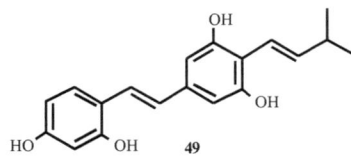
**49**

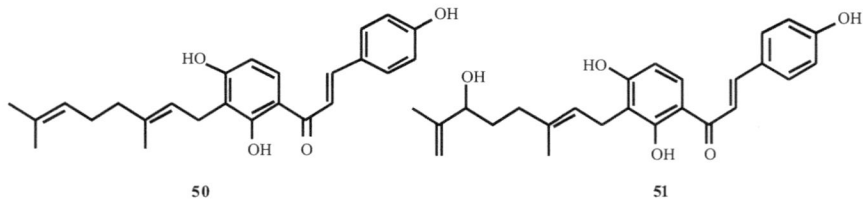
**50**

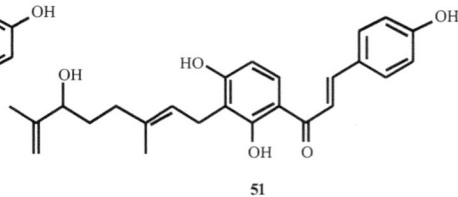
**51**

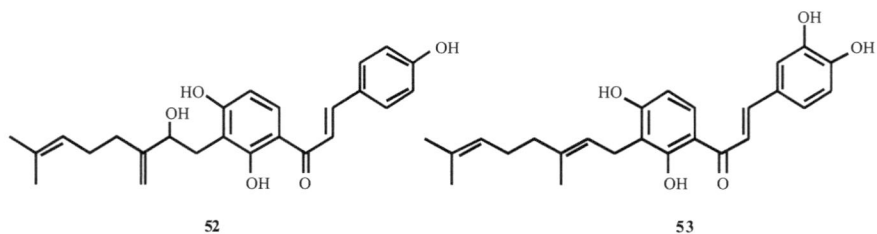
**52**

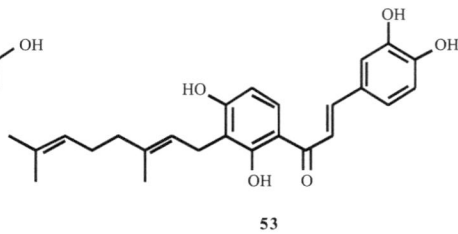
**53**

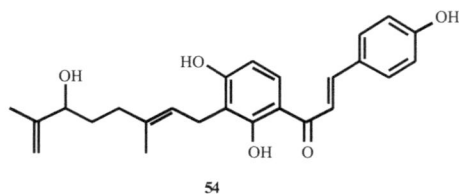
**54**

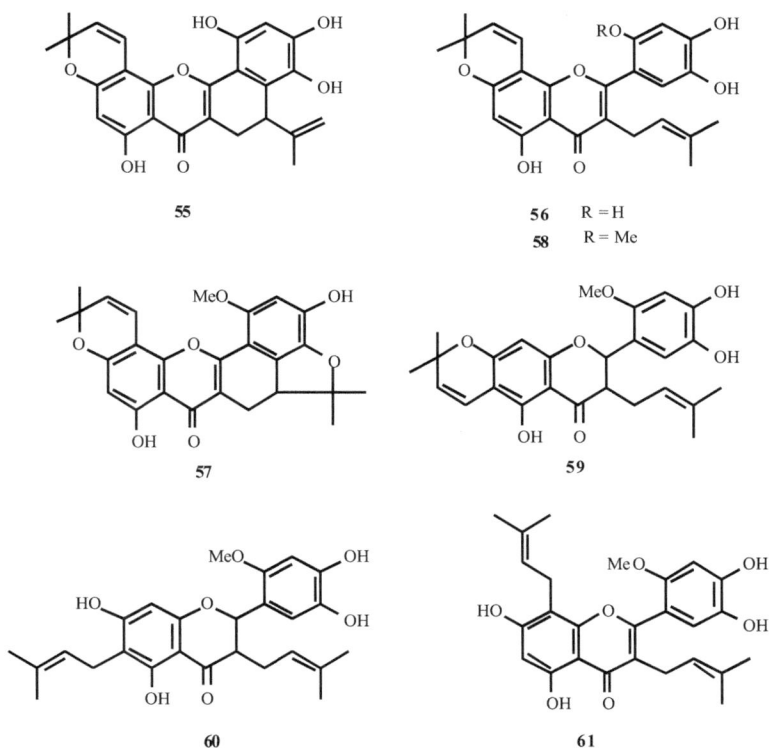

55

56 R = H
58 R = Me

57

59

60

61

Antifungal activity guided fractionation of the *n*-butanol extract from the methanol extract of the leaves of *A. nobilis* furnished 2',4',4-trihydroxy-3'-geranylchalcone (**50**), 2',4,4'-trihydroxy-3'-[6-hydroxy-3,7-dimethyl-2(*E*),7-octadienyl]chalcone (**51**), 2',4', 4-trihydroxy-3'-[2-hydroxy-7-methyl-3-methylene-6-octaenyl]chalcone (**52**), 2',3,4,4'-tetrahydroxy-3'-geranylchalcone (**53**), 2',3,4,4'-tetrahydroxy-3'-[6-hydroxy-3,7-dimethyl-2(*E*),7-octadienyl]chalcone (**54**). The chalcones **52** and **54** are new natural products, whereas **50** and **51** are reported for the first time from the family Moraceae. All these compounds **50-54** showed fungicidal activity at **50** (5 μg/spot), **51** (5 μg/spot), **52** (5 μg/spot), **53** (2 μg/spot) and **54** (15 μg/spot) against *C. cladosporioides* on TLC bio-autography method. Compounds **50-54** exhibited strong radical scavenging property (active at 1 μg/spot) towards DPPH radical when assayed by TLC bio-autography method [31].

Chromatographic separation of the *n*-butanol extract from the methanol extract of the root bark of *A. nobilis* furnished four new prenylated flavonoids, artonine E 2'-methyl ether (**58**), isoarotonine E 2'-methylether (**59**), dihydroisoarotonine E 2'-methyl ether (**60**) and artonin V 2'-methyl ether (**61**), together with known artobiloxanthone (**55**), artonine E (**56**) and cycloartobiloxanthone (**57**). All these compounds showed strong radical scavenging properties towards DPPH radical[32].

## ACKNOWLEDGEMENTS

We gratefully acknowledge the contributions of the members of our research group Ms. B.M.M. Kumarihamy, Mr. A.G.D. Bandara, Ms. C.P. Jayasooriya, Ms. B.A.I.S. Balasooriya

(Institute of Fundamental Studies), Mr. N. Hara (Tokyo Institute of Technology) and all others whose names appear in the reference section and the acknowledgement sections of the relevant references.

## REFERENCES

[1]     Bandaranayake, W.M.; Sultanbawa, M.U.S.; Weerasekera, S.C.; Balasubramaniam, S.; A glossary of sinhala and tamil names of the plants of Sri Lanka, *The Sri Lanka Forester*, **1974**; **XI**, 67.
[2]     Abeywickrama, B.A.; *Proc. Workshop on Natural Products*, Colombo, Sri Lanka. **1975**.
[3]     Chopra, R.N.; Nayar, S.L.; Chopra, I.C.; In Glossary of Indian Medicinal Plants, Council of Scientific and Industrial Research, New Delhi. **1956**, pp. 72 and 99
[4]     Miller, R. W.; Clardy, J.; Kozlowski, J.; Mikolajczak, K. L.; Plattner, R. D.; Powell, R. G.; Smith, C. R.; Weisleder, D.; Qi-Tai, Z.; *Planta Medica*, **1985**, *51*, 40–42.
[5]     Shah, V.C.; D'Sa, A.S.; De Souza, N.J.; *Steroids,* **1989**, *53*, 559-565.
[6]     Bandara, B.M.R.; Jayasinghe, L.; Karunaratne, V.; Wannigama, G.P.; Bokel, M.; Kraus, W.; Sotheeswaran, S.; *Phytochemistry*, **1989**, *28*, 1073 – 1075.
[7]     Jayasinghe, U.L.B.; Wannigama, G.P.; Balasubramaniam, S.; Nasir, H.; Atta-ur-Rahman; *Journal of the National Science Council of Sri Lanka*, **1992**, *20*, 187 - 190.
[8]     Bandara, B.M.R.; Jayasinghe, U.L.B.; Karunaratne, V.; Wannigama, G.P.; Bokel, M.; Sotheeswaran, S.; *Planta Medica*, **1990**, *56*, 290-292.
[9]     Bandara, B.M.R.; Jayasinghe, L.; Karunaratne, V.; Wannigama, G.P.; Kraus, W.; Bokel, M.; Sotheeswaran, S.; *Phytochemistry*, **1989**, *28*, 2783-2785.
[10]    Jayasinghe, U.L.B.; Wannigama, G.P.; MacLeod, J.K.; *Natural Product Letters*, **1998**, *2*, 249-253.
[11]    Jayasinghe, U.L.B.; Wannigama, G.P.; MacLeod, J. K.; *Journal of the Chemical Society of Pakistan*, **1998**, *20*, 131-137.
[12]    Jayasinghe, L.; Kumarihamy, B.M.M.; Arundathie, B.G.S.; Dissanayake, L.; Hara, N.; ; Fujimoto, Y.; *Steroids*, **2003**, *68*, 447-450.
[13]    Jayasinghe, L.; Hara, N.; Fujimoto, Y.; *Phytochemistry*, **2003**, *62*, 563-567.
[14]    Jayasinghe, U.L.B.; Balasooriya, B.A.I.S.; Fujimoto, Y.; *Proceedings, Sri Lanka Association for the Advancement of Science (SLAAS)*, Colombo, **2003**, p.216.
[15]    Jayasinghe, U.L.B.; Fujimoto, Y. **2004**, (Manuscript submitted).
[16]    Jayasinghe, L.; Jayasooriya, C. P.; Oyama, K.; Fujimoto, Y.; *Steroids*, **2002**, *67*, 555-558.
[17]    Jayasinghe, U.L.B.; Jayasooriya, C.P.; Fujimoto, Y.; *Proceedings, Sri Lanka Association for the Advancement of Science (SLAAS)*, Colombo, **2003**, p.220.
[18]    Jayasinghe, U.L.B.; Jayasooriya, C.P.; Fujimoto, Y.; *Fitoterapia*, **2002**, *73*, 424-427.
[19]    Jayasinghe, L.; Jayasooriya, C.P.; Hara, N.; Fujimoto, Y.; *Tetrahedron Letters*, **2003**, *44*, 8769 - 8771.
[20]    Jayasinghe, L.; Shimada, H.; Hara, N.; Fujimoto, Y.; *Phytochemistry*, **1995**, *40*, 891 - 897.
[21]    Jayasinghe, U.L.B.; Fujimoto, Y.; Hostettmann, K.; *Natural Product Letters*, **1998**, *12*, 135 - 138.
[22]    Jayasinghe, U.L.B.; Fujimoto, Y.; *Fitoterapia*, **1999**, *70*, 87 - 88.
[23]    Jayasinghe, U.L.B.; Bandara, A.G.D.; *Proceedings, Sri Lanka Association for the Advancement of Science (SLAAS)*, Colombo, **1997**, p.338.
[24]    Jayasinghe, U.L.B.; Bandara, A.G.D.; Hara, N.; Fujimoto, Y.;*Fitoterapia*, **2001**, *72*, 737-742.
[25]    Jayasinghe, U.L.B.; Balasooriya, B.A.I.S.; Bandara, A.G.D.; Fujimoto, Y.; *Natural Product Research*, **2004**, (in press).
[26]    Jayaweera, D.M.A.; In Medicinal plants used in Ceylon, Part II. *The National Science Council of Sri Lanka*, Colombo, **1982**.
[27]    Jayasinghe, L.; Kumarihamy, B.M.M.; Jayaratne, K.H.R.N.; Udishani, N.W.M.G.; Bandara, B.M.R.; Hara, N.; Fujimoto, Y.; *Phytochemistry*, **2003**, *62*, 637-641.
[28]    Homans, A.L.; Fuchs, A.; *Journal of chromatography*, **1970**, *51*, 327–329.
[29]    Sultanbawa, M.U.S.; Surendrakumar, S.; *Phytochemistry*, **1989**, *28*, 599–605.
[30]    Jayasinghe, U.L.B.; Puvanendran, S.; Hara, N.; Fujimoto, Y.; *Natural Product Research*, **2003**, (in press).
[31]    Jayasinghe, L.; Balasooriya, B.A.I.S.; Padmini, W.C.; Hara, N.; Fujimoto, Y., *Phytochemistry*, **2003**, *65*, 1287–1290.
[32]    Jayasinghe, L.; Samarakoon, T.B.; Kumarihamy, B.M.M.; Fujimoto, Y.; **2004** (Manuscript submitted).

Atta-ur-Rahman/Choudhary/Khan (Eds.) *Frontiers in Natural Product Chemistry, Vol. 1*

# Chemical and Bioactive Constituents from Formosan *Zanthoxylum* Species

Ih-Sheng Chen[1,*] and Che-Ming Teng[2]

*[1]Graduate Institute of Pharmaceutical Sciences, College of Pharmacy, Kaohsiung Medical University, Kaohsiung 807, Taiwan, [2]Pharmacological Institute, College of Medicine, National Taiwan University, Taipei 100, Taiwan*

**Abstract:** There are approximately 100 species of *Zanthoxylum* in the tropical and subtropical regions, and 10 of them are indigenous to Taiwan. For the last 10 years, our laboratory has examined six species of *Zanthoxylum* in Taiwan (*Z. ailanthoides*, *Z. integrifoliolum*, *Z. nitidum*, *Z. pistaciiflorum*, *Z. schinifolium* and *Z. simulans*) for their chemical and bioactive compounds. This research has led to the isolation of 59 new compounds and around 200 known compounds. The structures of the new compounds were established by spectroscopic data and chemical evidence. These new compounds showed diversity of structures including benzo[*c*]phenanthridine, 2-phenyl-1-*N*-methylphthaliamide, pyrano-quinoline, 2-quinolone, isobutylamide, indolopyridoquinazoline, aporphine, phenylacetonitrile, coumarin, phenylpropanoid, lignan, and flavonoid. Several isolates showed antiplatelet aggregation activity *in vitro*.

## INTRODUCTION

*Zanthoxylum* is a unique genus of Rutaceae, usually prickly in the stem or trunk, and with imparipinnate leaves having pellucid dots. Its fruit usually dehisces into 2 valves, in which there is a shiny black seed. In earlier time, *Zanthoxylum* plants were divided into two genera based on the number of perianth in their morphology: bisseriate in *Fagara* and uniseriate in *Zanthoxylum*. Recently, however, many chemical studies on *Fagara* and *Zanthoxylum* plants have provided evidence that these two taxons are meaningless. The currently used *Zanthoxylum* is in a broad sense, including the former *Fagara* and *Zanthoxylum*. The term *Xanthoxylum* is equivalent to *Zanthoxylum* and is currently used in Japan.

Chemical researches on *Zanthoxylum* became popular partly from the use of *Zanthoxylum* plants as folk medicines, and partly from the discovery of antitumor benzo[*c*]phenanthridine alkaloids, nitidine [1], and fagaronine [2], isolated from *Fagara macrophylla* and *Fagara xanthoxyloides*, respectively. Thereafter, many total syntheses of benzo[*c*]phenanthridine alkaloids have also been accomplished.

There are about 100 *Zanthoxylum* species [3] in tropical and subtropical regions. Ten wild species are distributed in Taiwan besides one cultivated species:

1. *Zanthoxylum ailanthoides* Sieb. & Zucc.

2. *Z. armatum* DC.

3. *Z. avicennae* (Lam.) DC.

---

*Corresponding author: E-mail: m635013@kmu.edu.tw

4.  *Z. beecheyanum* K. Koch (cultivated)

5.  *Z. integrifoliolum* (Merr.) Merr.

6.  *Z. nitidum* (Roxb.) DC.          *endemic species

7.  *Z. pistaciiflorum* Hayata*

8.  *Z. scandens* Blume

9.  *Z. schinifolium* Sieb. & Zucc.

10. *Z. simulans* Hance

11. *Z. wutaiense* Chen*

The chemical study of Formosan *Zanthoxylum* species was initiated by Ishii and our research group, with the isolation of a new phenylpropanoid, cuspidiol [4] from the wood of *Z. scandens* (*Z. cuspidatum*) in 1973. Successive investigation of the bark of the same species has led to the isolation of four new alkaloids [5], des-*N*-methylavicine, arnottianamide, isoarnottianamide and base X-C-1. Further examination of the root wood [6] of *Z. integrifoliolum* has led to the isolation of two new alkaloids, integriamide and integriquinolone. From the root wood of *Z. wutaiense* [7], four new compounds, including 3 optically active phenylpropanoids: wutaiensol, wutaiensal, and methyl demethoxy-wutaiensate, and a related compound, wutaialdehyde were isolated and structurally established. In 1984, a new oxybenzo[*c*]phenanthridine alkaloid, oxyterihanine [8] was obtained from the bark of *Z. nitidum*.

Inspired by the discovery of several antiplatelet principles from Chinese Medicine, such as osthole from *Angelica pubescens*, denudatin B and veraguensin from *Magnolia fargessii*, honokiol and magnolol from *Magnolia officinalis*, panaxynol from *Panax ginseng*, we have tried to search for antiplatelet constituents from Formosan plant *via* random screening *in vitro*. Consequently, several species of *Zanthoxylum* in Taiwan have been found to exhibit inhibitory activity on platelet aggregation *in vitro*. Thus, three species, *Z. simulans*, *Z. schinifolium* and *Z. integrifoliolum* were chosen to study for their antiplatelet and chemical constituents, and 3 other species, *Z. nitidum*, *Z. pistaciiflorum* and *Z. ailanthoides* were studied for their chemical constituents. In this symposium, we report on the new compounds and antiplatelet constituents isolated from six Formosan *Zanthoxylum* species during the last ten years.

### Z. simulans

Sixteen new compounds were isolated by means of phytochemical survey of *Z. simulans*: compounds 1~3 and 8~12 from the root bark [9-12], a dimeric 2-quinolone, 5 from the root wood [13], compounds 4, 6, 7 and 13 from the stem bark [14], and compounds 14~16 from the stem wood [15]. The presence of pyranoquinoline alkaloids with a side chain of 5 C in this plant can be distinguished it from other *Zanthoxylum* species.

### Z. schinifolium

Examination of the bark [16,17] and root bark [18,19] of *Z. schinifolium* led to the isolation of a new 3-methoxy coumarin, 17, and seventeen new 7-terpenyloxy coumarins, mainly with or without a methoxy group at C-8. These new coumarins are comprised of compound 18~34. Half of the isolates of leaves [20] are the same as those obtained in the bark and root bark, and only one new compound was recognized as *cis*-fagaramide (35). Comparing the leaves' constituents of the *Zanthoxylum* species, *Z. schinifolium* is

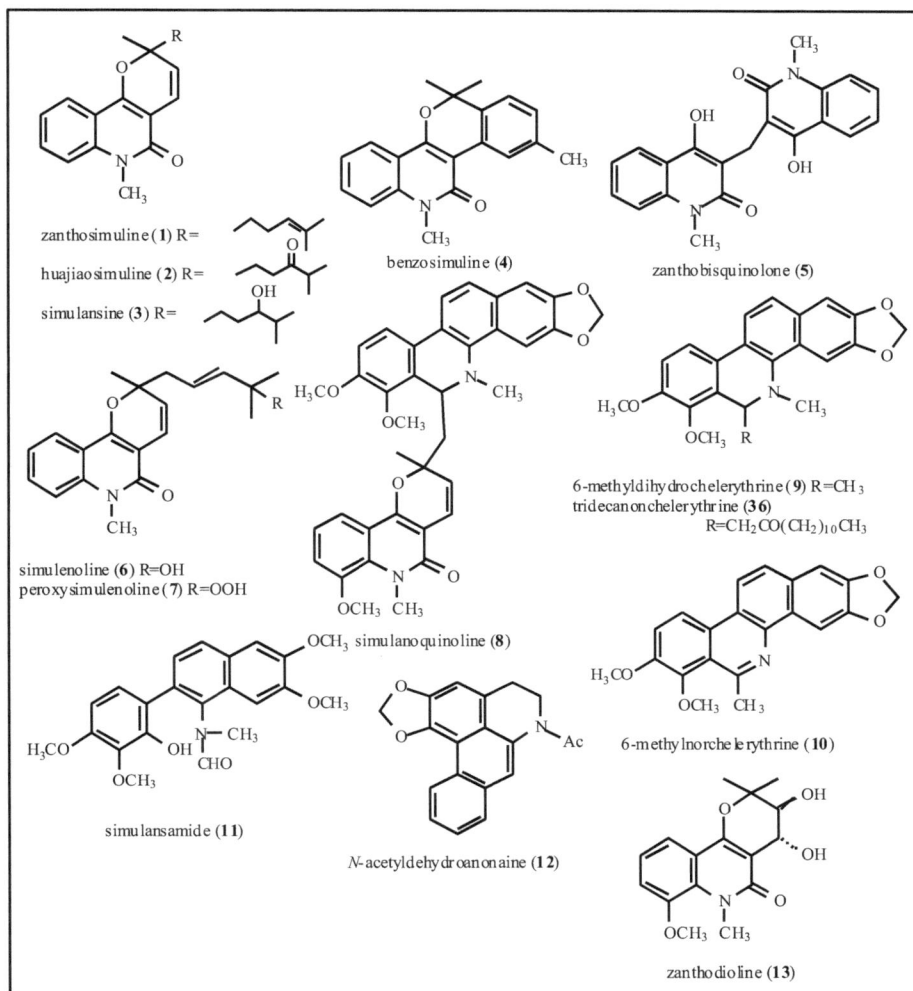

zanthosimuline (1) R=
huajiaosimuline (2) R=
simulansine (3) R=

benzosimuline (4)

zanthobisquinolone (5)

simulenoline (6) R=OH
peroxysimulenoline (7) R=OOH

6-methyldihydrochelerythrine (9) R=CH₃
tridecanonchelerythrine (36)
R=CH₂CO(CH₂)₁₀CH₃

simulanoquinoline (8)

simulansamide (11)

N-acetyldehydroanonaine (12)

6-methylnorchelerythrine (10)

zanthodioline (13)

distinguishable from other *Zanthoxylum* species due to the presence of a lot of 7-geranyloxy coumarins.

### Z. integrifoliolum

Successive investigation of the stem bark [21] afforded two new compounds, **36** and a phenylpropanoid, **37**. Its fruit has a strong anesthetic taste. Examination of the fruit [22-25] led to the isolation of 12 new compounds, including **38~40**, a flavonoid, **41**, six isobutylamides, **42~47**, **48** and **49**. The aliphatic unsaturated isobutylamides isolated from the fruits of this species carry predominantly an unsubstituted *N*-isobutyl group unlikely *Z. bungeanum* [26,27] and *Z. piperitum* [28], which have a predominantly hydroxy-substituted *N*-isobutyl group.

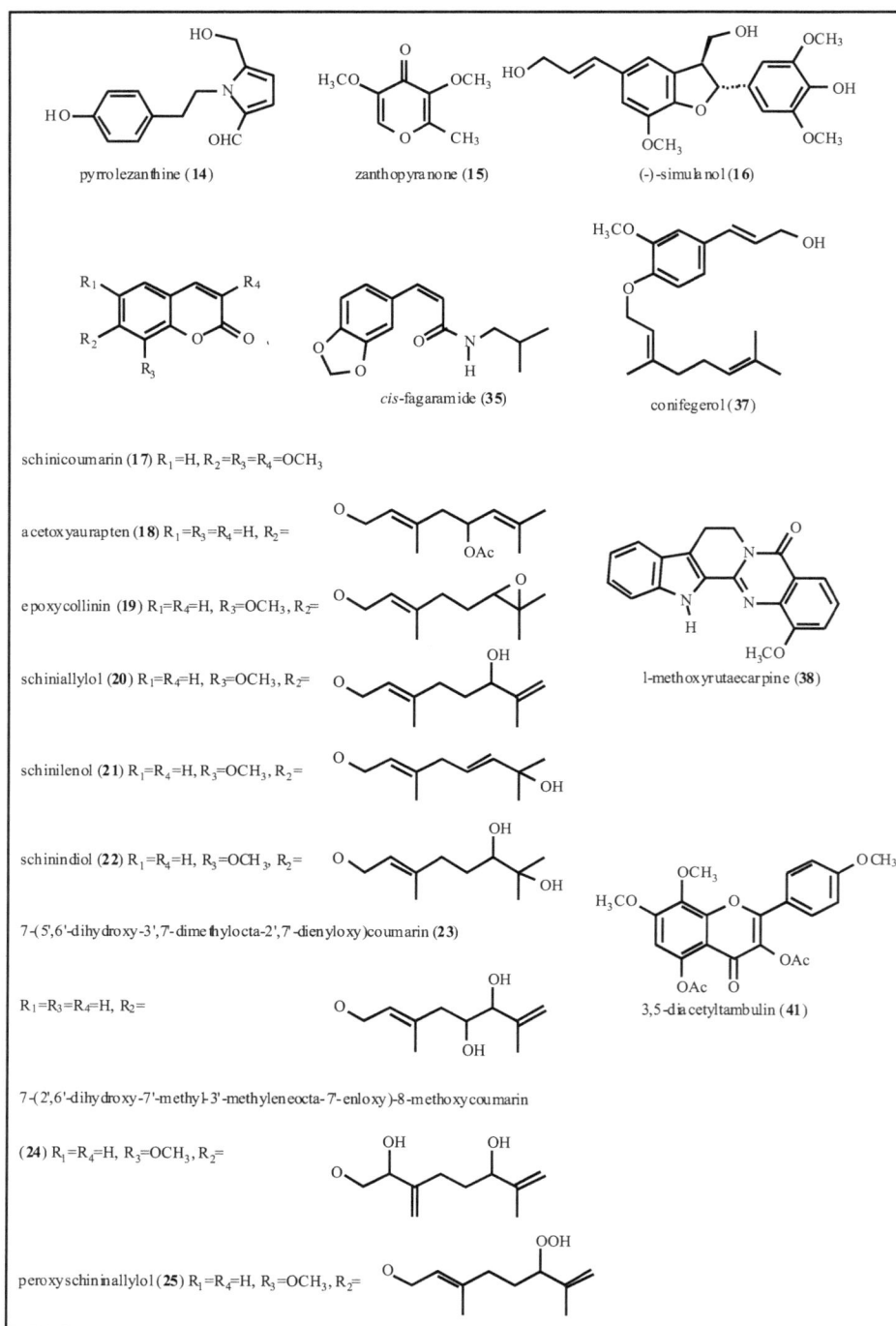

pyrrolezanthine (**14**)

zanthopyranone (**15**)

(-)-simulanol (**16**)

*cis*-fagaramide (**35**)

conifegerol (**37**)

schinicoumarin (**17**) R$_1$=H, R$_2$=R$_3$=R$_4$=OCH$_3$

acetoxyaurapten (**18**) R$_1$=R$_3$=R$_4$=H, R$_2$=

epoxycollinin (**19**) R$_1$=R$_4$=H, R$_3$=OCH$_3$, R$_2$=

schiniallylol (**20**) R$_1$=R$_4$=H, R$_3$=OCH$_3$, R$_2$=

schinilenol (**21**) R$_1$=R$_4$=H, R$_3$=OCH$_3$, R$_2$=

schinindiol (**22**) R$_1$=R$_4$=H, R$_3$=OCH$_3$, R$_2$=

7-(5',6'-dihydroxy-3',7'-dimethylocta-2',7'-dienyloxy)coumarin (**23**)

R$_1$=R$_3$=R$_4$=H, R$_2$=

l-methoxyrutaecarpine (**38**)

7-(2',6'-dihydroxy-7'-methyl-3'-methyleneocta-7'-enloxy)-8-methoxycoumarin

(**24**) R$_1$=R$_4$=H, R$_3$=OCH$_3$, R$_2$=

3,5-diacetyltambulin (**41**)

peroxyschininallylol (**25**) R$_1$=R$_4$=H, R$_3$=OCH$_3$, R$_2$=

(Compound 2. Contd....)

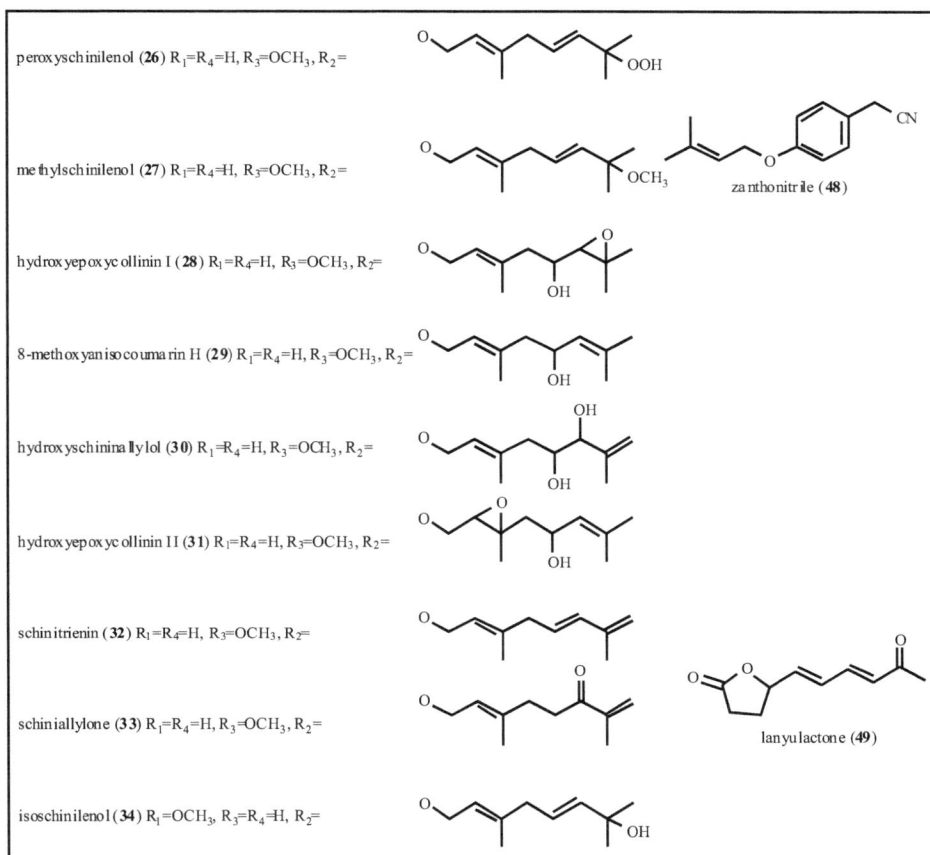

peroxyschinilenol (**26**) R$_1$=R$_4$=H, R$_3$=OCH$_3$, R$_2$=

methylschinilenol (**27**) R$_1$=R$_4$=H, R$_3$=OCH$_3$, R$_2$=

zanthonitrile (**48**)

hydroxyepoxycollinin I (**28**) R$_1$=R$_4$=H, R$_3$=OCH$_3$, R$_2$=

8-methoxyanisocoumarin H (**29**) R$_1$=R$_4$=H, R$_3$=OCH$_3$, R$_2$=

hydroxyschininallylol (**30**) R$_1$=R$_4$=H, R$_3$=OCH$_3$, R$_2$=

hydroxyepoxycollinin II (**31**) R$_1$=R$_4$=H, R$_3$=OCH$_3$, R$_2$=

schinitrienin (**32**) R$_1$=R$_4$=H, R$_3$=OCH$_3$, R$_2$=

schiniallylone (**33**) R$_1$=R$_4$=H, R$_3$=OCH$_3$, R$_2$=

lanyulactone (**49**)

isoschinilenol (**34**) R$_1$=OCH$_3$, R$_3$=R$_4$=H, R$_2$=

Since 1979, bishordeninyl terpene alkaloids have been isolated from the leaves of *Zanthoxylum* species by Stermitz *et al*. [29]. Examination of the leaves of this species has also led to the isolation a new bishordeninyl alkaloid, **50** [30].

### Z. nitidum

The wood of Formosan *Z. nitidum* was examined by Ishikawa *et al.* [31]. Three new compounds including two phenylpropanoids, **51** and **52**, and a benzodioxane type lignan, **53**, have been obtained. But **52** should be a known compound–4'-(3''-methyl-4''-hydroxybutyloxy)-3-phenylpropanol, due to the first isolation was done by Reisch *et al.* [32].

Oxyterihanine [8], a phenolic oxybenzo[*c*]phenanthridine alkaloid has been isolated from the bark of Formosan *Z. nitidum*. The occurrence of oxyterihanine was suppose to occur *via* the *in vivo* oxidation from a predicted phenolic quanternary benzo[*c*]-phenanthridinium alkaloid, terihanine (**54**). Because phenolic benzo[*c*]phenanthridinium alkaloids are difficult to obtain using the traditional partition method, we employed preparative paper chromatography on the benzo[*c*]phenanthridinium alkaloids-containing

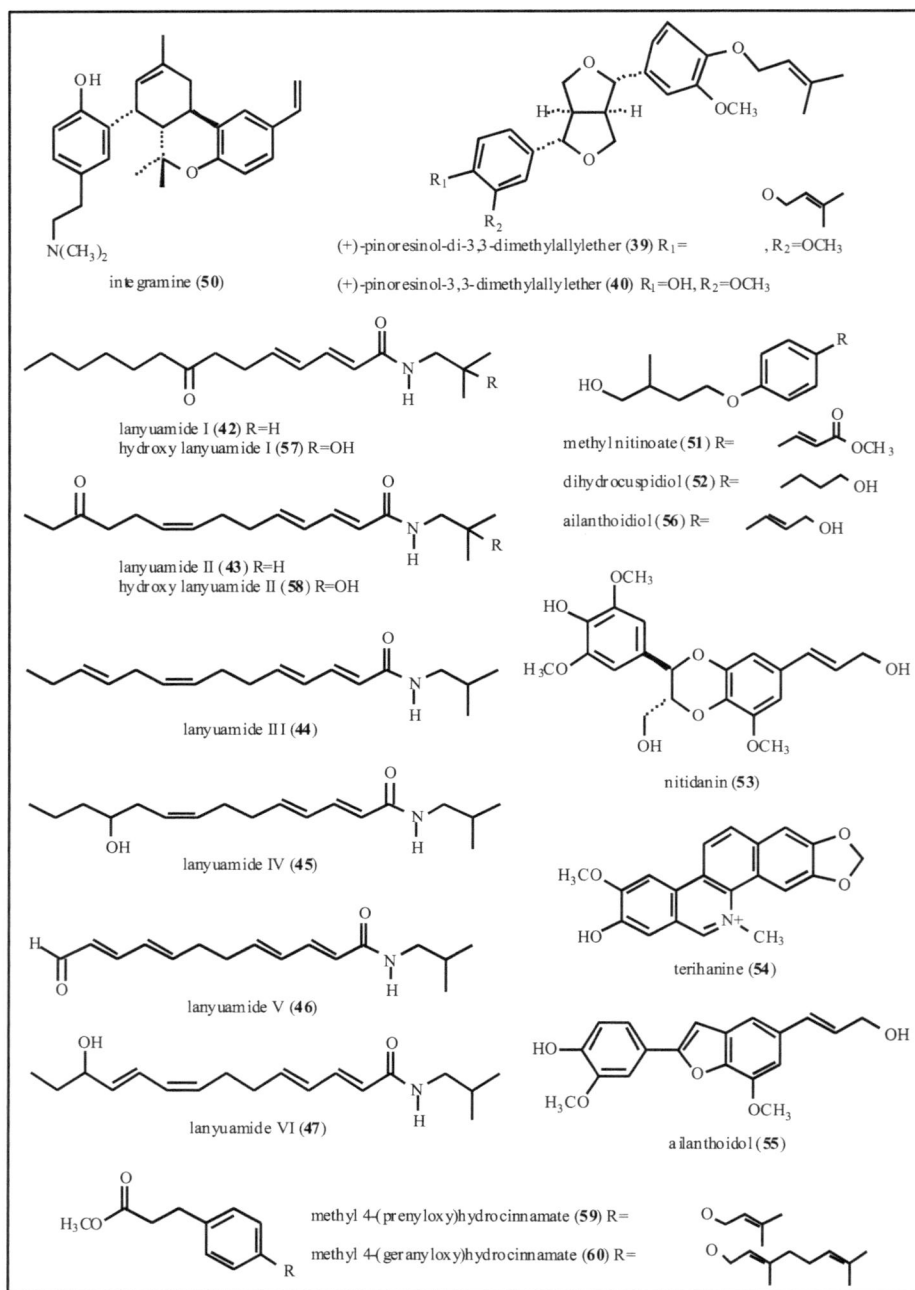

integramine (50)

(+)-pinoresinol-di-3,3-dimethylallylether (39) R₁=          , R₂=OCH₃

(+)-pinoresinol-3,3-dimethylallylether (40) R₁=OH, R₂=OCH₃

lanyuamide I (42) R=H
hydroxy lanyuamide I (57) R=OH

methyl nitinoate (51) R=

dihydrocuspidiol (52) R=

ailanthoidiol (56) R=

lanyuamide II (43) R=H
hydroxy lanyuamide II (58) R=OH

lanyuamide III (44)

nitidanin (53)

lanyuamide IV (45)

terihanine (54)

lanyuamide V (46)

lanyuamide VI (47)

ailanthoidol (55)

methyl 4-(prenyloxy)hydrocinnamate (59) R=

methyl 4-(geranyloxy)hydrocinnamate (60) R=

fraction of the root of this species. Consequently, 8-hydroxy-2,3-methylenedioxy-9-methoxy-5-methylbenzo[c]phenanthridinium was separated and was further identified by comparison with the synthetic terihanine [33]. Thus, the existence of **54** [34] in nature is confirmed.

### *Z. ailanthoides*

One new nor-neolignan, **55**, and one new phenylpropanoid, **56**, were isolated from the stem wood [35] of Formosan *Z. ailanthoides*. Examination of the root bark of Formosan *Z. ailanthoides* led to the isolation of 110 known compounds and two new isobutylamides, **57** and **58** [36].

### *Z. pistaciiflorum*

This plant grows only in a limited region of Pingtung County, Taiwan. Two new esters, **59** and **60** [37], have been isolated from the stem bark of this species.

## ANTIPLATELET AGGREGATION ACTIVITY

Platelet aggregation was measured by the turbidimetric method [38]. Active principles with antiplatelet aggregation activity, isolated from several species of Formosan *Zanthoxylum*, comprised of huajiaosimuline [10], simulansamide [12], (–)-*N*-acetylanonaine [13], haplopine [13], γ-fagarine [13], (–)-*N*-acetyldehydroanonaine [14], (–)-*N*-acetylnornuciferine [14], aesculetin dimethyl ether [14], arborinine [14], benzosimuline [14], decarine [14], skimmianine [14], simulenoline [14], zanthobungeanine [14], (–)-balanophonin [15], acetoxyaurapten [16], acetoxycollinin [16], aurapten [16], collinin [16], schinicoumarin [16], schininallylol [16], l-hydroxyrutaecarpine [22], l-methoxyrutaecarpine [22], rutaecarpine [22], atanine [23], 3,5-diacetyltambulin [24], hydroxy γ-sanshool [23], a mixture of (2*E*,4*E*,8*Z*,11*Z*)- and (2*E*,4*E*,8*Z*,11*E*)-2'- hydroxy-*N*-isobutyl-2,4,8,11-tetradecatetraenamide [23], lanyuamide I [23], lanyuamide II [23], prudomestin [23], γ-sanshool [23], tetrahydrobungeanol [23], 6-acetonyldihydrochelerythrine [35], dictamnine [35], dihydroalatamide [35], 4-methoxy-1-methyl-2-quinolone [35], and chelerythrine [39]. These active principles showed completely inhibitory activity on platelet aggregation induced by AA, collagen, thrombin or PAF at the 100 µg/mL or below. Of these, l-hydroxyrutaecarpine [22], isolated from the fruit of *Z. integrifoliolum*, exhibited strong antiplatelet activity induced by AA and showed an IC$_{50}$ of *ca.* 1~2 µg/mL. The action mechanism on antiplatelet aggregation of chelerythrine [39], isolated from the root bark of *Z. simulans*, was clarified as an inhibition of the thromboxane formation and PI breakdown.

## ACKNOWLEDGEMENTS

These studies on *Zanthoxylum* were financially supported by the National Science Council of the Republic of China.

## REFERENCES

[1]    Wall, M.E.; Wani, M.C.; Tayler, H.L.; Abstracts of Papers,162nd National Meeting of American Chemical Society, Washington, D.C., Sept. 1971, MEDI 34; Abstract of Papers, The 3rd International Congress of Heterocyclic Chemistry, Sendai, Japan, **1971**, B. p.29.

[2]    Messmer, W.M.; Tin-Wa, M.; Fong, H.H.S.; Bevelle, C.; Farnsworth, N.R.; Abraham, D.J.; Trojánek, J.; *J. Pharm. Sci.*, **1972**, *61*, 1858-1859.

[3]    Chang, C.E.; Hartley, T.G.; Editorial Committee of the Flora of Taiwan, Taipei, **1993**, III, 510-544.

[4]    Ishii, H.; Ishikawa, T.; Chen, I.S.; *Tetrahedron Lett.*, **1973**, 4189-4192.

[5]    Ishii, H.; Ishikawa, T.; Lu, S.T.; Chen, I.S.; *Yakugaku Zasshi*, **1976**, *96*, 1458-1467.

[6]    Ishii, H.; Chen, I.S.; Akaike, M.; Ishikawa, T.; Lu, S.T.; *Yakugaku Zasshi*, **1982**, *102*, 182-195.

[7]    Ishii, H.; Ishikawa, T.; Chen, I.S.; Lu, S.T.; *Tetrahrtron Lett.*, **1982**, *23*, 4345-4348.

[8]    Ishii, H.; Ishikawa, T.; Akaike, M.; Tohjoh, T.; Toyoki, M.; Ishikawa, M.; Chen, I.S.; Lu, S.T.; *Yakugaku Zasshi*, **1984**, *104*, 1030-1042.
[9]    Wu, S.J.; Chen, I.S.; *Phytochemistry,* **1993**, *34*, 1659-1661.
[10]   Chen, I.S.; Wu, S.J.; Tsai, I.L.; Wu, T.S.; Pezzuto, J.M.; Wu, M.C.; Chai, H.; Suh, N.; Teng, C.M.; *J. Nat. Prod.*, **1994**, *57*, 1206-1211.
[11]   Chen, I.S.; Wu, S.J.; Leu, Y.L.; Tsai, I.W.; Wu, T.S.; *Phytochemistry*, **1996**, *42*, 217-219.
[12]   Wu, S.J.; Chen, I.S.; Chern, C.Y.; Teng, C.T.; Wu, T.S.; *J. Chin. Chem. Soc.*, **1996**, *43*, 195-198.
[13]   Chen, I.S.; Wu, S.J.; Lin, Y.C.; Tsai, I.L.; Seki, H.; Ko, F.N.; Teng, C.M.; *Phytochemistry*, **1994**, *36*, 237-239.
[14]   Chen, I.S.; Tsai, I.W.; Teng, C.M.; Chen, J.J.; Chang, Y.L.; Ko, F.N.; Lu, M.C.; Pezzuto, J.M.; *Phytochemistry*, **1997**, *46*, 525-529.
[15]   Yang, Y.P.; Cheng, M.J.; Teng, C.M.; Chang, Y.L.; Tsai, I.L.; Chen, I.S.; *Phytochemistry*, **2002**, *61*, 567-572.
[16]   Chen, I.S.; Lin, Y.C.; Tsai, I.L.; Teng, C.M.; Ko, F.N.; Ishikawa, T.; Ishii, H.; *Phytochemistry*, **1995**, *39*, 1091-1097.
[17]   Chang, C.T.; Doong, S.L.; Tsai, I.L.; Chen, I.S.; *Phytochemistry*, **1997**, *45*, 1419-1422.
[18]   Tsai, I.L.; Lin, W.Y.; Chang, C.T.; Chen, I.S.; *J. Chin. Chem. Soc.*, **1998**, *45*, 99-101.
[19]   Tsai, I.L.; Lin, W.Y.; Teng, C.M.; Ishikawa, T.; Doong, S.L.; Huang, M.W.; Chen, Y.C.; Chen, I.S.; *Planta Med.*, **2000**, *66*, 618-623.
[20]   Cheng, M.C.; Yang, C.H.; Lin, W.Y.; Tsai, I.L.; Chen, I.S.; *J. Chin. Chem. Soc.*, **2002**, *49*, 125-128.
[21]   Jen, C.M.; Tsai, I.L.; Horng, D.J.; Chen, I.S.; *J. Nat. Prod.*, **1993**, *56*, 2012-2019.
[22]   Sheen, W.S.; Tsai. I.L.; Teng, C.M.; Ko, F.N.; Chen, I.S.; *Planta Med.*, **1996**, *62*, 175-176.
[23]   Chen, I.S.; Chen, T.L.; Chang, Y.L.; Teng, C.M.; Lin, W.Y.; *J. Nat. Prod.*, **1999**, *62*, 833-837.
[24]   Chen, I.S.; Chen, T.L.; Lin, W.Y.; Tsai, I.L.; Chen, Y.C.; *Phytochemistry*, **1999**, *52*, 357-360.
[25]   Tsai, I.L.; Lin, W.Y.; Huang, M.W.; Chen, T.L.; Chen, I.S.; *Helv. Chim. Acta*, **2001**, *84*, 830-833.
[26]   Xiong, Q.; Shi, D.; Yamamoto, H.; Mizuno, M.; *Phytochemistry*, **1997**, *46*, 1123-1126.
[27]   Mizutani, K.; Fukunaga, Y.; Tanaka, O.; Takasugi, N.; Saruwatari, Y.; Fuwa, T.; Yamauchi, T.; Wang, J.; Jia, M.R.; Li, F.Y.; Ling, Y.K.; *Chem. Pharm. Bull.*, **1998**, *36*, 2362-2365.
[28]   Yasuda, I.; Takeya, K.; Itokawa, H.; *Phytochemistry*, **1982**, *21*, 1295-1298.
[29]   Caolo, M.A.; Stermitz, F.R.; *Tetrahedron*, **1979**, *35*, 1487-1492.
[30]   Liu, S.L.; Tsai, I.L.; Ishikawa, T.; Harayama, T.; Chen, I.S.; *J. Chin. Chem. Soc.*, **2000**, *47*, 571-574.
[31]   Ishikawa, T.; Seki, M.; Nishigaya, K.; Miura, Y.; Seki, H.; Chen, I.S.; Ishii, H.; *Chem. Pharm. Bull.*, **1995**, *43*, 2014-2018.
[32]   Reisch, J.; Wickramasinghe, A.; Kumar, V.; *Phytochemistry*, **1989**, *28*, 3242-3243.
[33]   Ishii, H.; Chen, I.S.; Ueki, S.; Akaike, M.; Ishikawa, T.; *Chem. Pharm. Bull.*, **1987**, *35*, 2717-2725.
[34]   Tsai, I.L.; Ishikawa, T.; Seki, H.; Chen, I.S.; *Chin. Pharm. J.*, **2000**, *52*, 43-49.
[35]   Sheen, W.S.; Tsai, I.L.; Teng, C.M.; Chen, I.S.; *Phytochemistry*, **1994**, *36*, 213-215.
[36]   Cheng, M.J.; Tsai, I.L.; Chen, I.S.; *J. Chin. Chem. Soc.*, **2003**, *50*, 1241-1246.
[37]   Chen, J.J.; Huang, H.Y.; Duh, C.Y.; Chen, I.S.; *J. Chin. Chem. Soc.*, **2004**, *51*, 659-663.
[38]   Teng, C.M.; Chen, W.Y.; Ko, W.C.; Ouyang, C.; *Biochim. Biophys. Acta*, **1987**, *924*, 375-382.
[39]   Ko, F.N.; Chen, I.S.; Wu, S.J.; Lee, L.G.; Hu, T.F.; Teng, C.M.; *Biochim. Biophys. Acta*, **1990**, *1052*, 360-365.

Atta-ur-Rahman/Choudhary/Khan (Eds.) *Frontiers in Natural Product Chemistry, Vol. 1*

# Effect of *Murraya paniculata* (L.) Jack Extract on the Adult Mortality of *Callosobruchus maculatus* F. (Coleoptera: Bruchidae)

J.U. Mollah and W. Islam*

*Institute of Biological Sciences, University of Rajshahi, Rajshahi 6205, Bangladesh*

**Abstract:** Leaf, stem and root of *Murraya paniculata* (L.) Jack was extracted in four different organic solvents (petroleum ether, ethyl acetate, acetone and methanol). The extracts were tested on the mortality of adult male and female of *Callosobruchus maculatus* F. All the evaluated extract was toxic to both the sexes. Males generally showed higher susceptibility compared to females. Petroleum ether extract was more toxic than others. It was in the order: pet. ether>EtOAc>acetone>MeOH extract. Leaf extract was most toxic in comparison to stem and root extracts. It was in order: Leaf>root>stem. Generally, 72 hours exposure exhibited lower $LD_{50}$ values compared to 24 and 48 hours.

**Key Words**: *M. paniculata, C. maculatus,* extract, mortality, leaf, stem, root and solvent.

## INTRODUCTION

Pulse is considered as one of the economically important cereal crops in Bangladesh. Pulses seeds, including blackgram, are a rich source of protein (20-30%) [1]. It has been widely known that during storage and also in other stages of post-harvest handling, the food grains are either damaged or lost due to various agents like insects, vertebrates, microorganisms and environmental conditions. Insects are considered as the most destructive among those agents causing significant post-harvest food losses, particularly in developing countries.

*Callosobruchus maculatus* F. is one of the most important and destructive pest of almost all kinds of pulses both in the field and storage. The damage in storage is more crucial than damage in the field. Gujar and Yadav [2] recorded 55-60% loss in seed weight and 45.50-66.30% loss in protein content due to damage by the pulse beetle. Maximum damage was recorded nearly 100% after 4 months by *C. maculatus* [3].

Control of this pest populations around the world is primarily depended upon continued applications of organophosphorus and pyrethroid insecticides and the fumigants, methyl bromide and phosphine, which are still the most effective means for the protection of stored food, feedstuffs and other agricultural commodities from insect infestation [4,5]. Although effective, their repeated use for decades has disrupted biological control by natural enemies and led to outbreaks of other insect species and sometimes resulted in the development of resistance. It has had undesirable effects on non-target organisms, environmental and human health concerns [6,7]. To combat these problems, there is need for the development of safe and selective insect-control alternatives. One alternative to synthetic insecticide are insecticidal plants. Many plant extracts and essential oils may be alternative sources of stored-product pest protection because they constitute a rich source of bioactive chemicals

---

*Corresponding author: E-mail: mwislam2001@yahoo.com

and many of them are largely free from adverse effect, often active against specific target insects, biodegradable and are potentially suitable for use in integrated pest management [6].

The plant *Murraya paniculata* (L.) Jack an evergreen shrubs or small trees belonging to the family **Rutaceae**. It is distributed to China, India, Australia, South and East Asia including Bangladesh [13, 9]. It is locally known as **Kamini** in Bengali and **Orange Jasmine** in English. In Bangladesh, it is widely grown in gardens and roadside as ornamental plant or for fencing the gardens in many areas of the country [9]. Leaves contain monoterpene and sesquiterpene rich oil [10]. A few reports have been published on the medicinal properties and insecticidal activities of *M. paniculata*. The leaves of *M. paniculata* are the source of monoterpene and sesquiterpene rich oil [10], which showed growth disrupting activity against insects [11, 9]. Oil of *M. paniculata* plays good role on the reduction of population of *C. maculatus* [12].

This paper describes a laboratory study to assess the potential of *M. paniculata* extracts in different solvents against adult male and female of *C. maculatus*.

## MATERIALS AND METHODS

### Extract Preparation

The collected plant parts were dried in an oven and made into fine dust in a hand grinding machine. The sufficient amount of dust of plant parts were extracted in four different organic solvents viz. petroleum ether (pet.ether), ethyl acetate (EtOAc), acetone and methanol (MeOH). The extracts were dried in a vacuum rotary evaporator at 40°C under reduced pressure.

### Preparation and Application of Doses

Four different doses i.e., 0.01875, 0.03750, 0.07500 and 0.15000gm for pet. ether and EtOAc; 0.025, 0.050, 0.10 and 0.20gm for acetone and MeOH extract were weighted by an electronic balance and dissolved in requisite amount of respective solvents. The doses were transferred to $\mu g/cm^2$ by measuring the dry-weight of extracted materials and divided by the surface area of Petri dish (9 cm. diam). The test insects were exposed to the residual film technique. Extract was dispersed into each Petri dish for each dose. After evaporating the solvent from the Petri dish, 30 same aged (0-24h old) adult male and female *C. maculatus* were released into each Petri dish. Control lines for male and female were maintained with respective solvents only. The experiments were replicated thrice. Mortality was recorded after 24, 48 and 72 hours exposure. The mortality was corrected according to Abbott's formula [13]. The recorded mortality was subjected to probit analysis according to [14] and [15]. The beetles were reared in blackgram (*Phaseolus mungo* L.) seeds in Petri-dish (15 cm. diam) at 30±1°C and 70% relative humidity.

## RESULTS AND DISCUSSION

The LD$_{50}$ values, 95% confidence limits, regression equations (Y), $\chi^2$-values with 2 degrees of freedom and correlation coefficient (r-value) for adult mortality of *C. maculatus* at different exposure time with different solvents extract have been shown in Table **1, 2** and **3.** The data provided comprehensive evidence that the extracts used in the experiment were effective against the both sexes of adult *C. maculatus*. The $\chi^2$-values showed no significant heterogeneity. Comparing LD$_{50}$ values from probit analysis, pt. spt. extracts were more toxic than other extracts. It was in the order: pet. ether>EtOAc>acetone>MeOH. Generally, 72 hours exposure exhibited lower LD$_{50}$ values than 24 and 48 hours. Males were more

**Table 1.**    $LD_{50}$, 95% Confidence Limits, Regression Equation, $\chi^2$ and r-values of *M. paniculata* Leaf Extracts Tested on Adult Male and Female *C. maculatus* in Different Exposure Time.

| Solvent | Sex | Exposure Time (h) | $LD_{50}$ Values ($\mu g/cm^2$) | 95% confidence limits | | Regression equation | $\chi^2$-values in 2 df | r- values |
|---------|-----|-------------------|--------------------------------|-------|-------|---------------------|-------------------------|-----------|
| | | | | lower | upper | | | |
| Pet. ether | Male | 24 | 1260.58 | 2424.961 | 65526.99 | Y=1.8857+0.7595X | 0.2954 | 0.9891 |
| | | 48 | 1343.499 | 934.3695 | 1931.773 | Y=1.9577+0.9725X | 0.9611 | 0.9849 |
| | | 72 | 351.5071 | 283.8438 | 435.2868 | Y=-0.4797+2.1523X | 2.6276 | 0.9697 |
| | Female | 24 | 23967.8 | 2437.942 | 235631.4 | Y=1.8835+0.7116X | 0.0532 | 0.9962 |
| | | 48 | 2650.096 | 1464.19 | 4796.515 | Y=1.8473+0.9210X | 0.0297 | 0.9996 |
| | | 72 | 437.0447 | 344.5526 | 554.3651 | Y=0.5765+1.6752X | 1.6403 | 0.9842 |
| EtOAc | Male | 24 | 27633.68 | 1544.753 | 494331.5 | Y=2.6002+0.5403X | 0.3566 | 0.9671 |
| | | 48 | 1139.338 | 813.1096 | 1596.452 | Y=2.0469+0.9661X | 1.6441 | 0.9686 |
| | | 72 | 373.1267 | 302.5792 | 460.1227 | Y=-0.4464+2.1177X | 2.0506 | 0.9825 |
| | Female | 24 | 69689.59 | 1247.162 | 3894146 | Y=2.4742+0.5215X | 0.1581 | 0.9886 |
| | | 48 | 1918.224 | 1153.927 | 3188.749 | Y=2.1553+0.8665X | 0.2538 | 0.9927 |
| | | 72 | 455.9676 | 358.8.42 | 579.4423 | Y=0.7098+1.6135X | 0.5852 | 0.9942 |
| Acetone | Male | 24 | 24719.61 | 2644.92 | 231031.2 | Y=2.2410+0.3280X | 0.2353 | 0.9830 |
| | | 48 | 2145.431 | 1434.856 | 3207.9 | Y=1.7425+0.9778X | 0.5575 | 0.9862 |
| | | 72 | 522.18 | 421.395 | 547.0696 | Y=-0.4188+1.9938X | 1.3226 | 0.9885 |
| | Female | 24 | 21671.18 | 3519.527 | 133438.4 | Y=1.6292+0.7774X | 0.0355 | 0.9972 |
| | | 48 | 3106.781 | 1708.041 | 5650.975 | Y=2.0790+0.8364X | 0.1808 | 0.9963 |
| | | 72 | 599.8454 | 465.7069 | 772.6202 | Y=0.7511+1.5295X | 0.6553 | 0.9929 |
| MeOH | Male | 24 | 20911.96 | 3182.541 | 137408.8 | Y=1.8945+0.7188X | 0.1345 | 0.9940 |
| | | 48 | 2133.051 | 1479.112 | 3076.106 | Y=1.4365+1.0704X | 0.3257 | 0.9963 |
| | | 72 | 556.4314 | 447.2685 | 692.2371 | Y=-0.1291+1.8683X | 0.4922 | 0.9977 |
| | Female | 24 | 43196.03 | 3012.164 | 619453.6 | Y=1.9173+0.6650X | 0.0300 | 0.9975 |
| | | 48 | 3080.635 | 1956.665 | 4850.252 | Y=1.1489+1.1039X | 0.0354 | 0.9995 |
| | | 72 | 696.4027 | 549.5798 | 882.4501 | Y=0.7229+1.5045X | 1.0650 | 0.9931 |

*Correlation coefficient = r < 0.01

susceptible than the females. Mortality was directly proportional to the level of dose and time. The correlation co-efficient (r) values were showed significant (P<0.01), positive correlation among doses, exposure time and mortality in all the cases. The probit regression lines showed that the insect mortality rate was positively dose and time dependent in all the cases.

**Table 2.** LD$_{50}$, 95% Confidence Limits, Regression Equation, $\chi^2$ and r-values of *M. paniculata* Stem Extracts Tested on Adult Male and Female *C. maculatus* in Different Exposure Time.

| Solvent | Sex | Expo sure Time (h) | LD$_{50}$ Values ($\mu g/cm^2$) | 95% confidence limits | | Regression equation | $\chi^2$-values in 2 df | r- values |
|---------|-----|------|------|------|------|------|------|------|
| | | | | lower | upper | | | |
| Pet. ether | Male | 24 | 12496.6 | 2577.519 | 60587.4 | Y=1.7529+0.7926X | 0.0451 | 0.9985 |
| | | 48 | 1617.061 | 1109.827 | 2356.121 | Y=1.6346+1.0488X | 0.0896 | 0.9997 |
| | | 72 | 379.6129 | 298.4989 | 482.7686 | Y=0.3246+1.8126X | 0.9496 | 0.9904 |
| | Female | 24 | 18961.1 | 2436.836 | 177536.8 | Y=1.9560+0.7116X | 0.0749 | 0.9879 |
| | | 48 | 2265.787 | 1330.684 | 3858.007 | Y=1.8941+0.9257X | 0.2383 | 0.9956 |
| | | 72 | 409.9367 | 313.9346 | 535.2963 | Y=0.9685+1.5430X | 1.2898 | 0.9880 |
| EtOAc | Male | 24 | 19953.94 | 1965.196 | 202605.9 | Y=2.3356+0.6196X | 0.2606 | 0.9822 |
| | | 48 | 1290.66 | 901.4572 | 1847.899 | Y=2.0051+0.9627X | 0.4119 | 0.9862 |
| | | 72 | 385.6062 | 308.5439 | 481.9157 | Y=-0.0083+1.9366X | 1.8319 | 0.9162 |
| | Female | 24 | 29532.2 | 2158.316 | 404088.4 | Y=2.0498+0.6610X | 0.1034 | 0.9944 |
| | | 48 | 1861.813 | 1207.49 | 2870.703 | Y=1.7333+0.9990X | 0.3200 | 0.9968 |
| | | 72 | 474.4847 | 391.0034 | 575.7902 | Y-0.2273+1.9532X | 4.4608 | 0.9640 |
| Acetone | Male | 24 | 20675.85 | 2782.907 | 153613 | Y=2.1489+0.6607X | 0.1945 | 0.9874 |
| | | 48 | 1767.047 | 1250.108 | 2497.75 | Y=1.7128+1.0123X | 0.1363 | 0.9991 |
| | | 72 | 505.1159 | 409.4969 | 623.0623 | Y=-0.6619+2.0943X | 2.6510 | 0.9793 |
| | Female | 24 | 23597.4 | 3102.775 | 179464.5 | Y=1.9214+0.7040X | 0.0790 | 0.9953 |
| | | 48 | 2898.052 | 1600.7 | 5246.899 | Y=2.2122+0.8052X | 0.2577 | 0.9936 |
| | | 72 | 542.695 | 419.1445 | 714.5605 | Y=0.7734+1.5436X | 1.2901 | 0.9880 |
| MeOH | Male | 24 | 17652.34 | 3262.829 | 95501.5 | Y=1.7960+0.7545X | 0.0959 | 0.9951 |
| | | 48 | 1938.845 | 1383.434 | 2717.237 | Y=1.3885+1.0985X | 0.0549 | 0.9997 |
| | | 72 | 520.5543 | 417.4939 | 649.0553 | Y=-0.2757+1.9421X | 2.0337 | 0.9825 |
| | Female | 24 | 73633.65 | 2358.197 | 2299178 | Y=2.1310+0.5895X | 0.0302 | 0.9959 |
| | | 48 | 4948.746 | 2305.266 | 10623.55 | Y=1.7475+0.8804X | 0.2836 | 0.9891 |
| | | 72 | 565.9026 | 427.9196 | 748.3787 | Y=1.0369+1.4397X | 0.5565 | 0.9959 |

*Correlation coefficient = r < 0.01

The results of the present study clearly showed that leaf, stem and root extract of *M. paniculata* possessed toxic effect against adult male and female *C. maculatus*. There is no available published information regarding *M. paniculata* leaf, stem and root extracts to

**Table 3.** LD$_{50}$, 95% Confidence Limits, Regression Equation, $\chi^2$ and r-values of *M. paniculata* Root Extracts Tested on Adult Male and Female *C. maculatus* in Different Exposure Time.

| Solvent | Sex | Expo. sure Time (h) | LD$_{50}$ Values ($\mu g/cm^2$) | 95% confidence limits | | Regression equation | $\chi^2$-values in 2 df | r- values |
|---|---|---|---|---|---|---|---|---|
| | | | | Lower | upper | | | |
| Pet. ether | Male | 24 | 17999.66 | 2058.771 | 157369.4 | Y=2.2707+0.6414X | 0.0521 | 0.9987 |
| | | 48 | 1510.999 | 1028.194 | 2220.513 | Y=1.8787+0.9818X | 0.1837 | 0.9973 |
| | | 72 | 385.478 | 310.9014 | 477.9427 | Y=-0.1903+2.0071X | 1.9264 | 0.9802 |
| | Female | 24 | 13198.16 | 2657.42 | 65549.09 | Y=1.6173+0.8209X | 0.0264 | 0.9984 |
| | | 48 | 1841.21 | 1221.307 | 2775.759 | Y=1.5727+1.0497X | 0.1429 | 0.9976 |
| | | 72 | 417.2481 | 318.1555 | 547.2036 | Y=1.0705+1.4995X | 2.6716 | 0.9763 |
| EtOAc | Male | 24 | 11718.98 | 2355.628 | 58300.54 | Y=1.9111+0.7592X | 0.0535 | 0.9969 |
| | | 48 | 1659.359 | 1196.471 | 2301.327 | Y=1.0437+1.2287X | 0.0022 | 0.9996 |
| | | 72 | 387.6098 | 312.4791 | 480.8048 | Y=-0.1647+1.9953X | 4.1705 | 0.9592 |
| | Female | 24 | 11067.08 | 2617.902 | 46785.66 | Y=1.5949+0.8420X | 0.0453 | 0.9994 |
| | | 48 | 1985.297 | 1326.663 | 2970.917 | Y=1.2987+1.1223X | 0.1381 | 0.9982 |
| | | 72 | 419.2606 | 318.6145 | 551.6993 | Y=1.1278+1.4765X | 0.5499 | 0.9937 |
| Acetone | Male | 24 | 22823.74 | 2537.209 | 205313.4 | Y=2.2849+0.6230X | 0.0776 | 0.9937 |
| | | 48 | 1628.298 | 1165.367 | 2275.124 | Y=1.7603+1.0087X | 0.0929 | 0.9978 |
| | | 72 | 515.9814 | 414.388 | 642.8688 | Y=-0.3110+1.9579X | 3.3677 | 0.9692 |
| | Female | 24 | 25337.58 | 3098.532 | 207192.8 | Y=1.9385+0.6952X | 0.1283 | 0.9916 |
| | | 48 | 2931.999 | 1735.138 | 4954.425 | Y=1.8079+0.9207X | 0.1108 | 0.9982 |
| | | 72 | 569.6025 | 440.5044 | 736.5352 | Y=0.7035+1.5592X | 0.9673 | 0.9923 |
| MeOH | Male | 24 | 13351.55 | 3703.908 | 48128.56 | Y=1.2376+0.9120X | 0.6089 | 0.9987 |
| | | 48 | 2597.866 | 1754.459 | 3846.716 | Y=1.1085+1.1397X | 0.1805 | 0.9978 |
| | | 72 | 533.8908 | 423.5731 | 672.9408 | Y=0.0470+1.8160X | 1.6138 | 0.9911 |
| | Female | 24 | 17377.44 | 3426.644 | 88125.79 | Y=1.5845+0.8056X | 0.0136 | 0.9996 |
| | | 48 | 3135.905 | 1894.128 | 5191.786 | Y=1.4851+1.0053X | 0.3627 | 0.9932 |
| | | 72 | 635.5005 | 508.5312 | 794.1714 | Y=0.2640+1.6896X | 0.1114 | 0.9985 |

*Correlation coefficient = r < 0.01

compare the present result. However, Huixin *et al*. [12] observed that the essential oils of *M. paniculata, Cinnamomum cassia, C. burmannii, Ocimum basilicum, Chenopodium ambrosioides, Carum carvi, Foeniculum vulgare, Zanthoxlum buneanum, Pelargonoum graveolens* and *Ageratum conyzoides* produced all over 90% population reduction, insect penetration of *C. maculatus* and weight loss of mungbean seeds after 45 or 115 days treatment. Mahal [16] observed the dust *M. paniculata*, *Nigella sativa*, *Datura metel*, *Jatropha curcas*, *Vitex negundo* and *Eucalyptus camaldulensis* produced 2.22 to 93.33% mortal effects in *R. dominica* at doses from 0.625 to 20% after 18 days of exposure. The males were more susceptible than the females. The toxicities were in order of *N. sativa* > *M. paniculata* >*J. curcas* >*E. camaldulensis* >*D. metel* >*V. negundo*.

## CONCLUSIONS

It is known that *Murraya* contains monoterpene and sesquiterpene rich oils [10], which exhibit growth disrupting activity against insects [11, 9]. The tested plant extracts having these components might be effective to cause mortality in *C. maculatus* even as crude form. However, the findings of the present experiments indicate the efficiency of extracts in killing *C. maculatus* adults.

## ACKNOWLEDGEMENTS

The authors gratefully acknowledge grants from The Third World Network of Scientific Organisations (TWNSO), Italy and the Director, Institute of Biological Sciences, Rajshahi University, Bangladesh for laboratory facilities.

## REFERENCES

[1]     Sharma, S. S.; *Bull. Grain Tech.* **1984**, *22*, 62-68.
[2]     Gujar, G. T.; Yadav, T. D.; *Indian J. Ent.* **1978**, *40*, 108-112.
[3]     Pandey, G.P.; Doharey, R. B.; Varma, B. K.; *Indian J. Agric. Sci.* **1981**, *51*, 910-912.
[4]     Kim, S. I.; Park, C.; Ohh, M. H.; Cho, H. C.; Ahn, Y. J.; *J. Stored Prod. Res.* **2003a**, *39*, 11-19.
[5]     Park, C.; Lee, S. G.; Choi, D. H.; Park, J. D.; Ahn, Y. J.; *J. Stored Prod. Res.* **2003b**, *39*, 375-384.
[6]     Kim, S. I.; Roh, J. Y.; Kim, D. H.; Lee, H. S.; Ahn, Y. J.; *J. Stored Prod. Res.* **2003b**, *39*, 293: 303.
[7]     Park, C.; Kim, S. I.; Ahn, Y. J.; *J. Stored Prod. Res.* **2003a**, *39*, 333-342.
[8]     Anon *The wealth of India*. A dictionary of Indian raw materials and industrial products. **1950**; vol. *VI*, pp. 447-448. CSIR, New Delhi, India.
[9]     Ghani, A. *Medicinal Plants of Bangladesh: Chemical Constituents and Uses*. Asiat. Soc. Bangladesh, Dhaka, Bangladesh. **1998**.
[10]    Li, Q.; Zhu, L. F.; But, P. P. H.; Kong, Y. C.; Chang, H. T.; Waterman, P. G.; *Biochem. Syst. Ecol.* **1988**, *16*, 491-494.
[11]    Slama, K.; Romanuk, M.; Sorm, F.; *Insect Hormones and Bioanalogues*. Springer-Verlag, New York, USA, **1974**, pp. 91.
[12]    Huixin, L.; Ruhai, L.; Mushan, W.; Pinyan, Y.; Zhiguo, K.; Yusheng, N. Effect of 25 plant essential oils against *Callosobruchus maculatus*. Proc. 7ᵗʰ Int. Working Conf. on Stored- product Protection **1998**, *1*, 849-851.14-19 October, Beijing, Peoples Republic of China.
[13]    Abbott, W. S.; *J. Econ. Entomol.* **1925**, *18*, 265-267.
[14]    Finney, D. J. *Probit analysis: a statistical treatment of the sigmoid response curve*. Cambridge University Press, London. **1947**.
[15]    Busvine, J. R. *A critical review of the techniques for testing insecticides*. Commonwealth Agricultural Bureau, London. **1971**, pp. 345.
[16]    Mahal, N.; *Biology and control of Rhyzopertha dominica (Fabricius) (Coleoptera: Bostrichidae)*. Ph. D Thesis, Institute of Biological Sciences, Rajshahi University, Rajshahi, Bangladesh. **2002**, pp. 1-329.

224

www.ingramcontent.com/pod-product-compliance
Lightning Source LLC
Chambersburg PA
CBHW050830220326

41598CB00006B/337